योगनिद्रा

YOGA-NIDRĀ

Ascent into the Subconscious

Its roots, traditional foundations and modern developments:
A comprehensive guide to the method developed
by Svāmī Satyānanda Sarasvatī

Nadeshda Stürzebecher
(saṃnyāsī Antarśuddhī)

Edited by
Georgi Krastev

PURPLE CLOUD PRESS

DISCLAIMER

We cannot provide specific information to individuals about their symptoms, diseases or treatment. This work is to be utilized by professionals with sufficient training and proper licensure in medicine, psychology, yoga-therapy and the *yoga-nidrā* method of Svāmī Satyānanda. It should serve as commentary for yoga teachers and practitioners who are interested in the subject of *yoga-nidrā* in its original and integral contexts for deepening and enriching their knowledge and understanding.

Library of Congress Control Number: 2025908505

Hardcover ISBN-13: 978-1-991081-22-3
Softcover ISBN-13: 978-1-991081-21-6

EDITOR, ACADEMIC ADVISOR & TRANSLATOR
Georgi Krastev

FRONT COVER ART & INTERIOR ILLUSTRATIONS
Drdha Vrata Gorrick • www.divyakala.com
COVER IMAGE: God Viṣṇu in the State of *yoga-nidrā*

COVER DESIGN
Anne-Marie Taranto • www.rhapsodica.com

INTERIOR DESIGN
Barabara Tada • www.pixelgardendesign.com

PUBLISHED BY PURPLE CLOUD PRESS
purplecloudinstitute.com • purplecloudpress@gmail.com

Purple Cloud Vision

Purple Cloud Press was founded on the principle that only by merging theoretical knowledge and practical experience is one able to gain true understanding and grasp the nuances of pertinent writings. Therefore, all publications by Purple Cloud Press are underpinned by this principle of scholar-physician and scholar-practitioner into the following threefold mission;

- to publish the works of the founders of the Purple Cloud Institute and other authors' finished works in the field of Eastern medicine, Asian religions and martial arts,
- to translate original ancient Asian texts into the European languages,
- to commission writings about masters' and teachers' lineage traditions.

Purple Cloud Press incentivizes authors and translators by guaranteeing them a large percentage of the royalties in order to encourage continued translation projects as well as by providing a platform to reach the largest possible readership. Purple Cloud Press strongly believes that this will help make accessible the profundity of treasures previously hidden from the non-Chinese speaking world.

purple cloud
press

In memoriam
Paramahaṃsa Satyānanda Sarasvatī

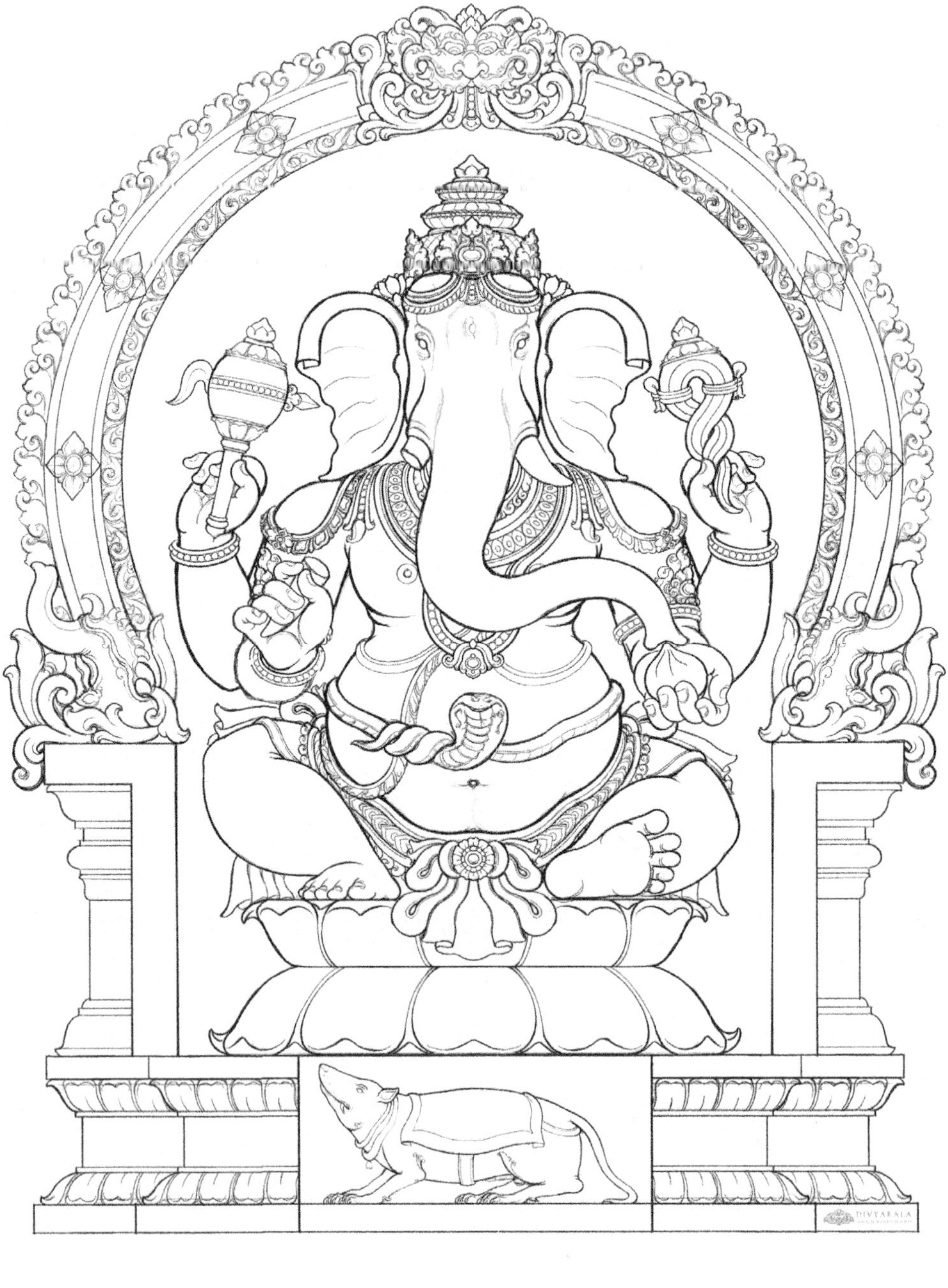
DIVYAKALA

॥ब्रह्मोवाच॥

विश्वेश्वरीं जगद्धात्रीं स्थितिसंहारकारिणीम् ।
निद्रां भगवतीं विष्णोरतुलां तेजसः प्रभुः ॥

त्वं स्वाहा त्वं स्वधा त्वं हि वषट्कारः स्वरात्मिका ।
सुधा त्वमक्षरे नित्ये त्रिधा मात्रात्मिका स्थिता ॥

अर्धमात्रा स्थिता नित्या यानुच्चार्या विशेषतः ।
त्वमेव संध्या सावित्री त्वं देवि जननी परा ॥

त्वयैव धार्यते सर्वं त्वयैतत्सृज्यते जगत् ।
त्वयैतत्पाल्यते देवि त्वमत्स्यन्ते च सर्वदा ॥

विसृष्टौ सृष्टिरुपा त्वं स्थितिरुपा च पालने ।
तथा संहृतिरुपान्ते जगतोऽस्य जगन्मये ॥

महाविद्या महामाया महामेधा महास्मृतिः ।
महामोहा च भवती महादेवी महेश्वरी ॥

प्रकृतिस्त्वञ्च सर्वस्य गुणत्रयविभाविनी ।
कालरात्रिर्महारात्रिर्मोहरात्रिश्च दारुणा ॥

त्वं श्रीस्त्वमीश्वरी त्वं ह्रीस्त्वं बुद्धिर्बोधलक्षणा ।
लज्जा पुष्टिस्तथा तुष्टिस्त्वं शान्तिः क्षान्तिरेव च ॥

खड्गिनी शूलिनी घोरा गदिनी चक्रिणी तथा ।
शङ्खिनी चापिनी बाणभुशुण्डी परिघायुधा ॥

सौम्या सौम्यतराशेषसौम्येभ्यस्त्वतिसुन्दरी ।
परापराणां परमा त्वमेव परमेश्वरी ॥

यच्च किञ्चित्क्वचिद्वस्तु सदसद्वाखिलात्मिके ।
तस्य सर्वस्य या शक्तिः सा त्वं किं स्तूयते तदा ॥

यया त्वया जगत्स्रष्टा जगत्पात्यत्ति यो जगत् ।
सोऽपि निद्रावशं नीतः कस्त्वां स्तोतुमिहेश्वरः ॥

विष्णुः शरीरग्रहणमहीशान एव च ।
कारितास्ते यतोऽतस्त्वां कः स्तोतुं शक्तिमान्भवेत् ॥

सा त्वमित्थं प्रभावैः स्वैरुदारैर्देवि संस्तुता ।
मोहयैतौ दुराधर्षावसुरौ मधुकैटभौ ॥

प्रबोधनं च जगत्स्वामी नीयतामच्युतो लघु ।
बोधश्च क्रियतामस्य हन्तुमेतौ महासुरौ ॥

इति श्रीमार्कण्डेयपुराणे सावर्णिकि मन्वन्तरे देवीमाहात्म्ये मधुकैटभवधो नाम एकाशीतितमो ऽध्याये ब्रह्मस्तुतिः ॥

Contents

PART TWO
Svāmī Satyānanda's *yoga-nidrā*-Method in Detail

PART THREE
Fields of Application of Satyananda Yoga Nidra in Today's Society

Part Four
Overview of the Contemporary Developments of yoga-nidrā in the Western Context

Part Five
Appendix

Preface

Yoga-nidrā is a means of contacting the source of self-knowledge and inspiration lying within each person. It is a technique of self-induced dreaming in which the treasure-house of our consciousness can be systematically illumined, explored and then used to enrich our daily live.[1]

Svāmī Satyānanda Sarasvatī

Yoga-nidrā, most often reffered to as 'yogic sleep', and described by Svāmī Śatyānanda as 'psychic sleep', is one of the most popular yet frequently misunderstood methods of yoga today. *Yoga-nidrā* operates by harnessing one's awareness as a tool to release the mind from the contents of the subconscious and unconscious. These contents can and often do inhibit the mind from entering deeper states of immersion. The term *yoga-nidrā* refers to both the specific state of consciousness sought after and the method employed to attain that state.

Svāmī Satyānanda Sarasvatī (1923–2009), the originator of the first contemporary *yoga-nidrā* method, was among the foremost disciples of Svāmī Śivānanda Sarasvatī (1887–1963), — a physician and Indian master — one of the pioneers who made yoga accessible to the general public in modern times.

Svāmī Śivānanda based his teachings on what is now referred to as an 'integral approach to yoga', which combines simple techniques from the classical paths of yoga. Svāmī Satyānanda continued the legacy of his spiritual master by greatly systematising and enriching his teachings. He accomplished this

1 Golden Jubilee Edition. (2013). *The Golden Collection* 3 – A collection of original publications from the Bihar School of Yoga Tradition. Munger: Yoga Publication Trust, p. 24.

by making almost lost or forgotten methods from the tantras[2] accessible for the wider public for the first time, integrating them into a profound yoga system developed through many years of intensive practice and study. In 1963, he founded the Bihar School of Yoga (BSY) in the north Indian city of Munger in the state of Bihar, which was recognised as the world's first yoga university by UNESCO. Hence, Svāmī Satyānanda's yoga system became widely known as 'Bihar Yoga' and later as 'Satyananda Yoga'. In this publication it will be referred to as Bihar Yoga.

In the early 1960s, Svāmī Satyānanda was the first to develop a practical *yoga-nidrā* method in the form of a systematically structured technique which could be effortlessly practised by people today. This method, now commonly known as 'Satyananda Yoga Nidra', achieves its purpose by integrating various tantric principles and techniques of immersion to refine the awareness[3] and perception. This approach enables interaction with the subconscious and tapping into the unconscious mind. In this process, tensions, blockages and latent impressions stored in the physical and subtle body, and mind can be released. The subtle connections between the body, vital energies, and mind are utilised for this purpose. Therefore, Svāmī Satyānanda's *yoga-nidrā* method embodies the essence of his extensive teachings and represents the jewel of his legacy within the Bihar School of Yoga.

According to Svāmī Satyānanda's conception, *yoga-nidrā* should not be regarded merely as a relaxation technique, despite its relaxing effects. This misconception is nowadays particularly prevalent in the West, where the method is often interpreted as merely a pleasant relaxation practice or, in the context of Western therapeutic approaches (such as psychotherapy), reduced to a focus solely on its relaxing and therapeutic benefits.

However, it is a challenge to put subtle experiences into words due to the inherent limitations and the genuine ambiguity of language. This is particularly difficult when it comes to profound concepts and terminology deeply alien to modern culture. A gradual introduction into *yoga-nidrā*'s original

---

2 In Indic traditions, 'tantra' first referred to any treatise on a specific topic (such as medicine), but later came to be used primarily for texts presenting comprehensive systems combining philosophy and ritual and often also yogic practice, often detailing specific practices, deity worship, mantras, techniques of immersion, and visualisations. Tantra evolved and was adopted by a multitude of Indian religious traditions, including Śaivism, Buddhism and Jainism.

3 The German original uses the word 'Gewahrsein' – signifying the 'state of being established in immersive awareness'.

context and its way of thinking about it, with practical experience remaining the natural centre of focus, is therefore appropriate. The focus of yoga teaching should be on the experience derived from one's own practice, and this is not something which can be replaced by knowledge gained from books, feelings or imagination. Regardless, it is essential to also become familiar with the systematics and background of the techniques in question.

This book is an attempt to explore the original *yoga-nidrā* method of Svāmī Satyānanda, staying as close as possible to its sources and its roots in the Indic traditions and placing it in the context of both the integral yoga approach and the more than two-thousand-year history of yogic philosophy and practice in India. Its focus is on the understanding of the meaning of the term *yoga-nidrā* in its original Indic contexts, and how these are integrated within the syncretic teaching of Svāmī Satyānanda. The differences in approach between the *interpretatio occidentis* and the *interpretatio orientis* will be discussed, and the concept, practice and method of yoga-nidrā will be presented in their entirety to the best of the author's ability. Likewise, *yoga-nidrā* should become recognisable as a path of profound spiritual growth, very much in contrast to its treatment as a mere exercise for the purpose of relaxation.

The book is divided into four parts:

Part One examines the traditional, philosophical and metaphysical background of *yoga-nidrā*, laying the foundation for a better understanding of *yoga-nidrā*'s historical appearance and context. It presents key concepts belonging to three of the main streams of thought and practice in India — Vedānta, Sāṃkhya and Tantra — and their practical application in yoga. On this foundation, the most important path of yoga for *yoga-nidrā* — *raja-yoga* — will be looked at from various angles in order to clarify important terms associated with *yoga-nidrā* within that framework. The term *yoga-nidrā* is also discussed historically.

In **Part Two**, Svāmī Satyānanda's *yoga-nidrā* method and its eight stages are presented in detail.

Part Three discusses the effects of *yoga-nidrā* and its areas of application in contemporary society, while drawing upon scientific findings from clinical studies dating from the 1970s to the present day which investigate and substantially support the therapeutic effectiveness of Satyananda Yoga Nidra.

Part Four deals with contemporary secularised developments of Satyananda Yoga Nidra in the West and concludes with an overview of contemporary literature concerned with Satyananda Yoga Nidra and selected other practices and methods, which claim to be based upon *yoga-nidrā*.

The **Appendix** provides a brief introduction to Bihar Yoga, on whose integral approach Svāmī Satyānanda's *yoga-nidrā* method is based, as well as an introduction to his successors and contemporary masters of this tradition. The Appendix also includes a systematic scientific literature review specifically of the research on Satyananda Yoga Nidra as well as a brief Sanskrit glossary.

At the back of the book, you will find a link to download three guided *yoga-nidrā* recordings by the author for your personal practice.

This book intentionally contains no chapter with scripts for delivering the technique to participants, as experience has shown that many yoga teachers often use such scripts without proper education or a thorough understanding of Svāmī Satyānanda's *yoga-nidrā* method and his integral yoga approach. Instead, they directly apply them in their yoga classes and even offer *yoga-nidrā* training. This is irresponsible and not only fails to uphold the professional delivery of the method, but is also dangerous, as it involves working with the subconscious and unconscious of the participants. Readers are encouraged to seek guidance from an authorised teacher in order to properly learn the method. Those interested in undertaking formal training should approach an authorised facilitator from the tradition of the Bihar School of Yoga. Such training should be conducted in person and extends over a sustained period of time, typically lasting more than six months.

The author does not speak on behalf of the institution of Bihar Yoga or the Bihar School of Yoga, but from her own experience and understanding gained during her study and practice within this tradition. The author hereby wishes to pay tribute to the teachings of Paramahaṃsa Satyānanda Sarasvatī, Paramahaṃsa Niranjanānanda Sarasvatī and Paramahaṃsa Satyasaṅgānanda Sarasvatī. The author is solely responsible for any errors and/or omissions.

For ease of reading, the names of the masters of the Bihar School of Yoga tradition are abbreviated: Svāmī Satyānanda (Paramahaṃsa Satyānanda

Sarasvatī) or those of his successors — Svāmī Nirañjanānanda (Paramahaṃsa Nirañjanānanda Sarasvatī) and Svāmī Satyasaṅgānanda (Paramahaṃsa Satyasaṅgānanda Sarasvatī).

Vienna, February 14th 2023

The original manuscript of this book was written in German following five years of research and was completed in 2023. Although the German version remains unpublished, this English edition constitutes its first official publication.

In cases where cited online sources are no longer accessible, readers may consult archived versions preserved in digital internet libraries.[4]

Vienna, December 5th 2025

4 For example, the Wayback Machine by Internet Archive: https://web.archive.org.

Acknowledgements

My deepest gratitude goes to my *guru*, Paramahaṃsa Niranjanānanda Sarasvatī, for his guidance and inspiration.

I would especially like to thank Georgi Krastev for his invaluable academic support, for meticulously correcting the Sanskrit terms and their translations into both German and English, and for the countless hours he dedicated to discussions and reflections. His tireless mental and emotional support, encouragement at every step of the writing process, and unwavering presence have been crucial.

I would also like to thank Frank Stürzebecher for undertaking the challenging task of making the first corrections in German and for his support throughout the entire process.

Special thanks go to Elisabeth Lexer for her editing of the German text, her talent in making the sentences flow effortlessly, and for engaging with the subject of this book with such empathy.

I am particularly grateful to clinical psychologist Mag. Stephan Schmidmeier for his contribution to Chapter 17. *Yoga-nidrā and Western Psychology*. My heartfelt thanks to Dr. Jakob Thannesberger for proofreading the medical content of this book. I extend my gratitude to psychotherapist Nikolas Hochstöger, Bakk. Phil., for sharing his professional insights and proofreading Chapter 15. *Effects of Stress and the Importance of Relaxation*, Chapter 16. *Absence of Tension Through śavasanā and yoga-nidrā* and Chapter 17. *Yoga-nidrā and Western Psychology*. Special thanks to Patrick Zeitlhuber, MA for proofreading of Part I.

My deep appreciation also goes to my classical Indian iconography teacher Drdha Vrata Gorrick, master artist and renowned *śilpa-śāstra* teacher, whose exquisite artwork enriches this book. His generous permission to include his art has added both beauty and depth to its pages.

My heartfelt thanks also go to my son, Immanuel Stürzebecher, for his constant support and the contribution of some of the figures in the book. I am deeply thankful to my mother, Julia Dimitrova, for her care and sympathy, to Svāmī Tarpanvidya and all my friends and colleagues who never doubted the successful completion of this manuscript, and who encouraged and supported me in my endeavours.

To all the practitioners and participants in the courses and trainings I have conducted—and continue to offer—your curiosity, dedication, and trust have supported and inspired me throughout the writing of this book.

This book would not have been possible in its current form without your help.

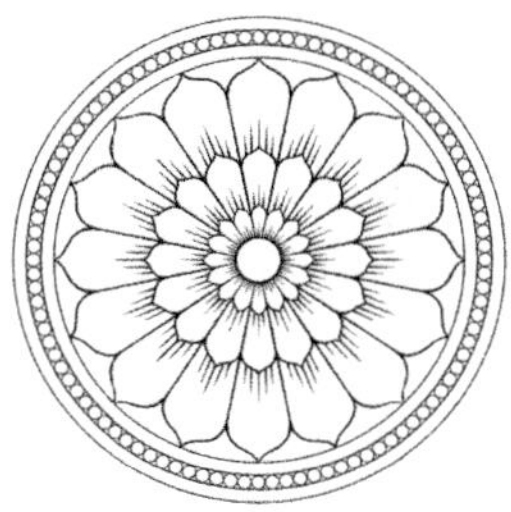

Part One

Yoga-nidrā from the Point of View of Classical Indian Philosophy

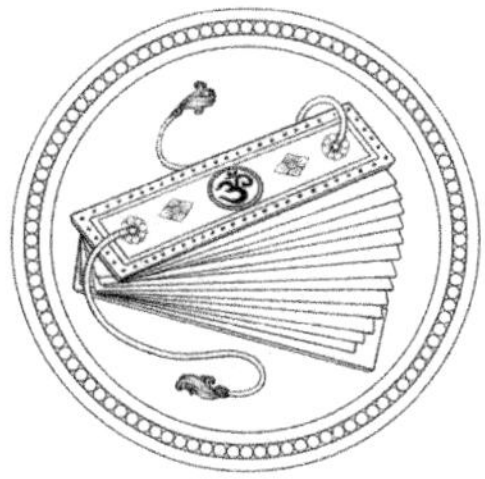

CHAPTER 1

Indian Schools of Thought

Although yoga is more concerned with practice than with theory, a basic idea of the philosophical aspects will help the practitioner to know what he is trying to do and achieve in yoga and how he will attain meditational states.[1]

Svāmī Satyānanda Sarasvatī

DESPITE COMMONLY HELD BELIEFS OF ITS UNITY, India's spiritual heritage consists of a broad range of ideas, philosophies and ways of life. These are mostly reflected in six main schools of thought usually referred to as the 'Six Points of View' or the 'Six Philosophies' (*ṣaḍ-darśana*). These are: Sāṃkhya, Nyāya, Vaiśeṣika, Pūrva Mimāṃsa, Vedānta and Yoga. Regardless of the fact that Tantra is not explicitly considered a *darśana* or an independent school of thought, its influence and varied currents are undoubtedly recognisable within and beyond the historical development of the six *darśanas*.

1 Saraswati, Satyananda, Swami. (2001). *Meditations from the Tantras*. Munger: Yoga Publication Trust. (reprint 2nd edition), p. 62.

These six *darśanas* are traditionally considered 'orthodox' in the sense that they ultimately derive their authority from the texts of the Veda — the oldest Indian corpus of ritual, philosophical and mythical texts, which they (at least formally), regard as the highest authority on both spiritual and earthly matters. Other prominent schools of thought and religion in India were considered semi-compliant with Brahmanical precepts (such as the non-transgressive initiatory Śaivism of the Atimārga), while others still were considered to be in complete break with Vedic authority (such as Buddhism, Jainism and antinomian schools of Śaivism such as the Kulamārga).

While the six 'orthodox' *darśanas* are nominally based on the authority of the Veda, they include both theistic and purely philosophical approaches. They are also not completely discrete traditions, nor are they uniform in their teachings as, like every tradition, they underwent change and development with time.

As reliant on the authority of the Veda in one way or another, seekers and scholars of earlier times did not see their own insights as ultimate answers to all questions. This was, however, contrary to the views of the Buddhists and the Jains, where direct (yogic) experience is the authoritative source of knowledge about Ultimate Reality and liberation (*mokṣa*). Many traditions, such as non-transgressive Śaivism, span a grey zone between being compatible with the Brahmanical framework of the Veda and stepping outside of it. For this reason, there have been and still are heated debates in India about the various paths to spiritual fulfilment.

One of the orthodox among the six paths is usually referred to as Yoga (योग).[2] Yoga as regarded as a separate school of thought has no datable beginning, nor does it have a definable founder. Particular traditions of yoga have legendary or mythical founders, such as the 10th century master Matsyendranātha or sometimes the god Śiva himself. There were and are many systems of Yoga belonging to many traditions and the continuity and intermixture between these is as important to the institutions of these traditions

2 This is to be understood in the sense of the non-Buddhist yoga traditions of India or yoga as a designation of the predominantly *rāja-* and *haṭha-yoga* currents. However, we have to note that almost all Indian traditions used the term yoga or 'yoking' with many different meanings ranging from the banal 'application' to the mystical 'union' and the word is by no means to be understood as always being the same or having the same referent in all contexts. The idea that there is one discrete, palpable, ancient, continuous and pan-Indian tradition called 'Yoga' is a modern conception. The same applies to a multitude of other Sanskrit terms.

as it is often contested and debated by scholars. The earliest systematic Yoga (as in the *Pātañjalayogaśāstra*) is arguably firmly Brahmanical in origin[3], though it has been reliably proven to have developed in dialogue with Buddhist thought.[4]

From a practitioner's point of view, it is perhaps most important to focus on studying the teachings belonging to the tradition of their choice, while educating oneself about the background and development of other traditions as well, in order to gain at least a general idea of the context of their practice. However, it is necessary to briefly discuss the use and meaning of terms such as 'yoga' and 'tantra' in the context of their historical use and development and the problematic and heterogenous nature of their modern usage.

Disambiguating 'Yoga' and 'yoga', 'Tantra' and 'tantra', *rāja-yoga*, haṭha-yoga, and Their Relation to Vedānta, Neo-Vedānta, and the New Age

What is meant by 'Yoga' in the context of the six classical philosophical systems (*ṣaḍ-darśana*) of Indian thought is the Yoga based on Patañjali's Yoga-sūtras. Known as '*rāja-yoga*' in later nomenclature, it was codified between the 3rd and 5th centuries CE and systematised further in its commentary—the Yoga-bhāṣya. It is a dualistic, Sāṃkhya-based system with rigorous metaphysics and epistemology, not simply a collection of practices. Classical Yoga's goal is to achieve absorption (*samādhi*) by isolating the individual Self (*puruṣa*) from external forces and neutralising the turbulations of the mind.[5] Within Vedāntic literature, Yoga as a *darśana* was recognised, but criticised. Advaita Vedānta rejected the dualistic ontology of Sāṃkhya and classical Yoga, asserting instead the non-duality (*advaita*) of the individual self (*ātman*) and the absolute (*brahman*). Thus, when speaking about Classical Yoga with a capital 'Y' in this book what is meant is Patañjali's system, not

---

3 Maas, Philipp, A. (n. d). *The Pātañjalayogaśāstra alias the Yogasūtra and the Yogabhāṣya*. Sahapedia. https://www.sahapedia.org/patanjalayogasastra-alias-yogasutra-and-yogabhasya (accessed on 22.10.2023).

4 Maas, Philipp, A. (2020). Sarvāstivāda Buddhist Theories of Temporality and the Pātañjala Yoga Theory of Transformation (pariṇāma). *Journal of Indian Philosophy*. 48.5: pp. 963–965. https://doi.org/10.1007/s10781-020-09450-1 (accessed on 22.10.2023).

5 Larson, G. J. (1969). *Classical Sāṃkhya: An interpretation of its history and meaning*. Delhi: Motilal Banarsidass, pp. 34–41 and Larson, G. J.& Bhattacharya, R. S. (1987). *Yoga: India's philosophy of meditation*. Delhi: Motilal Banarsidass, pp. 52–63.

its later re-interpretations. Consequently, 'yoga' with a miniscule 'y' will be used to refer to the particular practices within a tradition, the general sense of 'union' or 'liberation', or modern yoga.

Later Vedāntic commentators and modern reformers, however, reinterpreted Patañjali's classical Yoga or *rāja-yoga* from an Advaita point of view, reading *samādhi* not as the isolation of *puruṣa*, but actually as the realisation of brahman.[6] The result was that classical *rāja-yoga* came to be viewed as a pathway of immersion within a broader non-dualist theology rather than as a dualist liberation philosophy in its own right. Thus, speaking of *rāja-yoga* in a Pātañjala context, on the one hand, and in Vedāntic and even Neo-Vedāntic context, on the other, actually deals with two epistemologically distinct approaches to liberation.

From about the time of Patañjali onwards (ca. 5th–6th centuries CE) what is generally referred to as 'Tantra' started to develop and gained momentum on the Indian religious, spiritual and ritual stage. Tantra was a new ritual system at the time and was also intended to be an alternative to the existing Brahmanical systems. Incorporating non-Brahmanical ritual practices of local origin with fire rituals and worship from that tradition, Tantra probably had a hand in the innovation of mystic formulae (*mantras*) for the purposes of liberation. Tantric traditions in their majority, be they Hindu, Buddhist or otherwise, are primarily initiatory. That means that liberation, whatever its ontological reality, is inaccessible without initiation by a proper *guru*. Most tantric traditions focused on a particular deity or set of deities, which later developed into complex, numerously populated systems of cosmology, epistemology and theoretics of liberation, as well as their respective accompanying practices. Tantric systems can be dualistic or monistic, depending on the tradition. The roots of the most well-known non-Buddhist 'tantric' practices and notions in modern times in the West can be traced back to Śaiva, Śaiva-Śākta, and Vaiṣṇava (Pāñcarātra) traditions. In the case of the broad category of modern yogic practices, this occurred via the medium of *haṭha-yoga* in the late incarnations of its historical development.

Originally used as a derogatory term for forceful yogic practices in the Kālacakra tradition of tantric Buddhism at the turn of the first millenium,

---

6 Maas, P. A. (2013). *A concise historiography of classical yoga philosophy*. In K. Baier, P. Maas & K. Preisendanz (Eds.). *Yoga in Transformation: Historical and Contemporary Perspectives* (pp. 57–87). Vienna: Austrian Academy of Sciences Press, pp. 60–63.

'*haṭha-yoga*' was only later adopted by the non-Buddhist tradition which came to bear that name long after it had already developed. Between roughly the 11th and 15th centuries CE, a body of yogic literature arose that also integrated tantric (especially Śaiva) and physiological practices, including, for the first time, a more pronounced use of physical yogic postures (*āsanas*). Texts such as the *Amṛtasiddhi* (ca. 11th century), *Haṭhapradīpikā* (15th century), Śiva-saṃhitā, and *Gheraṇḍa-saṃhitā* define '*haṭha*' not merely as 'force' (as the term was used in Buddhist yoga of the Kālacakra tradition) but as the disciplined activation of the subtle body through techniques involving the physical body like gestures (*mudrā*), contractions/holds (*bandha*), and breathing practices (*prāṇāyāma*). The goal of these methods was to awaken a presumed dormant energy within the body (*kuṇḍalinī*) for the purpose of achieving liberation. While drawing conceptually upon Patañjali's meditative goals, this later haṭha tradition grounded itself in Śaiva and Buddhist tantric cosmology, seeking non-dualist '*rāja-yoga*' in the above-mentioned modified sense through the medium of bodily alchemy.[7]

The relationship between *haṭha-yoga* and Vedānta also evolved historically through assimilation. Initially, *haṭha* was not Vedāntic; its literature is almost entirely Tantric in orientation. Yet from the 15th century onwards, Advaitic renunciate orders, particularly the *daśanāmī-saṃnyāsins*[8], absorbed *haṭha* methods into their practice, recasting them yet again, this time as preparatory techniques for realising non-dual awareness.[9] By the 19th century, Advaita's metaphysical monism came to dominate Indian religious discourse, and *haṭha-yoga* was mostly reinterpreted as a physical path to Vedāntic realisation rather than a tantric discipline.

A decisive moment in this process occurred with Svāmī Vivekānanda's publication of *Rāja Yoga* in 1896. Drawing upon both Patañjali's system *and* Advaita Vedānta, Vivekānanda redefined 'yoga' as a universal spiritual science grounded in reason and introspection, which, ironically, fits within the

---

7 Mallinson, J. & Birch, J. (2017). *The Yoga of the Haṭhapradīpikā: A critical edition and translation*. Oxfordshire: Routledge, pp. 21–24 and Mallinson, J. (2020). Haṭha Yoga's early history: From Vajrayāna to Śaivism. *Journal of the American Oriental Society*, 140(1). 1–28, pp 2–9. https://doi.org/10.7817/jameroriesoci.140.1.0001 (accessed on 28.10.2025).

8 The ten monastic orders will be explained below.

9 Mallinson, J. (2020). Haṭha Yoga's early history: From Vajrayāna to Śaivism. *Journal of the American Oriental Society*, 140(1), 1–28. P. 16–17. https://doi.org/10.7817/jameroriesoci.140.1.0001 (accessed on 28.10.2025).

Western conception of 'meditation', but in reality applies the approach of the so-called 'yoga of knowledge' (*jñāna-yoga*) — a term used both by monistic Vedānta and dualistic Sāṃkhya — and the introspective approach found in Patañjali, to a hybrid non-dual metaphysics. He translated Patañjali's dualistic *kaivalya* into the idiom of non-dual realisation and presented that 'yoga' as a method for perceiving the divine unity of existence. This re-interpretation — central to what later came to be called Neo-Vedānta — merged intellectual Vedānta with yogic practice, proposing that the world's religions were convergent paths toward a single Truth.[10] While being strongly influenced by Vivekānanda's liberationist framework, modern 'yoga', under several further influences, was presented as a practical, physical tradition, rather than as any one of the systems aimed at liberation it was derived from, cloaking the goal of liberation into nebulous New-age terminology, which blurred its spiritually-oriented origins and made it possible to practice derivatives of techniques and practices originally aimed at spiritual, religious and even magical goals in a modern, secularised environment. This modern 'yoga', with a small 'y', drew selectively from *haṭha* techniques while integrating Western physical culture and medical discourse. Masters such as Svāmī Śivānanda and Śrī Aurobindo further imbued it with Neo-Vedāntic ideals, presenting 'yoga' as the practical aspect of Vedānta — the embodiment of divine consciousness through ethical living and disciplined action.[11]

In this transnational form, 'yoga' became the vehicle of a 'global' spirituality which blended Indian monism with Western esotericism and humanistic psychology, where concepts such as *prāṇa*, *cakras*, and self-realisation were recast within a psycho-spiritual framework oriented toward self-actualisation rather than liberation from rebirth.[12] The dialogue between Indian thought and Western philosophy had already been established in the 18th and

10 De Michelis, E. (2004). *A history of modern yoga: Patañjali and Western esotericism*. New York: Continuum, pp. 41–45; Halbfass, W. (1988). *India and Europe: An essay in understanding*. New York: SUNY Press, pp. 233–238 and King, R. (1999). Indian philosophy and Western intellectuals: The problem of Orientalism. Oxfordshire: Routledge, pp. 84–92.

11 Singleton, M. (2010). *Yoga body: The origins of modern posture practice*. Oxford University Press, pp. 45–48 and Alter, J. S. (2004). *Yoga in modern India: The body between science and philosophy*. Princeton University Press, pp. 52–59.

12 Urban, H. B. (2003). *Tantra: Sex, secrecy, politics, and power in the study of religion*. Berkeley: University of California Press, pp. 112–117; Hanegraaff, W. J. (1996). *New Age religion and Western culture: Esotericism in the mirror of secular thought*. Leiden: Brill, pp. 388–395 and Strauss, S. (2005). *Positioning yoga: Balancing acts across cultures*. New York: Routledge, pp. 69–73.

19th centuries, when thinkers such as Schopenhauer, Goethe, and Nietzsche drew inspiration from early translations and studies of Indian texts on metaphysics. This intellectual interest later extended into psychology, most notably through Jung's 1932 seminar *The Psychology of Kundalini Yoga*, which initiated a discussion on the relation between Indic metaphysics and Western psychotherapy. Within this broader environment, the boundaries between Yoga as a *darśana*, tantric yogic practice, and modern spiritual disciplines have gradually blurred, resulting in the 'global yoga' phenomenon,—an increasingly heterogenous phenomenon, which often mutates far beyond even the 20th century reinterpretations of its roots.

It was within this context that, from the mid-20th century onwards, Svāmī Satyānanda developed his syncretic integral system of yoga, drawing primarily on three of these *darśanas*—Advaita Vedānta, Sāṃkhya, and Classical Yoga, as well as on the traditions of Śaiva-Tantra and mature *haṭha-yoga*. He integrated their philosophical principles and practical techniques into a comprehensive spiritual system aimed at addressing all levels of the individual—physical, perceptual, intellectual, emotional, psychological, and metaphysical—in a synergistic way. Svāmī Satyānanda's lectures and writings were clearly oriented toward the needs of modern practitioners. He distilled the essence of these complex systems of thought into accessible language and practical methods applicable to everyday life, irrespective of cultural or religious background. Despite his innovative reformulation approach, a close examination of his works through the lens of historical development reveals the depth of their philosophical foundations and their firm rootedness in traditional sources.

Svāmī Satyānanda's contribution to the modern practitioner lies in his systematic revival and recontextualisation of historical techniques, particularly those related to reaching the state of *pratyāhāra*, one of which is his method of *yoga-nidrā*. He also integrated many tantric practices and principles into his master Svāmī Śivanānda's system, relying on formidable tantric scriptures. Texts such as the *Vijñānabhairva-tantra*, for example, were not taught by any other pupils of Śivanānda's, but are now in wide circulation through the teachings and publications of the Bihar School of Yoga.

Through this approach, Svāmī Satyānanda bridged the gap between classical yogic theory and experiential application, allowing practitioners to engage with subtle aspects of mind and awareness that had largely been neglected in modern, primarily physically-oriented yoga movements. Furthermore, his interest in Western scientific research and psychology led him to interpret traditional yogic concepts in a way that resonated with contemporary understandings of the human psyche, thereby creating a dialogue between ancient wisdom and modern science.

Vedānta, Sāṃkhya and Tantra — Non-duality and Duality

> *[...] in the practical application of yoga, we see the combination of Samkhya, Tantra and Vedanta. In fact, one cannot be a yogi without the knowledge of these three systems.*[13]
>
> Svāmī Nirañjanānanda

Among the six 'orthodox' Indian philosophies, we find three which are relevant to the topic of Satyananda Yoga Nidra which share many views, regardless of their different characteristics. These are Advaita Vedānta, Sāṃkhya and the Classical Yoga of Patañjali.

Advaita, or 'Non-dual' Vedānta advocates that there is a Supreme Reality or Universal Self (*brahman*) which is one and the same as the individual Self (*ātman*), which are, however, seemingly divided as a result of ignorance/non-knowledge (*a-vidyā*). A seeker's goal is, therefore, to free oneself from ignorance, which is the cause of all suffering, and experience the transcendent reality of the *brahman*, thus realising the non-difference between *ātman* and *brahman*. Various schools developed within Vedānta over the course of time, but the most important to the current discussion is the Advaita or 'non-dualist' school.

Another form of Vedānta, some tantric currents, and the Sāṃkhya school, on the other hand, are *dvaita* — dualistic schools of thought. They recognise two equal and eternal principles of the universe. In Sāṃkhya, these are referred to as 'consciousness' (*puruṣa*, which is multiple and eternal) and

13 Saraswati, Niranjanananda, Swami. (1999). *Yoga Sadhana Panorama*. Volume 1. Munger: Yoga Publication Trust, p. 70.

'energy/chaos/nature' (*prakṛti*, which is singular and also eternal), while in Hindu Tantra they are most commonly called *śiva* and *śakti*[14]. Both assume that the existence of the universe is not possible or cannot be maintained without these two principles and/or their proximity/interaction.

Vedānta — the 'End of Perceivable Knowledge'

The emergence of the earliest texts (Vedas), which form the basis for the later development of Vedānta, can be attributed to a period from approx. 1500 to approx. 1000 BCE. Each Veda is composed of several parts, the last of which is the Upaniṣads. The Upaniṣads are a collection of early philosophical writings dating to the late Vedic period (from ca. 700 to ca. 200 CE). They are often also called Vedānta, as they are traditionally placed at the end of the Vedic texts and are seen as the end and fulfilment of the Vedas, as well as summarising their contents. There are, however, even later Upaniṣads, composed all the way up to the 10th century CE. The ones of particular interest here are those available at the time of Advaita Vedānta's presumed founder — Śaṅkara, around the 8th century CE. It is the teachings first crystallised in these texts that form the basis of Vedāntic philosophy.

The main theme of Śankara's Advaita Vedānta is that *cit* or *brahman* is the Supreme Reality beyond the mutable world. The task of the seeker is to recognise this Supreme Reality and to identify with the individual Self (*ātman*) rather than with the transient world. Like other philosophical traditions in India, Vedānta also recognises the principle of the connection between cause and effect (*karman*), though it regards this law as operating only within cyclical existence (*saṃsāra*), not in the ultimate reality of the *brahman*.

> When Indian religious and philosophical thought started to gain popularity in the West through figures such as Svāmī Vivekānanda and the perennial philosophy of Helena Blavatsky's Theosophy it took on a life of its own. Nowadays, the wider Western public's perception of 'spirituality', including what is thought of as 'Indian spirituality' has also been influenced by 'esoteric' New Age thinking, such as that characteristic of Blavatsky's

---

14 Many tantric currents (e.g., Kashmir Śaivism/Trika) are, however, also explicitly non-dual.

student—Alice Bailey, whose influence has permeated even into seemingly secular Western approaches to education (e.g. Social Emotional Learning). Perennialism, New Age thinking, as well as liberationist offshoots thereof, such as the Hippie movement, together with the rising popularity of trends such as modern postural yoga[15] in the 20th century, have created a distorted image of Indian religion and philosophy in the popular imagination. Therefore, Western views of Indian philosophy and religion sometimes have very different points of prominence when compared to those still present on the Subcontinent itself, which have their own historical and contemporary dynamics. Thus, historically, it is important to point out that when something is particularly famous in the West, that does not mean it had a correspondingly important role in the history and development of religion and philosophy in India. In fact, many of the most influential figures in the history of Indian religion and philosophy are largely, if not completely unknown to the Western public, with the exclusion of a minority of scholar-specialists.

A poignant case relating to the historical developments within Vedānta, for example, is the fame of Śaṅkara—the well-known propounder of Advaita Vedānta, when contrasted with the equally, if not greater influence of the famous philosopher of Viśiṣṭādvaita Vedānta and propounder of Śrīvaiṣṇavism from the 12th century CE—Rāmānuja, or the founder of dualistic (*dvaita*) Vedānta from the 13th century CE—Mādhava, as well as many others. While Śankara is extremely well-known in the West, technically, Rāmānuja's qualified non-dual theistic stance emphasizing devotion (*bhakti*) and Mādhava's strict dualism had an incredibly strong impact on Indian religious attitudes and practice, much of which can still be felt today.

A key terminological example of 'esoteric'-ised 20th century syncretism is the case of the English term 'meditation'. Coming from Old French *meditacion*—'thought', 'reflection', 'study', it originated in the Latin *meditationem*, from the verb *meditari*—'to think over', 'to prepare'. So, the term was used mostly in the sense of rational contemplation. In the 20th century, however, it has become an English umbrella term encompassing a vast category of practices and states, ranging from visualisation, concentration, breath

15 De Michelis, Elisabeth. (2004). *A history of modern yoga: Patañjali and Western esotericism*. London & New York: Continuum.

awareness, immersion and trance, to contemplation, active imagination, 'mindfulness', daydreaming, fantasy journeys, and so on.[16] In Sanskrit, however, there is no such umbrella term, as different practices and states are each referred to by exact, specific terminology. If one were to invent a word for 'meditation' and went to discuss it with the philosophers and masters of ancient India, it is very likely they would not even recognise the concept.

The Upaniṣads

From every page [of the Upaniṣads] we come across profound, original, and sublime thoughts, whilst a lofty and sacred earnestness pervades the whole. [...] With the exception of the original text, it is the most profitable and sublime reading that is possible in the world; it has been the consolation of my life and will be that of my death.[17]

Arthur Schopenhauer

The Upaniṣads are considered to be a collection of revelatory writings which offer explanations and discourses on the topics of the Vedas. They are traditionally placed as the last sections of each of the four Vedas (*Ṛg-*, *Yajur-*, *Atharva-*, and *Sāmaveda*), and together with the *Brahma-sūtras* and the Bhagavad-gītā section of the *Mahābhārata* they form the central texts of the Vedāntic tradition. What are thought of as the nine main Upaniṣads deal with the questions of the identity of the nature of the Supreme Reality and the innermost essence of each individual, with the cause of creation, what was there before, and with the essence and meaning of existence or what happens after death.[18]

16 Halbfass, Wilhelm. (1988). *India and Europe: An Essay in Understanding*. New York: SUNY Press.

17 Schopenhauer, Arthur. (2000). *Parerga and Paralipomena: Short Philosophical Essays (1976–1987)*. Volume II. (1st published 1974). Oxford: Oxford University Press, p. 398.

18 Thieme, Paul. (1999). *Upanischaden*. Ditzingen: Reclam-Verlag, p. 90.

Key Elements of Advaita Vedānta[19]

- ***brahman* and *īśvara***

Svāmī Nirañjanānanda defines Vedānta's *brahman* as 'the ever-expanding consciousness', as the absolute or the highest consciousness.[20] It has no qualities and is unimaginable, therefore undefinable. *Brahman* is the one true reality that exists beyond the conditioned, limited and manifest world of *māyā*—the deceptive appearance of reality as dualistic. The universe appears to be real in its existence, yet, according to Advaita Vedānta (henceforth 'Vedānta'), this appearance is impermanent. Through the veil of *māyā*, the one is subject to dualism—experiencing the ultimate as separate from oneself—while in truth, the individual Self (*jīvātman*) is identical with *brahman*. Consequently, they are one and the same. In Vedānta, *īśvara*, or the personal deity[21] who is the first to possess this quality, is said to arise directly from *brahman*. *Īśvara* is described and understood as the omnivalent, omnipotent, omniscient intelligence of the universe.

- ***ātman* and *jīva***

Ātman is defined in the Upaniṣads as the true individual Self, as the principle of life and sentience—not just that of humans, but of every being, including animals. *Ātman* is the innermost, eternal core, the Self, which is immortal. *Ātman* and *brahman* are one and the same; therefore, in the event of Advaita-Vedāntic liberation, one realises the non-duality of *ātman* and *brahman*.[22]

Jīva (often translated as 'soul', but more precisely meaning 'individual') describes the nature of a living being, the bearer of the individual personality, which is incarnated again and again according to the doctrine of rebirth. One can experience the joy of the bliss of the Self and attain liberation while existing as a body. He is then referred to as 'liberated while living'—*jīvan-mukta*.

---

19 Saraswati, Niranjanananda, Swami. (1999). *Yoga Sadhana Panorama*, Volume 1. Munger: Yoga Publication Trust, p. 79–85.

20 Ibid., p. 80.

21 I.e., not the deity of any particular person, but the Divine with a person, a personality, whereas *brahman* is supreme and impersonal.

22 Technically, there is never any 'return' as the two were originally never two and never separate. It is important to point out, that in Rāmānuja's Viśiṣṭādvaita Vedānta, liberation is, by contrast, achieved through the grace of the Supreme Deity – Nārāyaṇa or Viṣṇu, as a result of devotion (*bhakti*) since the individual Self (*ātman*) is not considered non-separate from the Ultimate (*brahman*).

• *māyā*, *avidyā* and *mokṣa*

Tangible existence in Vedānta is considered to be *māyā*—the deceptive appearance of reality as dualistic—it veils the reality of the *brahman*, on the one hand, and projects the world of appearance, on the other, so that when one engages with the world, one cannot comprehend its true reality and remains caught in duality.[23]

It is important to note, that it has become a common and widespread belief in both India and among modern practitioners in the West that *māyā* is synonymous with 'illusion' and carries an intrinsically negative connotation. However, that is not so in the original doctrines presented by Śaṅkara. In his commentary (*bhāṣya*) on the *Brahma-sūtra* the word *māyā* itself is employed to convey various meanings. Possible translations in the respective contexts are 'deception', 'magic (trick)', or 'the wondrous power of God'. A frequently cited comparison from the *Brahma-sūtra-bhāṣya* (2.1.14) is that just as the magician is not affected by his own magic trick, so *brahman* always remains untouched by the phenomenal world. Furthermore, *māyā* is used attributively in the sense of 'illusory', for example to characterize the phenomenal world in this way.

In contrast to later Vedāntins such as Sureśvara, Śaṅkara does not conceive of *māyā* as something substantial. The world is neither made out of a substance called *māyā*, nor was it created from it. Thus, *māyā* is also not synonymous with *avidyā*, even though Śaṅkara's disciples presented it that way. Despite its use in similar contexts, the terms and concepts *avidyā*, *nāmarūpe*, and *māyā* must not be understood as synonyms. In Śaṅkara, with the exception of certain chains of identification, they are kept strictly distinct terminologically. The causal ignorance (*avidyā*) conditions the arising of the undifferentiated primal matter (*avyākṛte nāmarūpe*), from which the phenomenal world (*vyākṛte nāmarūpe*) and the cycle of existence (*saṃsāra*) are produced—these, in turn, are characterized by the description 'illusory' (*māyā*).[24]

---

23 Torwesten, Hans. (1985). Vedanta: Herz des Hinduismus, Chapter: Maya, die indische Sphinx. Walter Verlag. Cited in *Vedanta-Heft*. 2, 2012. Wiesbaden: Vedanta-Zentrum, p. 43.

24 Summarised from Hacker, Paul. (1950). Eigentümlichkeiten der Lehre und Terminologie Śaṅkaras: Avidyā, Nāmarūpa, Māyā, Īśvara. *Zeitschrift der Deutschen Morgenländischen Gesellschaft*. 100, N. F. 25, p. 246–286. Thanks to Patrick Zeitlhuber for providing this passage.

Cosmic ignorance (*avidyā*) allows the divine to emerge in countless different forms, obscuring its undivided unity. It is the individual experience of *māyā* and results in misidentification. The means of liberation is therefore the knowledge of reality (*vidyā*). Once reality is realised as undivided, non-reality and duality cease to exist. The entirety of existence is then seen as an expression of Ultimate Reality. This knowledge is, however, not intellectual knowledge—it is the result of direct experience.

Mokṣa (from the root √*muc* 'to free') is a term used in most Indian spiritual traditions to describe the liberation of the individual from the shackles of cyclic existence (*bhava* or *saṃsāra*). Depending on the interpretation of this liberation in the various traditions, the exact meaning of what *mokṣa* entails can vary.

The Concept of Creation in Vedānta

In Vedānta, Ultimate Reality and the universe are fundamentally identical. While from a worldly point of view *īśvara* is the Creator, that Ultimate Reality is pure consciousness—*brahman*—beyond cause and effect, encompassing both the Creator and the Creation simultaneously.

Vedānta and Yoga

In a Vedānta context, the spiritual aspirant's goal of attaining *mokṣa* comprises the final dissolution of the perceived *ātman-brahman* duality. The essential practice of Vedānta consists of identifying with *brahman* and seeing and recognising it in everything—in other words: with the knowledge that everything is one, the Self and the world are experienced, and thus one interacts with the world in a completely conscious way. Similarly, all yoga practices, as varied as they are, are ultimately aimed at the experience of return to, identity, or oneness with true reality. According to Svāmī Satyānanda, there is, therefore, no difference between *dvaita* and *advaita*—Duality and Non-duality. *Dvaita* is the foundation of *sādhana*—practice for the sake of accomplishment. In the realisation of union, *advaita* becomes a reality and is the basis of experience.[25]

Sāṃkhya

Sāṃkhya is mainly translated as 'enumeration', 'enumerative philosophical method' or 'that which describes something in detail'. However, recently Philipp Maas translated it more convincingly as 'all-embracing insight'[26] — in other words those who hold it possible to perceive (*-khya*) the universe comprehensively (*sāṃ-*). He asserts that this is the philosophy par excellence of India, and it is crucial to familiarise oneself with it if one wishes to engage seriously with Indian philosophy. Svāmī Nirañjanānanda utilises the following translations: 'perfect knowledge of the entire process of manifestation, evolution and absorption' and 'a methodology of reasoning that results in spiritual knowledge, leading to liberation.'[27]

Sāṃkhya explains the elements which determine the structure of reality and emphasises that knowledge (*jñāna*), which is attained by distinguishing between the eternal and the impermanent, is the only path to liberation. The main period of Sāṃkhya's prominence is considered to be from 400 to 800 CE. The formulation of the essence of the Sāṃkhya is attributed to the *Sāṃkhya-kārikā* of Īśvarakṛṣṇa, however, other significant texts featuring different paradigms of Sāṃkhya are the seminal *Yoga-sūtras* of Patañjali and its adjacent commentary — the *Bhāṣya*, as well as texts like the famous medical treatise of Caraka — the *Caraka-saṃhitā*.

25 Satyanana, Swami. (n. d.). Yogic Concepts. In *Yoga Magazine*. (2008). Munger: Bihar School of Yoga. (11/12). http://www.yogamag.net/archives/2000s/2008/0811/0811ygcn.html (accessed on 12.01.2020).

26 Maas, Philipp. (2021). YSP 21: *What is Sāṅkhya Philosophy?*. [Yogic Studies] https://www.youtube.com/watch?v=11cnO7ADq3M&t=1829s (accessed on 10.10. 2022).

27 Saraswati, Niranjanananda, Swami. (2008). *Samkhya Darshan*. Munger: Yoga Publication Trust, p. 12.

Sāṃkhya

25 Elements of the Universe

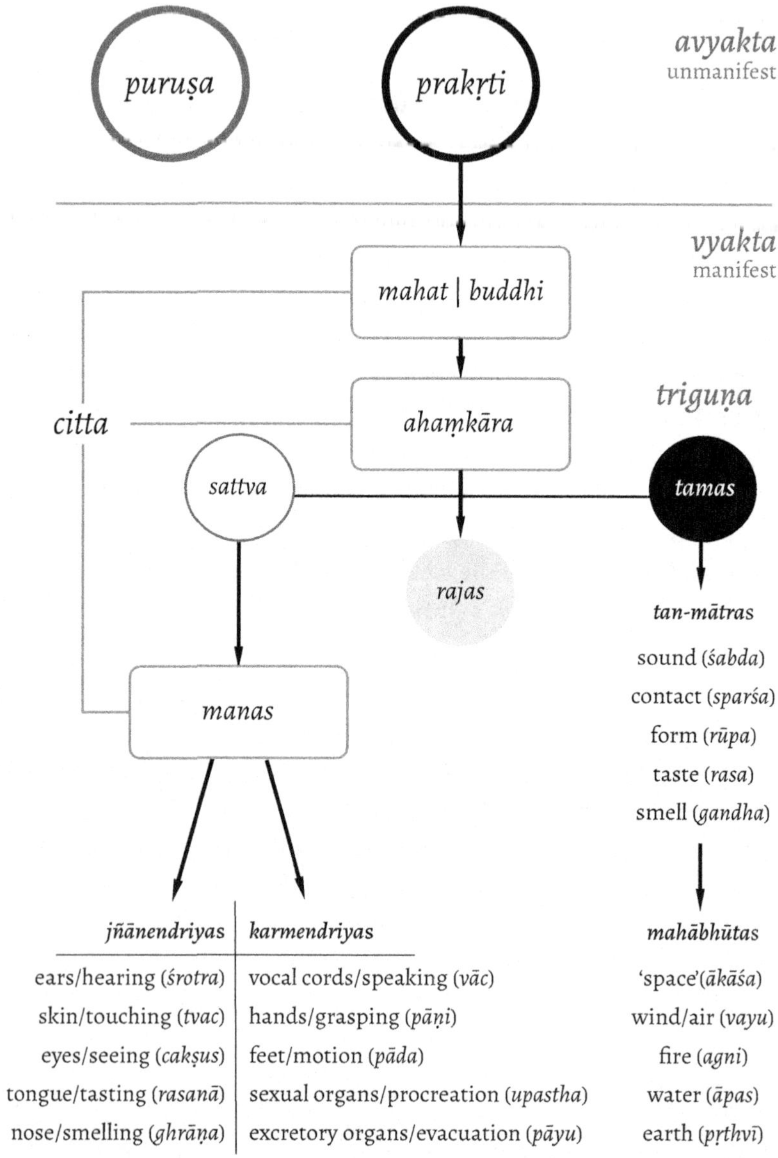

FIGURE I[28]

Key Elements of Sāṃkhya

Sāṃkhya encompasses both the description of the origin of the universe and the explanation of the functioning of the human mind. This view of the world is therefore closely related to the state of the individual mind (see Fig. 1 on the Sāṃkhya model).[29]

- *puruṣa* and *prakṛti* — *consciousness* and *primordial* matter

The Sāṃkhya doctrine deals with the interplay of the two eternal principles *puruṣa* — the inert, observing consciousness, the subject of experience, who is free from all content of consciousness — and *prakṛti* — the observed, the primordial matter, the creative energy, without properties but with its three inherent constituent qualities (*guṇas*).[30] Sāṃkhya explores the evolution and involution of all levels of consciousness and matter, of the macrocosm and microcosm.

- *tri-guṇa*

The tri-guṇa are the three qualities of nature: inertia/darkness/stability (*tamas*), restlessness/activity/ movement/energy (*rajas*) and purity/clarity/ goodness/harmony (*sattva*). These three qualities are in a balanced relationship with each other as long as the primordial matter *prakṛti* is in a state of equilibrium as potential. As soon as *prakṛti*, initiated by the mere presence of the *puruṣa*, becomes active through the interplay of the three *guṇas*, the first evolutes of reality (*tattvas*) begin to develop.[31]

- *mahat* (*buddhi*) — **the highest intelligence**

Mahat (also known as *buddhi*) is the first evolute of *prakṛti*. It and all the other twenty-two levels of manifestation (adding up to a total of twenty-five) are subject to the three *guṇas* into which *prakṛti* develops and are therefore

28 Figure 1. The origin of the world and the human mind according to Sāṃkhya as presented by Svāmī Nirañjanānanda. Ibid., p. 51.

29 The order of the stages of emergence in the Sāṃkhya teachings and their explanations presented here follows that given by Svāmī Nirañjanānanda in *Samkhya Darshan*. (2008).

30 Saraswati, Satyananda, Swami. (1989). Teachings of Swami Satyananda Saraswati. Volume III. In *Yoga Magazine*, Raja Yoga. 2016 (8). http://www.yogamag.net/archives/2010s/2016/1608/1608raja.html (accessed on 25.03.2020).

31 Saraswati, Niranjanananda, Swami. (2008). *Samkhya Darshan*. Munger: Yoga Publication Trust, pp. 29–34

conditioned. According to Svāmī Satyānanda, the role of the *mahat* is to activate *prakṛti* and to recognise and analyse its potential.[32]

- ***ahaṃkāra* — individuation[33], and *manas* — the interactive mind faculty**

Ahaṃkāra — the principle of individuation (*Sāṃkhya-kārikā* 24) by which the distinct qualities and characteristics of each entity in the world are formed, gives rise to the multiplicity of existence. It arises as next, both through the realisation of the conditioned *prakṛti* and through identification with it. It is the starting point of a threefold emanation — one with predominating *sattva*-, another predominating *rajas*- and the third where *tamas guṇa* predominates. According to Svāmī Nirañjanānanda, from *ahaṃkāra* with predominance of the *sattva* quality evolve the following evolute faculties of the human being: the process of thinking or analysing (*manas*), the faculty of perception or the organs of knowledge (*jñānendriya*[34]) and also the five organs of action/perception (*karmendriya*). These manifestations are capable of perception, they enable knowledge and understanding, resulting from their interaction with each other and from engagement with the outside world. After the organs of action, from *ahaṃkāra* with predominance of the *tamas* quality evolve the entities of the 'outside' world, expressed in the arising of the five subtle elements (*tanmātra*) and the five gross elements (*mahābhūta*), which then give rise to the gross, physical universe. In this process of creation, *manas* plays no causal role since these are the solid, stable and inherent properties of each element of existence.[35]

Within the classical Sāṃkhya system as reflected in Īśvarakṛṣṇa's Sāṃkhya-kārikā, there are three distinct mental faculties: *buddhi*, *ahaṃkāra* and *manas*. Patañjali in his *Yoga-sūtras*, however, uses *buddhi*, *manas* and *citta* — a term, which can have many meanings depending on the context — interchangeably for 'mind' without distinction.

---

32 Ibid., p. 49–50.

33 The term 'individuation' has been proposed by Philipp Maas as a translation of *ahaṃkāra*.

34 Most often termed *buddhīndriya*.

35 Saraswati, Niranjanananda, Swami. (2008). *Samkhya Darshan*. Munger: Yoga Publication Trust, pp. 50–58.

- *indriya*

Indriyas or 'organs' consist of the five sense faculties (*jñānendriyas*) and their functions and the five organs of action (*karmendriyas*). The *jñānendriyas* are the ears/hearing (*śrotra*), the skin/touching (*tvac*), the eyes/seeing (*cakṣus*), the tongue/tasting (*rasanā*), the nose/smelling (*ghrāṇa*). The *karmendriyas* are the vocal cords/speaking (*vāc*), the hands/grasping (*pāṇi*), the feet/motion (*pāda*), the sexual organs/procreation (*upastha*) and the excretory organs/evacuation (*pāyu*). The *karmendriyas* refer more to the function or ability inherent in the organ than to the actual organ itself.

According to Svāmī Nirañjanānanda, they arise from the sattvic *ahaṃkāra* (*Sāṃkhya-kārikā* 26–27) and are the instruments of the *manas*. Furthermore, the *jñānendriyas* are the means by which the *tri-guṇa*, *mahābhūtas* and the *antaḥkaraṇa* are expressed and experienced.[36]

- *tan-mātra*

The *tan-mātras* are the five subtle elements or sense experiences: sound, touch, form, taste and smell. They represent the subtle essence of the elements which, according to Svāmī Nirañjanānanda, unfold from the tāmasic *ahaṃkāra*, in which there is no aspect of conscious awareness. They are connected to the *jñānendriya*—organs of knowledge. Their interaction enables them to experience *prakṛti* and use them as 'tools' of experience in their field of existence.[37]

- *mahābhūta*

Mahābhūta refers to the five gross elements which emerge from the tanmātras with defined properties, qualities and attributes. They also arise from the tāmasic *ahaṃkāra*. They are: space (*ākāśa*), air/dynamism (*vāyu*), fire/form (*agni*), water/fluidity (*āpas*) and earth/solidity/stability (*pṛthvī*). Through the *ahaṃkāra*, the ego, the essence of the *tan-mātras* is experienced through the organs of knowledge (*jñānendriyas*) as sound, touch, form, taste, and smell.[38]

---

36 Ibid., p. 59.
37 Ibid., p. 59.
38 Ibid., p. 57–58.

Each *tan-mātra* is connected to one *jñānendriya* and one *mahābhūta*:

jñānendriyas	*tan-mātras*	*mahābhūtas*
ears/hearing (*śrotra*)	sound (*śabda*)	'space' (*ākāśa*)
skin/touching (*tvac*)	contact (*sparśa*)	wind/air (*vayu*)
eyes/seeing (*cakṣus*)	form (*rūpa*)	fire (*agni*)
tongue/tasting (*rasanā*)	taste (*rasa*)	water (*āpas*)
nose/smelling (*ghrāṇa*)	smell (*gandha*)	earth (*pṛthvī*)

TABLE 1: Key elements of Sāṃkhya.

- ***kaivalya*** **— liberation, autonomy**

Although they appear as two distinct principles, it is through the 'content' of *prakṛti* that *puruṣa* (the individual) gains experiences, evolves, and ultimately achieves liberation — *kaivalya* (*Sāṃkhya-kārikā* 68). *Prakṛti* is regarded as real and serves the purpose of guiding *puruṣa* away from the cycle of rebirth towards liberation, either through involvement with the material world or through detachment from it.[39]

Sāṃkhya and Yoga

The yoga based on Patañjali's *Yoga-sūtras* is essentially a system for the practical application of a Sāṃkhya-based philosophy.[40] In Sāṃkhya, Yoga, and Tantra, in contrast to Vedānta, active engagement with existence is viewed as a path to liberation. One is simply in a state of ignorance (*avidyā*), which obscures the recognition of both oneself and the diverse existence around oneself as being identical with the higher reality. This ignorance is the root of suffering.

The *Bhagavad-Gītā* (5.4–5) says on this matter:

---

39 Maas, Philipp. (2021). YSP 21: *What is Sāṅkhya Philosophy?*. [Yogic Studies] https://www.youtube.com/watch?v=11cnO7ADq3M&t=1829s (accessed on 10.10. 2022).

40 Feuerstein, Georg. (2008). *The Yoga Tradition – Its History, Literature, Philosophy and Practice* (3rd edition). Arizona: Hohm Press, p. 542.

> *The foolish declare that Sāṃkhya and yoga are separate, not the wise. He who performs even one of them correctly obtains the fruit of both.* (5.4) *The state attained by followers of Sāṃkhya is that reached by yogins, too. Sāṃkhya and yoga are one: who sees this [truly] sees.* (5.5)[41]

One could say that a metaphysical understanding of Sāṃkhya is to be found in the *Yoga-sūtras* of Patañjali and that yoga, with special emphasis on immersion, opens the way to it.

The Sāṃkhya doctrine is dualistic in nature, without explicitly denying the existence of a single source. This source could be considered to be the *īśvara* that Patañjali speaks about — the personal omnipresent divine, or, the creator, sustainer and destroyer, if looked at in more Śaiva terms. The Yoga-sūtras postulate the necessity of recognising the single origin of existence, so that self-realisation (or liberation — *kaivalya*) becomes possible. Nevertheless, one should focus on what is accessible at the experiential level, namely the expressions of *prakṛti*, without which, according to Sāṃkhya, nothing exists. According to Svāmī Nirañjanānanda, *puruṣa* and *prakṛti* are the creative extension of *īśvara*. Therefore, they are the two essential principles on which the practice of yoga is based. Sāṃkhya is not focused on the worship of deities but on the practice of continuous expansion of individual awareness, leading to profound realization.[42]

Non-dual Śaiva Tantra

The history of practices that can today be considered 'tantric' likely predates the Vedas, though the surviving written texts belonging to various tantric traditions themselves date only from around 600 to 1200 CE. Unlike Vedānta and Sāṃkhya, the more transgressive aspects of the tantric traditions had pioneers of the teaching who also came from the lower castes of society. Feuerstein suggests that this was possible because in many tantric traditions the practitioner should not renounce the mundane but experience it fully. Wallis explains, however, that, while early Sāṃkhya asserts the singleness

41 Mallinson, J. and Singleton M. (2017). *Roots of Yoga*. London: Penguin Classics, p. 25.

42 Saraswati, Niranjanananda, Swami. (2008). *Samkhya Darshan*. Munger: Yoga Publication Trust, p. 82.

(*ekatva*) and separateness (*pṛthaktva*) of the conscious self from the body (probably based on similar notions in the *Caraka-saṃhitā*) whereby they do not come into contact, this is 'in direct opposition of the tantric doctrine, which conceives the soul as an "experiencer" (*bhoktṛ*) not a "witness" (*draṣṭṛ*), which actually contacts (*sparśa*) the world through the expansion of its faculties'.[43] The concept of the 'observer' will henceforth be referred to by its Nominative form (*draṣṭā*) as it that is most common in modern yoga parlance, unlike the citation form (*draṣṭṛ*).

Furthermore, in Tantra the processes of the world and the processes of liberation or enlightenment are seen as a continuum rather than as oppo sites. The intention is to integrate physical existence into spiritual reality.[44] These tantric principles are very close to our everyday life today. While they share some similarities, it is noteworthy to point out that traditions such as mature *haṭha-yoga* aim rather at achieving liberation by means of the body in an ascetic manner.

The term *tantra* comes from the Sanskrit root √*tan* and means, among other things: 'loom', 'warp on a loom', or also: 'expansion', 'extension', 'liberation', 'continuum' or 'that by which knowledge/understanding is extended, spread out'.[45] Svāmī Satyānanda also traces the term back to the root √*tan* and connects it to the verb *tanoti* (to expand), which shares the same root. This interpretation emphasizes the 'expansion of the individual's consciousness'. He further relates the Sanskrit suffix *-tra*, typically indicating a 'tool', to *trāyate* (from the root √*trai*, to guard, protect, save), interpreting it as 'to liberate', 'to free from bondage'. According to Svāmī Satyānanda, this understanding of tantra as deriving from 'to expand' and 'to free' suggests a meaning of 'liberating the inner, subtle and dormant energy (*kuṇḍalinī-śakti*)' hidden in everything, thus describing the process of a *sādhana*, where limited consciousness is expanded and conditioned energy is liberated[46] — a decidedly tantric interpretation, which is more popular in the West through its somatocentric *haṭha-yoga* incarntion.

---

43 Wallis, Christopher, D. (2014). *To Enter, to be entered, to merge: The role of religious experience in the traditions of Tantric Shaivism*. Dissertation. Berkeley: University of California.

44 Feuerstein, Georg. (2008). *The Yoga Tradition – Its History, Literature, Philosophy and Practice* (3rd edition). Arizona: Hohm Press, p. 542–543.

45 Ibid., p. 512.

46 Saraswati, Niranjananda, Swami. (2013). *Tantra Darshan*. Munger: Yoga Publication Trust, p. 4.

In the course of time, many tantric currents emerged—from Mantramārga Śaivism to the Buddhist *kriya*, *cārya*, *yoga* and *yoganiruttara* Tantras or from the Vaiṣṇava Pāñcarātra tradition to the late, non-Buddhist Saurya, Gāṇapatya, Gāyatrī tantras and many more. This book will deal primarily with the non-Buddhist Śaiva and Śākta tantra traditions, which have also influenced the teachings of Svāmī Satyānanda and those of his successors—Svāmī Nirañjanānanda and Svāmī Satyasaṅgānanda.

Nondual ŚaivaTantra

36 elements of the Universe

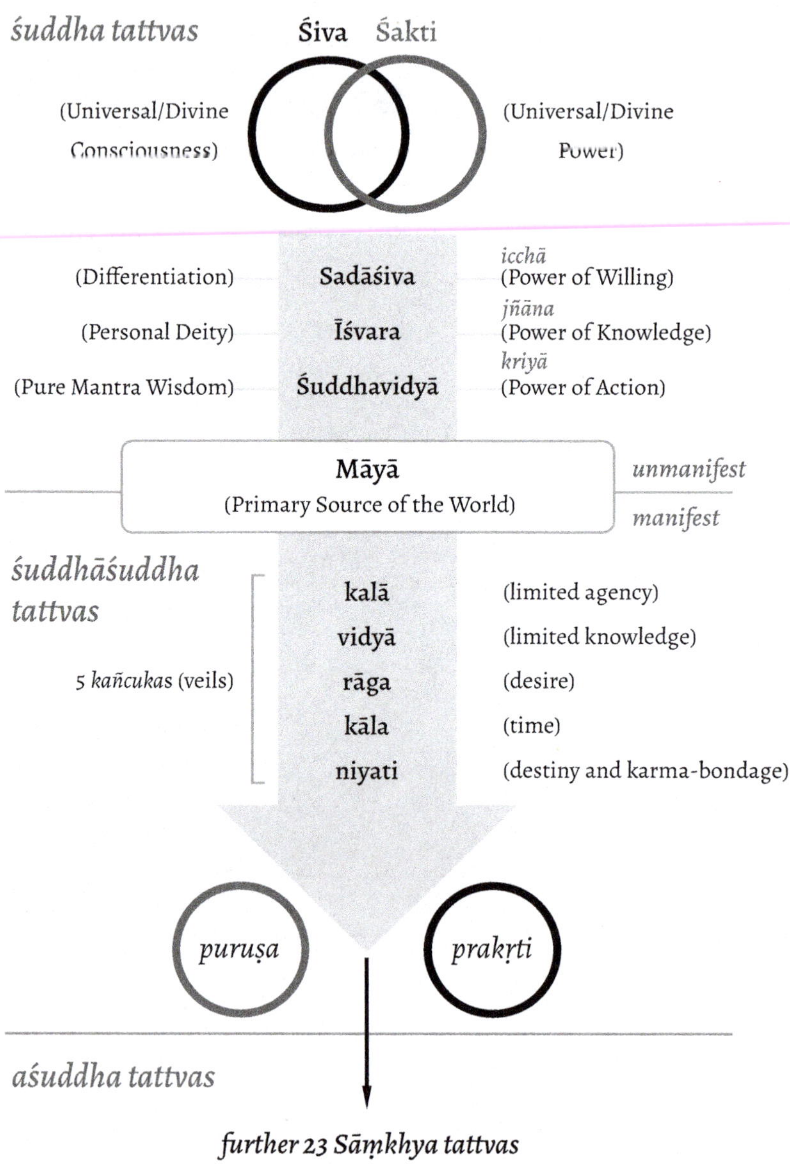

FIGURE 2

Key Elements of Śaiva Tanta

- *śiva* and *śakti*

According to Svāmī Satyasaṅgānanda, Śaiva-Śākta tantric philosophy (a subset of Śaiva Tanta) holds that the universe emerges as creation through *śakti*, the original nature. *Śiva*, or consciousness, remains passive in this process of creation and merely observes the play of creation. Although these two equal principles would then appear to be separate, they are seen as eternally coexisting and together form a whole.[47] This concept of Ultimate Reality is visualised in the unifying form of Ardhanārīśvara—who is represented as half-Śiva and half-Śakti (Figure 3).

Within some Śaiva systems, with the beginning of the unfolding of existence, evolution brings forth the 36 *tattvas* (elements) which make up the manifest and non-manifest world. *Tattva* is defined as an aspect of reality, a layer, or level. This idea overlaps to some extent with that of the Sāṃkhya philosophy (see Figure 1), whose conception of existence is based on 25 *tattvas*,[48] to which Śaivism adds an extra 11.

In later tantric approaches, some of which have also influenced the teachings of Svāmī Satyānanda, the aim is to dissolve the duality and to unite *śakti* with *śiva*, the individual with the universal. He posits that individual energy and consciousness are limited and 'trapped' according to that system. However, it is possible to discover how to utilise the individual energy (*śakti*) and use it to expand the awareness through tantric methods.

> Tantra has often been associated with sexuality, especially in the West since the 1960s. This is a misunderstanding and a confusion of Tantra with the Indian arts of love (*kāmaśāstra*). In fact, in some traditions of Tantrism, among other things, sexual practices are seen as a possible (and in some cases even necessary) path to liberation, whereby the ordinary erotic experience is transformed into a transcendental experience. Consequently, many tāntrikas (the practitioners of a certain Tantra) rejected the exclusivist views of other teachings and instead included the physical, the prāṇic, and the

47 Saraswati, Satyasanganānda, Swami. (2005). *Tattwa Shuddhi*. Munger: Yoga Publication Trust, p. 41.
48 Saraswati, Niranjanananda, Swami. (2013). *Tantra Darshan*. Munger: Yoga Publication Trust, p. 36.

mental dimensions in the spiritual quest.[49] However, while the *Śākta* tantric attitude was meant to be accessible to all, the specific sexual practices are generally only meant for advanced practitioners who are initiates—those who had already reached the stage of spiritual experience where their mind was able to dwell beyond sensual pleasure. Many tāntrikas were actually persecuted for these practices and consequently only performed them in secret.

49 Feuerstein, Georg. (2008). *The Yoga Tradition – Its History, Literature, Philosophy and Practice* (3rd edition). Arizona: Hohm Press, p. 543.

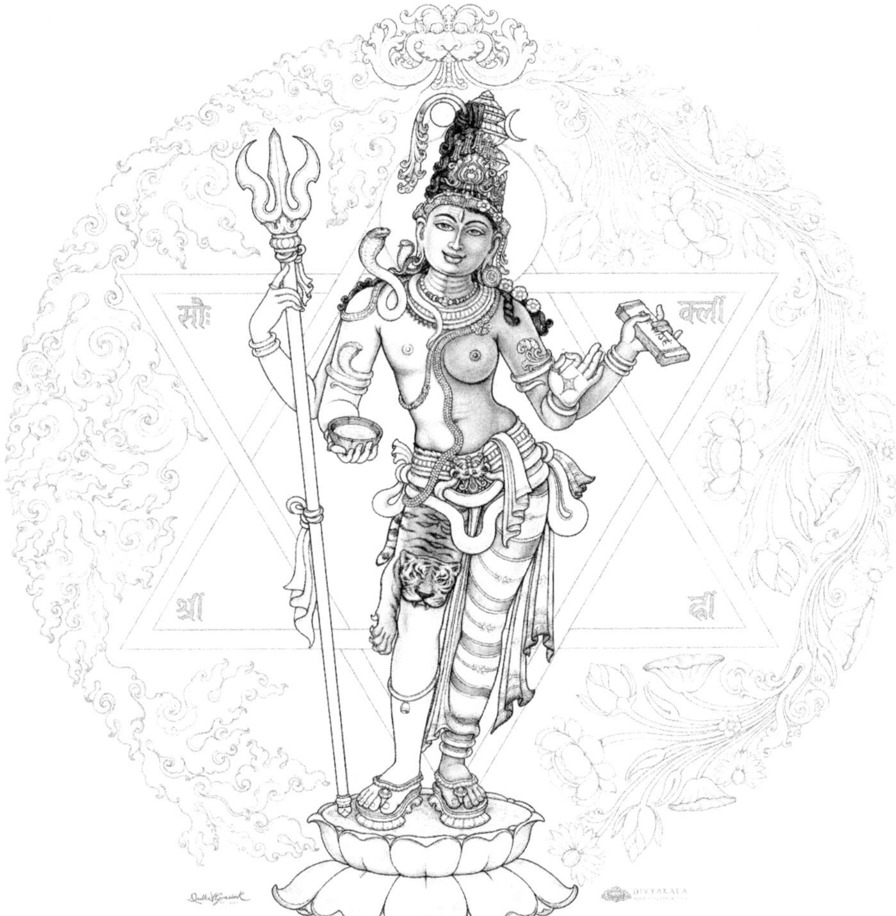

FIGURE 3: Ardhanārīśvara — Ultimate Reality represented as half-Śiva and half-Śakti.

The Tools of Tantra — Mantra, *yantra*, *maṇḍala* and *vidhi*

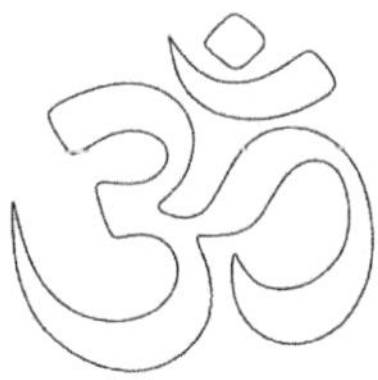

Mantra is one of the most important tools of the tantric traditions. 'The term "mantra" typically designates a short formula that is composed in Sanskrit and is considered to have a special power or efficacy.'[50] In the first millennium CE, mantras began to be prolifically used for magical and soteriological purposes, becoming ubiquitous across Indic traditions. Svāmī Nirañjanānanda defines mantra as follows: 'The power through which one can liberate the mind from its obsessions is mantra'.[51] The science of mantra in this context deals with the sound vibration which is used to harmonise and focus the scattered mental energies so that one is able to harmonise one's individual vibration with the Universal and experience one's true Self.

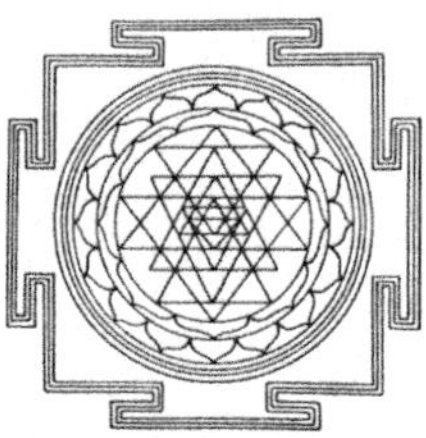

Yantras — geometric representations of tantric principles — are a tool, an instrument or means which lead to liberation. Svāmī Nirañjanānanda describes them as 'maps of consciousness'. Such drawings are traditionally made of coloured powders, strings or painted on cloth, birch bark or paper, and later embossed or etched into metal plates, most often gold or copper. However, this type of image has traditionally been more permanent. In Tantra, geometric shapes are most commonly used, representing the patterns of creation, deities, universal and unconscious psychic forces. In Bihar Yoga *yantra* is usually seen as the materialised vibration of a mantra and is therefore advised to be practiced together with the respective *mantra*. In that regard, *mantra* can be said to be the essential principle or energy, and the *yantra* — the body. Without the *mantra*, the *yantra* remains a beautiful form without much content.[52]

---

50 Haas, Dominik, A. (2025). *New Directions in Mantra Studies: Exploring the Emergence of Mantra Repetition*. ARGOS. https://doi.org/10.26034/fr.argos.2025.8033 (accessed on 28.10.2025).

51 Saraswati, Niranjanananda, Swami. (2013). *Tantra Darshan*. Munger: Yoga Publication Trust, p. 111.

52 Ibid., p. 117; Figure 5.: *Śrī yantra* is regarded as one of the holiest and most important *yantras*.

Despite its cosmic meanings a yantra is a reality lived. Because of the relationship that exists in the Tantras between the outer world (the macrocosm) and man's inner world (the microcosm), every symbol is ambivalently resonant in inner-outer synthesis, and is associated with the subtle body and aspects of human consciousness.[53]

Madhu Khanna

Maṇḍala symbolises the microcosm and macrocosm. A *maṇḍala* is a circle which contains a pictorial representation serving as a focal point to contain and channel subtle powers.[54] *Maṇḍalas* are usually more temporary images constructed out of powders and strings for the purpose of a particular ritual.

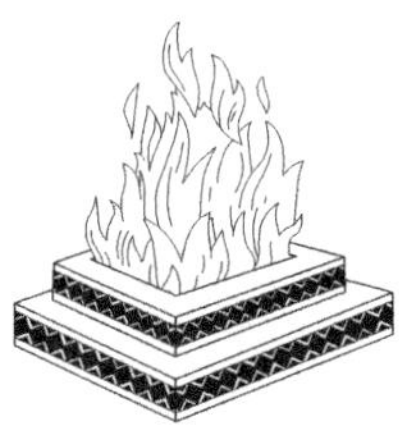

The fourth tool of Tantra, the 'ritual' (*vidhi*) stands for an action which is intended to establish a connection with the Divine in manifest or visualised form with a particular aim — worldly or soteriological. In traditions which deal with the subtler layers of being, an external ritual serves to evoke an extraordinary experience, bring about accomplishment and/or liberation.[55]

Tantra and Yoga

Tantra is a practical philosophy to bring the individual from the mundane state of being to the transcendental without suppressing the subconscious and unconscious tendencies of the personality, but through purifying them. This purification (or, in some cases, 'refinement' in the alchemical sense) can take place through *sādhana*, successive initiation and/or deity embodiment.

According to Svāmī Satyānanda, Tantra and Yoga have the same goal of their practice, namely — to transcend the material world and provide deep immersive experiences. Certain tantric and yogic systems focus on

53 Khanna, Madhu. (2003). *Yantra: The Tantric Symbol of Cosmic Unity*. Vermont: Thames & Hudson, p. 21.
54 Saraswati, Niranjanananda, Swami. (2013). *Tantra Darshan*. Munger: Yoga Publication Trust, p. 123.
55 Ibid., p. 130.

stimulating the cakras—the psycho-energetic centres of the body—through the experiences of daily life and by practising systematically structured yoga practices with that focus. The techniques should be adapted to each individual and neither over- nor under-challenge the practitioner. The individual begins practising at the point in life at which they currently find themselves.[56]

Short Overview of the Systems of Thought

> *Yoga is a practical system. Tantra is a system which emphasises acceptance of one's natural lifestyle and mentality, and alteration of the natural vṛttis.*[57] *Once that is attained, then Vedānta emphasises the experience of oneness, unity. If we are able to combine Yoga with Tantra and Vedānta, then the process becomes complete.*[58]
>
> Svāmī Nirañjanānanda

According to Svāmī Nirañjanānanda, Tantra, Sāṃkhya and Vedānta arose from five identical, fundamental questions:[59]

- What is this human body made of? How does it work?
- What is the life energy (*prāṇa*)? What is the relationship between the *prāṇa* and the physical, material dimension of the body? How does the *prāṇa* interact with the material body?
- What is the cause of *prāṇa* in different forms, and what is the cause of the creation of matter and the other elements?
- What is the individual Self (*ātman*)? How can it be experienced?
- How can one attain transcendence, enlightenment and freedom?

Tantra, Sāṃkhya, and Vedānta all aim to uncover the mechanisms behind an individual's conditioning, thereby allowing one to experience how this limits

56 Saraswati, Satyananda, Swami. (2001). *Meditations from the Tantras*. (2nd edition, reprinted). Munger: Yoga Publication Trust, p. 95–97.

57 *vṛtti* (f.) – movement, (circular) behaviour; tortion.

58 Saraswati, Nirajanananda, Swami. (1999). *Yoga Sadhana Panorama*, Volume 1. Munger: Yoga Publication Trust, p. 14.

59 Saraswati, Nirajanananda, Swami. (2002). *Yoga Darshan*. (1st edition, reprinted with corrections). Munger: Yoga Publication Trust, p. 6–7.

their perception of True Reality. Through practice and/or self-study, these systems provide methods for understanding how our conditioned states of consciousness and how we can constructively engage with them. Each of these three major systems offers a distinct, complete, and self-contained path, yet they were flexible enough to interact with other schools of thought.

Comparison Between Advaita Vedānta, Sāṃkhya and Śaiva Tantra

Advaita Vedānta	Sāṃkhya	Śaiva Tantra
	The Foundation	
Non-dualistic—*brahman* (highest reality) is the same as *ātman* (the individual soul), which sameness is obscured by ignorance (*avidyā*).	Dualistic—*puruṣa* and *prakṛti*. The world arises from the emanations of *prakṛti*, while *puruṣa* is the passive principle—the two never touch.	*Śiva* and *śakti* as the two inseparable, complementary forces of the universe—non-dualistic on the highest level.
	The Highest	
Conceptionless *brahman* is the Highest, absolute Reality. The Personal Divine (*īśvara*) is subsidiary to the impersonal highest *brahman*.	No concept of an ultimate personal God, just unmanifest (*avyakta*) Reality, composed of *puruṣa* and *prakṛti*.	A supreme Reality is identified with the tutelary deity of the respective tantric system. This deity may be a singular entity—male and female, or a union of two.
	The Means	
The practice of awareness with regard to the Self (ātma-jñāna) aims to remove ignorance and thus achieve the direct realisation of beginningless liberation. Liberation is already a fact, it must only be realised.	Knowledge is the means and the path to liberation. Liberation must be achieved through study and practice.	Harnessing the powers of experience through rituals, initiation, yoga, *mantra*, *yantra* and *maṇḍala* for the purpose of liberation. Liberation is achieved through *mantra* practice, initiation, theurgy, ritual, or a combination of the above.

continued »

Advaita Vedānta	Sāṃkhya	Śaiva Tantra
	The Path	
One strives to recognise (*jñāna*) the sameness of *ātman* and *brahman* through renunciation of the physical world, the study of the scriptures (*svādhyāya*), and knowledge of *brahman*, rather than through ritual or meditation.	One strives for liberation through the cultivation of discrimination (*viveka*) and the understanding that *puruṣa* and *prakṛti* are autonomous and separate. This can also be achieved through yogic practices and immersion such as those in Patañjali's system.	One strives to approach liberation through ritual and the personalisation of various aspects of the universe as deities and/or self-identification with them. Non-renunciation of the material world and integration of its elements within the Path to Liberation, while maintaining special tantric observances (*samaya*). Integration of the micro- and macrocosm—physical existence and spiritual reality.
	The Process	
Progressively realising the non-separation and non-difference between the individual and the Ultimate. *tat tvam asi*—You are 'that'.	Personal experience and study contribute towards progressively increased knowledge of the true nature of Existence.	Going through repeated initiation (*dīkṣā*) and ritual and/or meditative practice (*sādhana*) leads to increasingly greater realisation of identification with the Ultimate in the form of a deity, or possessing its power often accompanied by the attainment of supernatural powers. This process is impossible without the power of *mantras*.
	The Attitude	
Knowledge (*vidyā*) and non-attachment (*vairāgya*).	Attitude of the observer (*draṣṭā*), Perseverance in practice (*abhyāsa*).	Observing the pledges (*samaya*) and proper performance of the practice (*sādhana*). Obedience to one's spiritual master (*guru*/*ācārya*) and observance of tantric vows (*vrata*).

TABLE 2: Comparison between Advaita Vedānta, Sāṃkhya and Śaiva Tantra

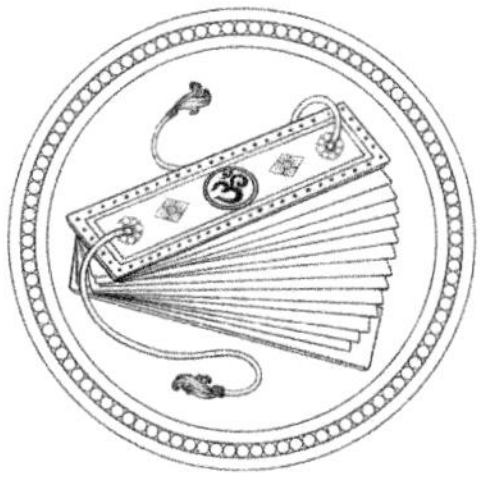

CHAPTER 2

Introduction to the Integral Approach to Yoga

[...] all forms[60] *[...] of yoga aim at bringing about the state of meditation. The reader should not assume, however, that one type of yoga should be practiced to the exclusion of all others. Though they are usually regarded as the different paths of yoga, a more realistic description would be to call yoga the path, and its various forms different lanes of the path. This can be compared to a piece of rope. In the same way, the different strands of each type of yoga, when performed in conjunction with each other, form the composite whole which takes one to meditation.*[61]

Svāmī Satyānanda

60 It is very important to point out here, that 'forms' here refers to the traditional branches or paths of yoga (i.e. *jñāna-*, *bhakti-*, *rāja-*, *kriyā-*, *karma-*, and *haṭha-*) and not to modern yoga 'styles' of the West.

61 Saraswati, Satyananda, Swami. (2001). *Meditations from the Tantras*. (2nd edition). Munger: Yoga Publication Trust, p. 84.

YOGA — DERIVES FROM THE nominal form of the root √*yuj* — means connection, but more precisely 'to yoke'. Within the system on which Svāmī Satyānanda's *yoga-nidrā* method is based, the purpose of yoga practices is to connect the mind with the physical body and to use this mind-body connection to reach higher levels of consciousness. Yoga therefore refers to both a physical and mental discipline, but also the path and the goal. The yoga schools known today in the West mostly originate from 20th century *haṭha yoga*-based systems, where the mind is secondary and practice is mostly focused on the body and breath, to the (sometimes complete) exclusion of immersive techniques.

> Svāmī Satyānanda's integral yoga system is not a contemporary yoga 'style' or a yoga 'type' he invented, but the approach to practising and experiencing yoga in its entirety in a systematic way.

Svāmī Satyānanda proposes a classification of six central yoga paths or yoga branches, which he describes as equal to each other in terms of the legitimacy of their methods for achieving yoga, and which should be practised in combination. Accordingly, all aspects of one's being are systematically addressed. Svāmī Satyānanda's integral yoga system includes the following six main yoga paths: the yogas of balancing the subtle energies of the body (*haṭha-yoga*), of mental management (*rāja-yoga*), of the psycho-physiological movements of the mind (*kriyā-yoga*), of action (*karma-yoga*), of emotional management (*bhakti-yoga*) and of study and inner realisation (*jñāna-yoga*). This assortment is to be understood as a syncretic approach integrating many varied traditions and practices.

Svāmī Satyānanda refers to yoga being a process which involves cultivating awareness and managing one's energies to realise and develop the mind's abilities in life as the 'integration of head, heart and hands', meaning that the mind is allowed to express itself freely and harmoniously through all three aspects. This process is not solely based on observances, physical exercises, breathing techniques, contemplation, or immersion, but also on the application of yogic principles in daily life.

Practitioners can integrate the appropriate techniques from the various yoga paths into their practice programme (*sādhana*) and into their lives in such a way, so that they fit their own personality, stage of life and their individual potential. Integrating the different yoga paths allows them to complement one another enabling increasing profound awareness and realisation.

Svāmī Satyānanda developed his *yoga-nidrā* method in the integral context of 'Bihar Yoga', sometimes also called 'Satyananda Yoga'. In the context of Bihar Yoga, 'yoga' is viewed as, among other things:

- Balancing the *prāṇa* in the *iḍā-* and *piṅgalā-nāḍīs*; (classical *haṭha-yoga*)
- Integration of the different aspects of the individual with and into everyday life—'Head, heart and hands.';
- The state of union of the individual with Universal Consciousness; (from the point of view of Vedānta—the realisation of the unity of *ātman* (the individual) with *brahman* (the Absolute), of Tantra—the union of *śakti* (the material world) with *śiva* (consciousness), the micro- with the macrocosm)
- Harmonious integration of the different paths of achieving and practicing yoga;
- A means—to achieve the goal of yoga;
- Attainment through personal experience;
- Path and journey back to the Origin.

Yoga-cakra — the Yoga-wheel of Bihar Yoga[62]

Bihar Yoga as an integral yoga system, classifies yoga paths into two categories—'outer' (*bahir-aṅga*) and 'inner' (*antar-aṅga*) paths. The former refers to the yoga paths which contribute to self-development, while the inner paths are those which lead to spiritual realisation.

The *bahiraṅga-yoga* paths aim to harmonise the body and mind as well as perception and behaviour. They prepare the practitioner for antaraṅga-yoga. The *antaraṅga-yoga* paths teach how to deal with the qualities inherent and genetically embedded in one's own personality and nature.[63] In this

62 More on Bihar Yoga in Part V. *Appendix 1. Introduction to Bihar Yoga*.

63 Saraswati, Niranjanananda, Swami. (2015). *Yoga Chakra – The Wheel of Yoga*. Munger: Yoga Publication Trust, pp. 102–152.

section, we will briefly look at each path within the framework of the Bihar Yoga system.

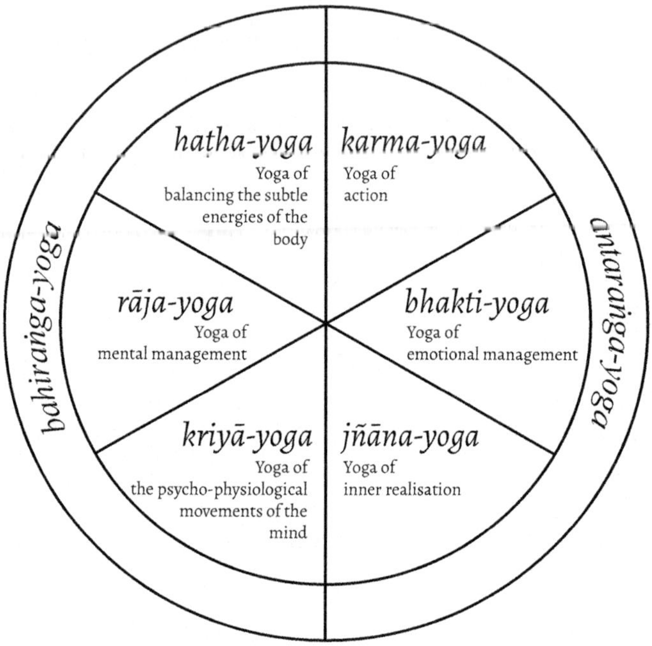

FIGURE 8: *Yoga-cakra* — the yoga-wheel of the Bihar Yoga[64]

The *bahiraṅga* (outer) paths of Bihar Yoga

• *haṭha-yoga* — the path of energetic balancing and purification

In modern times *haṭha-yoga* is often reduced exclusively to its physical aspects. However, one of the main purposes of the *haṭha-yoga* path is to balance *iḍā* and *piṅgalā* conceptualised as the mental and vital energies (*prāṇas*).

The postures and breathing techniques of *haṭha-yoga* — *āsana* and *prāṇāyāma*, which are dynamic in nature[65], help to correct the imbalances in the flow of *prāṇa* in the body and in the mind. When the balance in our body

64 Figure 8. *Yoga-cakra – the yoga-wheel of the Bihar Yoga*. Source: Ibid., p. 152.

65 In contrast to Patañjali's conception of *āsanas* as more akin to 'meditation postures'. This will be discussed in more detail below.

is restored, health and mental problems are reduced. There is an improvement in breathing, cardiovascular, nervous and digestive function. In this way, the body gradually reaches a state of well-being through the practice of *haṭha-yoga*. This harmonisation of *prāṇa* enables a shift of focus towards the management of the mind, which constitutes the domain of *rāja-yoga*, following *haṭha-yoga* within this approach.

- ***rāja-yoga*** **— the path of mental management**

This refers to the *rāja-yoga*, the eight-limbed yoga, which can be traced back to Patañjali's *Yoga-sūtras* and will be discussed in more detail below.[66]

- ***kriyā-yoga*** **— the path of the psycho-physiological movements of the mind**

The origin of *kriyā-yoga* in the Bihar Yoga tradition lies in tantric principles. In this context, *kriyā-yoga* consists of a sequence of certain *āsanas*, *prāṇāyāmas*, *mudrās* (energy-directing positions of the body and particularly of the hands, 'seals') and *bandhas* (contractions of specific muscle groups to direct the life energy in certain regions of the body, 'bindings'), but while in *haṭha-yoga* these form a sequential discipline: *āsana* → *prāṇāyāma* → *mudrā*/*bandha* → *samādhi*, in *kriyā-yoga* they are integrated into dynamic cycles combining all elements simultaneously. Another difference is that classical *haṭha* aims at the stabilisation of *prāṇa* leading to *rāja-yoga*/*samādhi*, while *kriyā-yoga* focuses on progressive immersion culminating in *dhyāna*[67]. This yoga path should not be confused with the term found in the *Purāṇas* or the *Yoga-sūtras*, nor with the *haṭha-yoga* or *kriyā-yoga* as expounded by Paramahaṃsa Yogānanda (1893–1952). Rather, *kriyā-yoga* in the Bihar Yoga tradition is a tantric-influenced system of practice for inner purification and focussing of the mind aimed at achieving the states of *pratyāhāra* (withdrawal from sensory perception), *dhāraṇā* (focused awareness) and *dhyāna* (prolonged immersive focused awareness).

66 See Part I., Chapter 03. *Introduction to Rāja-yoga: The Yoga-Sūtras of Patañjali* and *Preparing for rāja-yoga*.

67 It must be noted that this is also different from Patañjali's *kriyā-yoga* (*Yoga-sūtra* 2.1), which is a triad of *tapas*, *svādhyāya*, and *īśvara-praṇidhānā*, as the Bihar Yoga system involves *āsana*, *prāṇāyāma*, etc. See below.

The *antaraṅga* (inner) paths of Bihar Yoga

• *jñāna-yoga*—the path of intuitive knowledge

Jñāna-yoga is not only concerned with exploring the subtle nature of an individual, but is also the gradual discovery of the multi-layered nature of the personality as directed by the higher intellect (*buddhi*). *Jñāna-yoga* is the process of transforming spiritual knowledge into practical wisdom. *Jñāna-yoga* is described by the Bihar Yoga tradition as a way to attain the highest meditative state and inner knowledge.

Jñāna literally means 'knowledge' or 'realisation'. In the understanding of Bihar Yoga, knowledge refers to the meditative awareness leading to ultimate wisdom. *Jñāna* should not, by any means, be understood as a method of trying to find rational answers to eternal questions, but as contemplation, which should lead to self-inquiry and subsequently to self-realisation.

• *bhakti-yoga*—the path of emotional management

Bhakti traditionally translates as 'devotion' and refers to the surrender to a personal deity (Īśvara, Kṛṣṇa, Viṣṇu, Śiva). Many people describe this path as the 'yoga of devotion' and associate it with a decidedly religious attitude. However, 'devotion' in the context of Bihar Yoga should not be taken to refer to reverence or worship in the religious sense, but to a personal, psychological, intellectual and emotional change which leads from a state of existence characterised by *tamas* (torpidity) to a far higher quality, to a pure *sattva* (balanced) state of existence.

According to the Bihar Yoga tradition, *bhakti-yoga* is not necessarily theistic—it is instead viewed primarily as the path of emotional management in which emotional energy is channelled in order to 'open the heart', thus leading to a recognition of the higher nature inherent in every human being.

Some important aspects of the practice of *bhakti-yoga* include, among others, immersion for the sake of recognising and channelling emotional energy, the recitation of mantras and the singing of praises (*kīrtana*), and experiencing more refined human qualities in everyday life.[68]

---

68 Saraswati, Satyananda, Swami. (2001). *Meditations from the Tantras*. (2nd edition). Munger: Yoga Publication Trust, p. 86–87.

- ***karma-yoga*** **— the path of action**

Karma-yoga in the Bihar Yoga tradition refers to seeking to attain realisation through action and detachment from the expectations originally associated with it, so that free expression can manifest itself in the act of action. The aim of *karma-yoga* is to switch from the unconscious to the conscious mode of behaviour. *Karma-yoga* is not a technique, but a spiritual discipline which can be practised 24 hours a day. It is an approach which develops our balanced immunity to the reactive and/or negative components of an action, and teaches us to take charge of our habits.

Conscious action leads to an increase in our ability to manage mental associations which take the form of desires, ambitions, the ego as well as other personality aspects. In Classical Indian terms, this means that the state of *karma-yoga* is best achieved through *sevā* (selfless engagement in all activities). In ancient India, it was believed that the disciple would learn and practice *karma-yoga* most effectively under the direct guidance of his master over the course of a long stay with him (usually for a period of about twelve years).

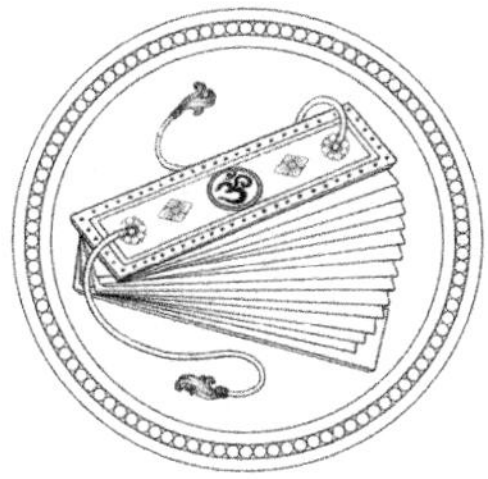

CHAPTER 3

Introduction to *Rāja-yoga*: the Path of the Sovereign

As a form of psychotechnology, Yoga deals first and foremost with the human mind or psyche. But, according to the yogic visionaries, our inner world parallels the structure of the cosmos itself. It is composed of the same fundamental layers that compose the hierarchy of the external world. Hence, the 'maps' put forward by Patañjali and other spiritual authorities are psychocosmograms, or guides to both the inner and outer universe. Their principal purpose, however, is to point beyond the levels, or layers, of psyche and cosmos, for the essential nature of the human being, the Self or Spirit, is held to be utterly transcendental.[69]

Georg Feuerstein

69 Feuerstein, Georg. (2008). *The Yoga Tradition – Its History, Literature, Philosophy and Practice* (3rd edition). Arizona: Hohm Press, p. 392.

THE SANSKRIT WORD *RĀJAN* IS usually rendered as 'king', though its most direct translation would be 'sovereign'. *Rāja-yoga* is therefore the 'sovereign yoga' or the highest yoga path and is considered one of the main paths of Yoga. Just as the king is the ruler over his kingdom, the *rāja-yogī* is no longer under the unconscious influence of his thoughts, feelings, moods and physical needs—but has sovereignty over them. Classical *rāja-yoga* starts being mentioned by name 'from the 11th or 12th century onwards and is usually identified with either the practices leading to *samādhi* or the state of *samādhi*'.[70] The term was only later retrospectively applied to the Classical Yoga of Patañjali. The main aim of *rāja-yoga* in the Bihar Yoga system is to transform the mind from a scattered to a focussed state and to awaken the dormant psychic potential of the human personality. In traditional Indian thought, numerous seekers have explored this fundamental theme of yoga and the individual layers of the mind during deep states of immersion. Such states are achieved through austerity (*tapas*), self-control, and deep immersion aimed at union (*yoga*) with the Universal. Such practices served as a methodical preparation for attaining liberation (*mokṣa*) and thus escaping suffering and the cycle of rebirths.[71] In this historical period, *rāja-yoga* was only accessible to scholars from the various philosophical schools of India and ascetics. The teachings later known as *rāja-yoga* were neither standardised nor systematically structured at this time.

---

70 Mallinson, J. and Singleton, M. (2017). *Roots of Yoga*. London: Penguin Classics, p. xxxix.

71 Ibid., p. xiv.

The *Yoga-sūtras* of Patañjali — an Overview

The ultimate goal of yoga is to always observe things accurately, and therefore never act in a way that will make us regret our actions later.[72]

T.K.V. Desikachar

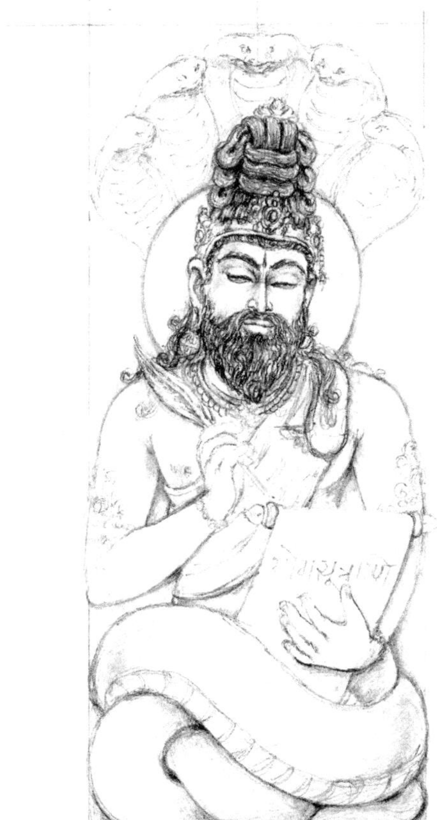

FIGURE 9: The scholar Patañjali.

72 Desikachar, T., K., V. (1999). *The Heart of Yoga: Developing a Personal Practice*. (2nd edition). Rochester: Inner Traditions Bear and Company, p.149.

The scholar Patañjali[73], believed to have lived between 200 BCE and 200 CE[74], summarised the essence of numerous yoga teachings and their associated techniques — proven through centuries of experience — in a text composed of concise guidelines presented as aphorisms (*sūtra*).[75] The text, however, has been traced by Philipp Maas as dating to sometime between 325 and 425 CE.[76] In this work, which became known as the '*Yoga-sūtra*s of Patañjali', Patañjali systematised the approaches of yoga and defined his Yoga as the 'teaching about the mind'.[77] With this work, he united various mystical yoga doctrines into a systematic yoga path and emphasised it as one of the leading schools of Indian philosophy. His text later aroused great interest among early Western scholars and became exceptionally prominent as the claimed basis for contemporary yoga in the West.[78] The existence of Patañjali has not been clearly proven historically and there is still speculation about it to this day. Regardless, the *Yoga-sūtra*s remain one of the most important texts in the history of philosophy and Yoga.

Although the *Yoga-sūtra*s were composed in the pre-Vedāntic period (prior to the 8th century CE) they share common Upaniṣadic vocabulary with Vedānta. Nevertheless, they are rooted in the philosophical framework of Sāṃkhya. In contrast to the Advaita Vedānta *rāja-yoga* approach, which is concerned with the fusion of the individual layers of the mind until complete dissolution into the Universal, Patañjali introduces the Sāṃkhya concept of the *draṣṭā* — the uninvolved observer — thus adopting a dualistic (*dvaita*) approach, at least in the initial stages of practice.[79]

The *rāja-yoga* outlined in the *Yoga-sūtra*s of Patañjali serves as a key element for understanding, classifying, and realising the goals and effects of *yoga-nidrā* within the broader context of Bihar Yoga.

---

73 Not to be confused with the eponymous grammarian.

74 Wolz-Gottwald, Eckard. (2016). *Yoga Philosophie-Atlas*. (5th edition). Petersberg: Verlag Via Nova, p. 109.

75 Eliade, Mircea. (2009). *Yoga – Immortality and Freedom*. Princeton: Princeton University Press, p. 7.

76 Maas, P. (2013). A Concise Historiography of Classical Yoga Philosophy. Pre-Print Version of the Article Published in: Eli Franco (Ed.), *Periodization and Historiography of Indian Philosophy. Publications of the De Nobili Research Library*, 37. Vienna: Sammlung De Nobili, 61, following Bronkhorst 1985: 194. https://doi.org/10.5281/ZENODO.8055379 (accessed on 20.10.2022).

77 Saraswati, Satyananda, Swami. (2013). *Four Chapters on Freedom*. (reprint). Munger: Yoga Publication Trust, p. 130.

78 Eliade, Mircea. (2009). *Yoga – Immortality and Freedom*. Princeton: Princeton University Press, p. 6.

79 Saraswati, Niranjanananda, Swami. (2017). *Raja Yoga Yatra 1 – Understanding Pratyahara*. Munger: Yoga Publication Trust, p. 5.

This subchapter is an overview of Patañjali's *Yoga-sūtras*, and the most important aspects and terms. It is intended to contribute to a deeper understanding of the mental processes which can be undergone during the Satyananda Yoga Nidra practice and provide helpful hints on the attitude towards practice. Even if one is already familiar with the *Yoga-sūtras* of Patañjali, it is important to revisit them again in the context of *yoga-nidrā*. The correct translation and interpretation of the *sūtras* is of particular importance. In popular contemporary literature, it is often observed that the *Yoga-sūtras* are interpreted freely, which results in a number of misunderstandings. The following pages aim to maintain the translation and interpretation of the terms and *sūtras* as precise and faithful to the original sources as possible, while also drawing on up-to-date scholarship and relating them to the interpretations found in Bihar Yoga. This approach provides the reader with clear guidance for applying these terms in the context of Svāmī Satyānanda's original *yoga-nidrā* method.

The *Yoga-sūtras* of Patañjali consist of 196 aphorisms (*sūtras*) and are divided into four chapters (*pādas*). They are generally regarded as difficult to understand and, like many other Indian philosophical texts, are accompanied by commentaries by other authors, making them more accessible to practitioners.

The *sūtras* describe inner processes and states which transcend worldly experiences. These descriptions arise from personal practice (*sādhana*) rather than intellectual understanding. Patañjali focused on the human psyche[80], its conditioning, and the various aspects of personality and their expression in daily life.

80 The psyche (psychic body) in Bihar Yoga, in contrast to western psychology, 'is the approximate borderline zone between the subconscious [subtle body] and unconscious [causal body] is known as the psychic body. [...] The psychic body is the zone where both the inner and outer experiences are visualised and experienced.' Saraswati, Niranjanananda, Swami. (2002). *Yoga Darshan*. (1st edition, reprinted with corrections). Munger: Yoga Publication Trust, p. 371–372.

The topics of the four chapters are:

Chapter 1—*Samādhi-pāda* (51 *sūtras*)

- definition of yoga and the *citta-vṛttis* (the patterns and modes of the mind)
- obstacles on the path
- methods with which to overcome those obstacles
- the highest stage—*samādhi*

Chapter 2—*Sādhana-pāda* (55 *sūtras*)

- *kriyā-yoga*
- definition of the *kleśas* (mental afflictions which cause suffering) and how they can be reduced
- concepts: *puruṣa* and *prakṛti*[81], *guṇas*, *māyā*
- 'limbs' 1–5 of the eightfold path (*yama, niyama, āsana, prāṇāyāma, pratyāhāra*)

Chapter 3—*Vibhūti-pāda* (55 *sūtras*)

- 'limbs' 6–8 of the eightfold path (*dhāraṇā, dhyāna, samādhi*), collectively referred to as *saṃyama*
- higher stages of awareness

Chapter 4—*Kaivalya-pāda* (34 *sūtras*)

- complete liberation (through isolation)
- *siddhis* (psychic/suprasensory abilities)
- *karman* and *saṃskāra* (impressions in the subconscious)
- theory of perception

---

81 'While [in Yoga] there are many *puruṣas*, both Sāṃkhya and Yoga agree that there is only one vast category called '*prakṛti*'. *Prakṛti* is the world of natural causes. *Prakṛti* in its manifest form contains three types of qualities, according to both Yoga and Sāṃkhya.' Ranganathan, Shyam. (2009). *Patañjali's Yoga Sūtra*. Black Classics. Delhi: Penguin Black Classics, p. 73–74.

Important aspects of Chapter 1 — *Samādhi-pāda*

The first five *sūtras* introduce the basics of Yoga and the entire scripture. They can be said to show the importance of the integral approach to yoga and make it understandable:

> *Sūtra* 1.1. *atha yoga-anuśāsanam* |
>
> Now, therefore (*atha*), [follow] complete instructions (*anuśāsanam*) regarding *yoga*.[82]

The 1st *sūtra* begins with a statement which presupposes that preparation has already taken place for embarking on the path of yoga. According to Svāmī Satyānanda, this means that the practitioner should have already achieved physical and mental purity and stability (e.g. by practising *haṭha-yoga*) in order to be able to continue their development with the next step.[83]

> *Sūtra* 1.2. *yogaś-citta-vṛtti-nirodhaḥ* |
>
> To block (*nirodhaḥ*)[84] the patterns (*-vṛtti*) of consciousness (*citta-*) is yoga.[85]

The 2nd *sūtra* can, accordingly, be seen as a definition of the goal of Yoga, namely the experience of unity as soon as the movements/fluctuations (*-vṛtti*) of the mind (*citta-*) have dissolved — i.e. the *puruṣa* is no longer affected by *prakṛti*. In this context, *citta-vṛtti* refers to different, states of consciousness — from the waking state through the dreaming state to deep sleep. Everyday mental activities are only a small part of this. These movements of the mind prove to be an obstacle to recognising and realising the original individual *puruṣa*. In Bihar Yoga this further refers to living out the actual and original potential of the mind. With regard to Satyananda Yoga Nidra,

---

82 Saraswati, Satyananda, Swami. (2013). *Four Chapters on Freedom*, (reprint). Munger: Yoga Publication Trust, p. 29.

83 Ibid., p. 31.

84 Probably basing his stylistic choice on the point that Patañjali's Yoga is a yoga of isolation, Svāmī Satyānanda renders *nirodha* as 'to block'. Perhaps it can also be understood as 'suppression', not in the modern sense such as in 'suppressing one's emotions', but rather in the sense of returning something which has unravelled to its previous state or neutralising it.

85 Ibid., p. 31.

it is only possible to experience, become aware of and dissolve the full range of *citta-vṛttis* if you can maintain your awareness throughout the three states, right into deep sleep (*nidrā*).

Sūtra 1.3. *tadā draṣṭuḥ svarūpe 'vasthānam* |

Then the seer (*draṣṭuḥ*) is established in his own essential nature.[86]

As soon as the mind is freed from any identification with the worldly, it is able to dwell in its true essence and recognise its Self.

DRAṢṬĀ — THE IMPARTIAL, NEUTRAL OBSERVER

Already in *sūtra* 1.3, Patañjali points to the necessary means which can help to detach oneself from identification. The *sūtra* deals with one of the most important approaches for achieving deep immersion (*dhyāna*), resulting in absorption (*samādhi*): the cultivation of the *draṣṭā* attitude — the state which enables you to step out of your own being as an impartial, neutral observer.

The *yoga-nidrā* method of Svāmī Satyānanda trains the awareness to cultivate the *draṣṭā* attitude and enables conscious dwelling in various states of consciousness. Through consistent practice, one can gradually penetrate the deeper and subtlest layers of consciousness. This mental stance is not only of great importance during yoga practice, but it should be maintained and cultivated above all in everyday life. It is an active attitude of accepting, realising and letting go. At the same time, the *draṣṭā* attitude refers to a state of being present which is not associated with any expectations, positive or negative. The focus is not on a future state or goal which we will achieve with practice one day, but on the here and now — and that is what the practice is about.

> 'Maintaining the stance of an observer' (*draṣṭā-bhava*) must not, however, be understood as 'mindfulness', as this is a loaded modern English term whose unsuitability for describing states of immersion we will discuss in some detail below. 'Observing' here should be understood as the non-judgemental, impartial awareness of something. The *draṣṭā* attitude

86 Ibid., p. 40.

> goes hand-in-hand with the expansion and deepening of awareness and the release of mental tensions. If the mind loses itself in tension, in identification with the world around it and in behavioural patterns, the practitioner cannot reach a deeper state of immersion. This process already begins with the practices of *āsana* and *prāṇāyāma*, which place precisely these aspects as the foundation of practice.

In Bihar Yoga, the path of deepening the *draṣṭā* stance and awareness follows a systematic progression from the external to the internal, from the gross to the subtle levels—moving from the physical, through the prāṇic, to the mental. One could also say that the path leads from the levels with stronger identification to the more subtle layers, where perception becomes increasingly refined.

In this system, the ability to observe is essential for achieving and maintaining a calm state of mind. This means the practitioner gradually becomes a pure witness, an impartial observer of what arises during practices like awareness of bodily sensations (such as breathing) and, more importantly, the distracting pull of associative thought streams. It is crucial not to judge, react, or get carried away by these thoughts, but to remain as the observer. When this happens, one connects with the inner nature of the event as an uninvolved, non-intervening witness—the unchanging, eternal Self.

By strengthening the observer attitude toward the processes of our own lives, we achieve, among other things:

- the uncoupling of perception from the distractions of sensory impressions (the subjects of unconscious attention) and the stream of thoughts. Through this detachment, one can attain the state of *pratyāhāra*—the fifth limb of Patañjali's eightfold path;
- 'The posture should be stable and comfortable.'[87] (*sūtra* 2.46. sthira-sukham *āsanam*), independent of the experiences that may arise during awareness practice, without becoming entangled in feelings of identification or related experiences;

87 Saraswati Satyananda, Swami. (2013). *Four Chapters on Freedom*. (reprint). Munger: Yoga Publication Trust, p. 206; Another approach to this *sūtra*'s meaning is 'A posture is what allows one to be still comfortably'.

- the purification of the individual field of awareness through the release of thoughts, emotions, and experiences that would otherwise remain buried within us, causing subconscious tension and distraction;
- develop a better understanding of the ego, mind and emotions through the ability to recognise their underlying patterns and expression in life.

The attitude of an observer is cultivated as a vital component of yoga practice. It is a fundamental aspect of all immersive techniques and,[88] when practiced correctly, becomes an integral part of everything we do with awareness in our lives.

Sūtra 1.4. *vṛttisārūpyam itaratra* |

Or[,] there is identification (*sārūpyam*) with the modifications [of the *citta*].[89]

Identification with the *citta-vṛtti*s chains us to duality and obstructs our ability to recognise and realise the intrinsic, original nature of the mind.

Sūtra 1.5. *vṛttayaḥ pañcatayyaḥ kliṣṭākliṣṭāḥ* |

[The m]odifications of mind are fivefold (*pañcatayyaḥ*); they are painful (*kliṣṭa*) or not painful (*akliṣṭa*).[90]

Whether the *vṛtti*s are painful or free from suffering, whether they bring us unhappiness or happiness, is ultimately unimportant. As soon as we attach ourselves to them, we identify with them, becoming trapped in the oscillation between the polarities of suffering and pleasure in our daily experiences.

In Svāmī Satyānanda's interpretation of Patañjali's Yoga as *rāja-yoga*, the five modifications of the mind (*citta-vṛtti*s; see below) are seen as the source of all experiences that give rise to both pleasure and pain. These modifications

88 Within the Bihar Yoga system, immersion techniques such as *yoga-nidrā*, *kāya-sthairyam* (body stillness), and *antar-mauna* (inner silence) are used to cultivate the observer stance (*draṣṭā-bhāva*).

89 Saraswati, Satyananda, Swami. (2013). *Four Chapters on Freedom*. (reprint). Munger: Yoga Publication Trust, p. 41.

90 Ibid., p. 42.

prevent us from becoming aware of ourselves and our true Self. They are therefore referred to as *māyā*—in the sense articulated by Sureśvara in later Vedāntic interpretation—as they distort our perception of true identity, creating conflict and confusion in our consciousness while scattering our energy and thoughts. The goal, then, is to bring these five modifications under control, directing and managing them to recognize and unleash the potential within us. The impact of the *vṛttis* intensifies as they intertwine with external aspects of the mind, such as ambition, egoism, and arrogance, which are connected to external circumstances through the senses.

We experience daily how our emotions shape a limited and egocentric world—our own *māyā*. We constantly oscillate between likes and dislikes, pleasure and displeasure in our everyday lives. These emotions are not simply states of mind; rather, they represent a scattered stream of energy that is constantly directed outward through the senses toward the material world. As soon as we see, smell, hear, or feel something, emotional associations and reactions linked to our attachment to the world arise. When emotions are focused on the external world, they become difficult to control. However, if they are suppressed, they can lead to blockages and unconscious stress. Fear, hatred, and love can often feel uncontrollable. They represent 'energy in its raw state', which shifts between various shades of negative and positive emotion, depending on the degree of our identification with the external world. Such potent energies can either guide us toward the material or spiritual dimensions. They may connect us to the gross material world, where their nature is selfish and egoistic, or they can detach us from the material and elevate us to a state of inner wisdom and spiritual being. Thus, energy can be seen as taking on two forms—*māyā* or *yoga*.

Role of the *citta-vṛttis* [91]

If we throw a pebble into a body of water, we will see ripples extending outwards towards the shore from the point where the pebble hit the water. Those circular ripples are manifestations of one single event, one single stone hitting the water and creating many ripples; it will not create just one ripple. In the same way, the vrittis give birth to many different expressions, attitudes and visions of life. They are the different coloured glasses through which we perceive the world. Sometimes the world looks very beautiful and pink, sometimes it looks very drab and dull. Sometimes we get carried away by the force and sway of a thought, or we begin to wonder about the rationality of a thought we have had. That is the role of vṛttis.[92]

Svāmī Nirañjanānanda

In *sūtras* 1.5 through 1.11 Patañjali describes the following five *citta-vṛttis*:

- *pramāṇa* — means of correct knowledge, evidence, proof from direct, unadulterated, objective perception;
- *viparyaya* — a wrong view, misconception, error due to lack of understanding or distorted, subjective perception, falsely understanding something as its opposite;
- *vikalpa* — imagination; false idea that has no relation to true reality;
- *nidrā* — deep sleep, a state of consciousness based on unconsciousness (neither the waking nor the dreaming state);
- *smṛti* — recollection, memory; the ability to store and recall (perceptions of the past).

1. *pramāṇa* — Correct Perception

Pramāṇas are the valid means of perception grounded in the direct experience or awareness of reality, based on the immediacy of evident facts, circumstances, or events, as well as inference or tradition. They do not create erroneous ideas in the mind.

---

91 Saraswati, Niranjanananda, Swami. (2002). *Yoga Darshan*. (1st edition, reprinted with corrections). Munger: Yoga Publication Trust, pp. 107–130.

92 Ibid., p. 7.

The following 'sub'-*vṛttis* can serve as sources of such knowledge:

- Direct perception (*pratyakṣa*) on the basis of directly experienced sensory impressions
- Inference (*anumāna*) is knowledge based on a cause. Analysing an event and reflecting upon it leads to a conclusion about a presumed fact.
- Testimony, tradition, scriptural knowledge (*āgama*) is knowledge which we acquire through the testimony of a trustworthy person or an authoritative text.

2. *viparyaya* — Wrong View, Misperception

Viparyaya can be understood as arising directly from, and as a manifestation of, *avidyā* or 'ignorance'. It is a distorted, limited or even reversed perception based on a false understanding of a fact or event or false means of knowledge.

3. *vikalpa* — Imagination

Vikalpa are all forms of cognition — imagination, ideas, beliefs or fantasies, which can arise or be conjured within the mind without any object or objective connection to reality. According to Patañjali, these are the expression of a limited, inert, self-centred mind. They arise as empty fantasies which disperse our focus, awareness and strength.

4. *nidrā* — Deep Sleep, Non-awareness

The nature of the first three *vṛttis* is directed outwards. The fourth — *nidrā* — represents a state of the mind turned inward, where external sensory perception is detached. In this state, there is neither conscious nor unconscious awareness of the external environment, the body, or the mind; the field of consciousness becomes inaccessible. *Nidrā* is a state which goes beyond waking and dreaming; it is a *vṛtti* usually characterised by *tamas*, mental non-activity and complete unconsciousness. This state arises spontaneously and, unlike immersion, is not self-directed or conscious. In contrast, achieving the transcendent state of *samādhi* requires a deliberate introversion of the mind, accompanied by complete awareness of the various levels of experience.

> According to the commentaries of Vyāsa and Vācaspati on the *Yoga-sūtras*, deep sleep (*nidrā*) is neither akin to the waking state nor to the dreaming state; rather, it resembles a state of 'one-pointedness' (*ekāgrya*). 'One-pointedness' is achieved by cultivating the pure sattvic quality of the mind (*Yoga-sūtra* 2.41), while in *nidrā*, all other *vṛttis* are absent, and the mind is influenced by *tamas*. Therefore, within the context of Patañjali, *nidrā* is considered a state to be transcended.[93]

5. *smṛti* — Recollection

Phenomenological recollection (*smṛti*) is generally rooted in sensory experiences stored within the memory aspect of the mind (*citta*)[94] and is brought to the surface in specific situations. The filtering, processing, and classification of such information are part of the subconscious activities of the intellect (*buddhi*).[95] While *smṛti* constitutes the non-cognitive memory of phenomena, *buddhi* perceives the abstract properties attributed to them by the other *vṛttis*, namely, the experiential action itself.[96] Everything we desire, like, or dislike is governed by impressions stored in the *smṛti* 'database'. The information we can consciously retrieve and analyse typically consists of memories held within the layers of the subconscious. However, some impressions are particularly challenging to understand when they arise, as they cannot be recognized or classified by the rational mind. These are known as *saṃskāras*, originating from the deeper layers of the unconscious. In Indian culture, *saṃskāras* can also encompass memories from past lives, and some memories may remain latent, never surfacing during one's lifetime.

Smṛtis play a crucial role in shaping thought and reaction patterns, significantly impacting our personality. They can become active even during the deepest states of absorption, drawing the mind back into the external world. Therefore, according to Svāmī Nirañjanānanda, *smṛti* is considered the most powerful of all *vṛttis* which need to be neutralised.[97]

---

93 Patañjali. (1998). *Patanjali's Yoga Sutras – with the Commentary of Vyāsa and the gloss of Vāchaspati Miśra, Prasāda, Rāma* (translation). New Delhi: Munshirm Manoharlal Pub Pvt. Ltd., p. 24.

94 Readers are reminded that Patañjali does not adhere to the strict division of the evolutes of *prakṛti* in the classical Sāṃkhya system.

95 Saraswati, Niranjanananda, Swami. (2002). *Yoga Darshan*. (1st edition, reprinted with corrections). Munger: Yoga Publication Trust, p. 126.

96 Patañjali. (1998). *Patanjali's Yoga Sutras – with the Commentary of Vyāsa and the gloss of Vāchaspati Miśra, Prasāda, Rāma* (translation). New Delhi: Munshirm Manoharlal Pub Pvt. Ltd., pp. 24–26.

What do we require in order to be able to overcome the *citta-vṛttis*?

Self-acceptance and Absence of Feelings of Guilt

In the understanding of Bihar Yoga, the first step in *rāja-yoga* is self-acceptance, which involves acknowledging the natural expressions of our personality. This can be achieved through self-analysis and an understanding of our characteristics. Exploring and becoming familiar with oneself is essential for progress on the spiritual path. The process should be systematic and constructive, characterised by mental clarity and awareness, and approached with a positive attitude (*ātma-bhava*), while avoiding entanglement in feelings of guilt. Guilt unconsciously obscures the truth of our actions and hinders the creative expression of our human nature.

Religious, social or moral principles shape our ideas of 'right' and 'wrong' from an early age, often contradicting our inherent nature, body, and mind. As a result, we tend to suppress emotions triggered by the outside world and become laden with a negative charge. This pent-up energy can manifest itself in the form of disharmonious and even pathological conditions on the physical or the mental level. Through the practice of yoga, we cultivate awareness of our personality and learn to transform feelings perceived as limitations — such as anger, rage, fear, and negativity — expressing them in a consciously permitted manner and form according to our own volition.[98]

Recognising and Following One's Own Innate Vocation (dharma)

The second aspect of *rāja-yoga* is to live in harmony with your innate vocation in life (*dharma*). *Dharma* involves allowing yourself to be who you truly are, ensuring that your actions, thoughts, and ambitions do not conflict with the realities of everyday life.[99] This does not necessarily mean conforming to every reality you encounter; rather, it entails not allowing yourself to be controlled by the illusion that any situation is insurmountable. The state of letting go creates the freedom to relinquish control and follow the natural flow of life without expectation. This can be achieved when your thoughts and actions, ambitions, everyday realities and desires are in harmony with

---

97 Saraswati, Niranjanananda, Swami. (2002). *Yoga Darshan*. (1st edition, reprinted with corrections). Munger: Yoga Publication Trust, p. 128.

98 Ibid., pp. 108–111.

99 Ibid., p. 111–112.

who you are and what you achieve or wish to achieve. In this way, actions and the qualities of life stand no longer in opposition. We learn to accept the circumstances of our lives without resistance and to change these circumstances while maintaining a stable, neutral inner position, recognising the nature of what is, as it is.

Vairāgya — Non-Attachment

'The word *vṛtti* [...] means 'circular movement'. [...] It [...] represents a beginning without an end, or an end without a beginning. One is always caught up in that circle. There is no escape until you use a sharp instrument to cut through it.'[100] Through identification, we are drawn towards pleasure (*ragā*) and develop aversion towards pain (*dveṣa*), even though these sensations, arising from sensory perception, are both impermanent. In order to cease (*nirodha*) being trapped in an endless cycle, we practise non-attachment (*vairāgya*).

Letting go can be regarded as a crucial prerequisite for attaining self-acceptance and dissolving identification with negative afflictions. As the degree of letting go increases, dependence on the pursuit of pleasure and the fear of pain gradually diminishes. Ultimately, the calm mind learns to remain unaffected by external circumstances. However, continuous practice (*abhyāsa*) is essential to achieve this state.

Abhyāsa — Continuity of Practice

Everyday life is typically experienced in a largely unconscious manner, making it strong and powerful. To achieve genuine change, regular conscious practice must counterbalance the entrenched habitual processes of daily life. This becomes particularly crucial during immersive practice, as it optimally supports the transformative processes initiated by it. By committing to practice at a specific time and place, we cultivate a quasi-mechanical habit that serves as a guide for our mind. Simultaneously, through immersion, we engage in a process that contrasts with our unconscious daily routines, working to dissolve the conditioned mechanics of automated life through heightened awareness and observation.

Abhyāsa refers to repetition, practice, or persistent engagement with a particular focus. It is characterised by two key aspects: firstly, a commitment to

100 Ibid., p. 114.

regular, long-lasting (*dīrghakāla*) and uninterrupted (*nairantarya*) spiritual practice aimed at achieving *citta-vṛtti-nirodha* (the cessation of the fluctuations of the mind). Secondly, it involves sincere reverence (*satkārā*) and confidence in the practice, which are essential for attaining the desired goal.

> *Sūtra* 1.12. *abhyāsa-vairāgyābhyāṁ tan-nirodhaḥ* |
>
> Dissolution (*nirodha*) occurs when non-identification and an attitude of equanimity towards the world (*vairāgya*) are harmoniously united with consistent practice (*abhyāsa*).

This synthesis of inner detachment from external influences and the active pursuit of regular practice encapsulates the essence of what yoga truly represents.[101]

Sādhana—Structured, Long-term Spiritual Practice

In *sūtra* 1.14, *sādhana* is described as a regular, structured spiritual practice that extends over a long period of time. It is characterised by trust in its efficacy (*śraddhā*), dedication, and an uninterrupted commitment.

For this reason, we should apply the above principles by integrating our practice into everyday life and striving to maintain as much conscious awareness as possible. If we happen to neglect our practice, we should not succumb to feelings of guilt or give up. Instead, we can gently set aside the inner critic and resume our practice at the next available opportunity. It can be beneficial to seek new sources of inspiration when faced with strong external distractions. Over time, we will likely observe that periods of inactivity become less frequent and shorter. The essential point is to continue practising and to accept these interruptions as a natural part of the process. Ultimately, a sense of inner stability will develop over time.

101 Saraswati, Satyananda, Swami. (2013). *Four Chapters on Freedom*. (reprint). Munger: Yoga Publication Trust, p. 58–59.

Important aspects of Chapter 2 — *Sādhana-pāda*

In chapter 2, Patañjali explains the importance of consistent and regular yoga practice (*sādhana*) and gives practical instructions.

> *Sūtra* 2.1. *tapaḥsvādhyāyeśvarapraṇidhānāni kriyā-yogaḥ* |
>
> Austerity (*tapas*), self-study of scriptures (*svādhyāya*) and surrender to the Godhead (*īśvarapraṇidhāna*) constitute *kriyā-yoga*.[102]

According to Vyāsa's commentary, *kriyā-yoga* encompasses the process of purifying the mind, followed by scriptural self-study (*svādhyāya*), and ultimately surrender to the higher or cosmic will (*īśvara*). This surrender serves to cultivate the motivation necessary for engaging in yoga practice.[103] In this section, Patañjali identifies three major areas of yoga practice under the umbrella of *kriyā-yoga*, each accompanied by specific techniques.

The first area focuses on purifying the mind from ignorance (*avidyā*) and *vāsanās*, a process referred to as *tapas* or 'austerity'. *Vāsanās* are the remnants of impressions stored in the subconscious, known as *saṃskāras*, and they embody the deepest wishes or desires, forming the core of the *kleśas* (afflictions). Specifically, *vāsanās* represent the aspects of past good or bad actions that leave an unconscious mark in the mind by past good or bad actions, causing pleasure or pain, respectively. They serve as psychic seeds that bind individuals to the world through desires, cravings, and expectations, keeping them entangled in it. The second practice of *kriyā-yoga* is self-study (*svādhyāya*), which involves either the study of texts on liberation (*mokṣa-śāstras*) or the recitation (*japa*) of purifying mantras, such as the mantra *oṃ*. Finally, the practice of *īśvara-praṇidhāna* trains the mind to recognise the immediate omnipresence of the universal principle.

According to Svāmī Satyānanda, if ignorance and unawareness (*avidyā*) are too great, the need arises to 'put the material impressions into the fire' through spiritual practice (*sādhana*). Then, purifying austerity (*tapas*) in this *sūtra* is not to be understood in the Christian sense of austerity or penance. Rather, it refers to the generation of a kind of physical, mental or spiritual heat

---

102 Ibid., p. 137.

103 Patañjali. (1998). *Patanjali's Yoga Sutras – with the Commentary of Vyāsa and the gloss of Vāchaspati Miśra, Prasāda, Rāma* (translation). New Delhi: Munshirm Manoharlal Pub Pvt. Ltd, p. 88.

through a specific practice which burns these mental impressions to the core. In other words: if undesirable habits need to be discarded, then such a habit must not only be given up at the conscious level, but the *saṃskāras* or their entire complex must be dissolved along with their psychic root in the layers of the subconscious. This is where yoga practice becomes essential. *Tapas* also means maintaining the heat and energy which arise from your practice.'[104]

In the interpretation of Svāmī Satyānanda, *svādhyāya* is the attempt to 'perceive your own self in different perspectives [...], *svādhyāya* means the detailed study of your own self, which includes study of the entire structure of your personality, which includes the physical, mental, emotional and spiritual aspects. In *kriya-yoga*, the different practices lead to perception of the self. It is the process of seeing your own consciousness. If you are trying to visualise a psychic smell, you perceive yourself in the form of smell.'[105]

Normally *īśvara-praṇidhāna* is interpreted as 'surrender to the Godhead', but according to Svāmī Satyānanda the term means 'placing [yourself] completely in innermost awareness, which means placing your consciousness completely or fusing it completely in inner awareness. *Īśvara* is inner awareness.'[106]

Kleśa: Tensions in the Mind which Bring About Suffering

According to Vyāsa, the aim of *kriyā-yoga* is, on the one hand, to attenuate the *kleśas* and, on the other, to reach *samādhi*.[107] In Patañjali's Yoga-*sūtras* 2.3–2.9, the *kleśas*—the five mental tensions which cause suffering—are listed. The mind identifies with them and thus becomes painfully bound to the gross material plane. These afflictions are the cause of the constraints and inner conflicts we feel on a daily basis. As soon as the *kleśas* are transcended, however, our normally sense-orientated identification is directed towards the

104 Saraswati, Satyananda, Swami. (2013). *Four Chapters on Freedom*. (reprint). Munger: Yoga Publication Trust, p. 137.
105 Ibid., p. 140.
106 Ibid., p. 138–139.
107 Patañjali. (1998). *Patanjali's Yoga Sutras – with the Commentary of Vyāsa and the gloss of Vāchaspati Miśra, Prasāda, Rāma* (translation). New Delhi: Munshirm Manoharlal Pub Pvt. Ltd., S. 90.

subtler, finer levels of our being. All *kleśas* are based on ignorance (*avidyā*) and contain a part of it.[108]

Svāmī Satyānanda explains that the *kleśas* arise in a certain sequence or order: from ignorance (*avidyā*) comes egotism (*asmitā*), from egoism comes attraction (*rāga*), from attraction comes aversion (*dveṣa*), from aversion comes love of life (the drive to live) together with the fear of death (*abhiniveśa*). 'If one is able to control *avidyā*, one will easily control all the other *kleśas*. The whole process of uprooting *avidyā* must start from the upper end. It is a process of involution. The process of evolution is from *abhiniveśa* to *dveṣa*, then to *asmitā*, then to *avidyā* and then to *vidyā* or enlightenment.'[109]

The *kleśas* have four forms of expression: dormant (*prasupta*), 'thin' (*tanu*), oscillating (*vicchinna*) and ascending (*udaraṇa*).[110]

---

108 Ibid., p. 92.

109 Saraswati, Satyananda, Swami. (2013). *Four Chapters on Freedom*. (reprint). Munger: Yoga Publication Trust, p. 143–144.

110 Patañjali. (1998). *Patanjali's Yoga Sutras – with the Commentary of Vyāsa and the gloss of Vāchaspati Miśra, Prasāda, Rāma* (translation). New Delhi: Munshirm Manoharlal Pub Pvt. Ltd., p. 91.

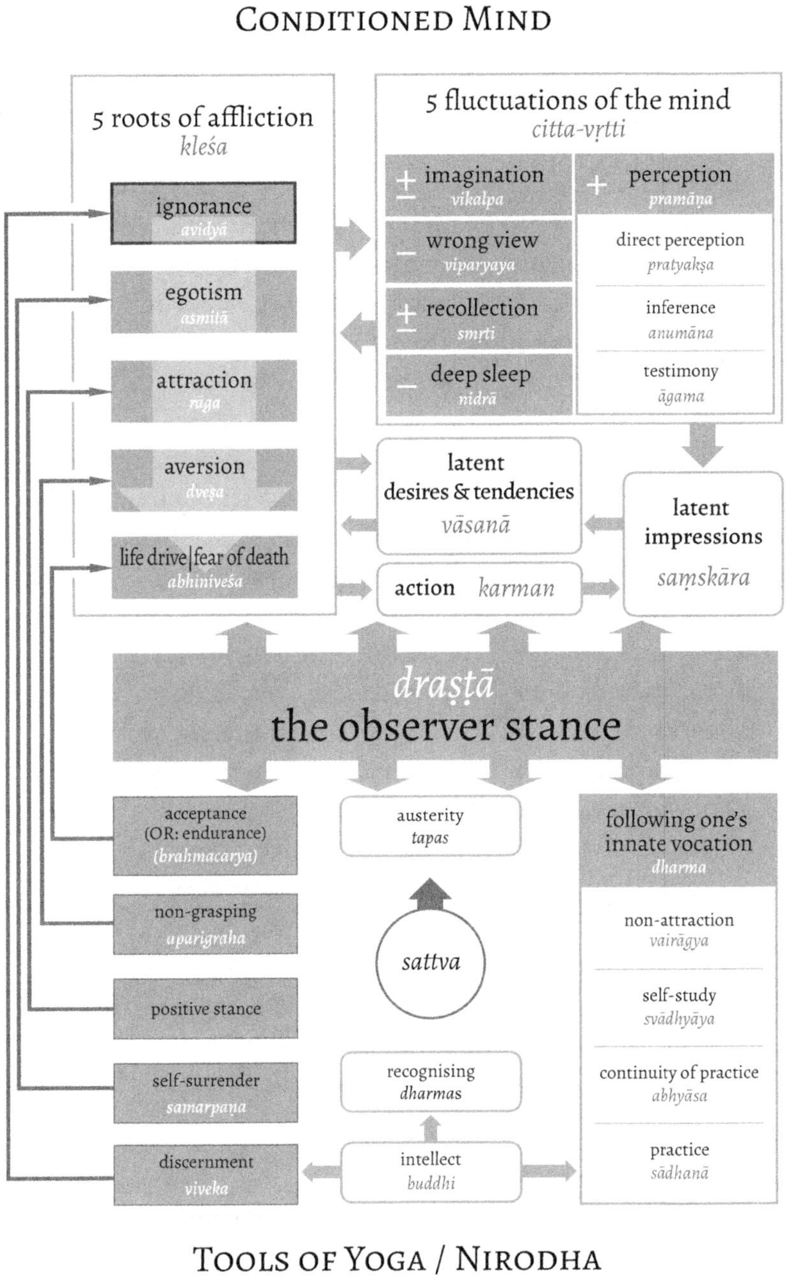

FIGURE 10: Overview of the connections between the *kleśas* and the other aspects of Yoga as emphasised by Patañjali in the *Yoga-sūtras* and interpreted in the context of Bihar Yoga.

Patañjali introduces the following five causes of suffering:

1. ***avidyā***—refers to the false identification (*khyāti*) of the non-eternal, impure, painful, and non-Self (*anātman*) as eternal, pure, pleasurable, and the Self (*ātman*). According to the 9th century commentator Vācaspati, *avidyā* can be understood as *viparyaya*[111]—the wrong way of recognising something as its opposite—and, according to Svāmī Satyānanda, with the late Vedāntic concept of *maya*, whereby cultivating *viveka* leads from *avidyā* to *vidyā* (wisdom)—a state in which one can distinguish between the body and the *atman*.[112]

2. ***asmitā***—According to *Yoga-sūtra* 2.6, *asmitā* is the conflation of the power of the observer and the power of the act of observation (*dṛk-darśaṇaśaktyor ekātmatevāsmitā*).[113] Vyāsa explains that *asmitā* is the confusion of the seer and the instrument of seeing—*puruṣa* and *buddhi*. Svāmī Satyānanda points out that *asmitā* is the active consciousness falsely identifying the individual consciousness (*puruṣa*) with its vehicle—the intellectual mind (*buddhi*). It is, however, the *ātman* or the individual *puruṣa* who performs the work of recognition, not the *buddhi*. The individual *puruṣa* transmits the power (*śakti*)[114] of seeing, thinking and hearing between the senses and the *buddhi*. *Asmitā* refers to the misidentification of the *buddhi* as the individual *puruṣa*/the *ātman*.[115] The same view is also held by Advaita Vedānta, where the Self can be misidentified with either the mind or the body.

   According to Svāmī Nirañjanānanda, *asmitā* can also refer to the false identification with the ego in any action. The entangled ego of the self-dramatising subject acts in a hostile world and keeps itself

---

111 Patañjali. (1998). *Patanjali's Yoga Sutras – with the Commentary of Vyāsa and the gloss of Vāchaspati Miśra, Prasāda, Rāma* (translation). New Delhi: Munshirm Manoharlal Pub Pvt. Ltd., p. 91.

112 Saraswati, Satyananda, Swami. (2013). *Four Chapters on Freedom*. (reprint). Munger: Yoga Publication Trust, p. 146–147.

113 Patañjali. (1998). *Patanjali's Yoga Sutras – with the Commentary of Vyāsa and the gloss of Vāchaspati Miśra, Prasāda, Rāma* (translation). New Delhi: Munshirm Manoharlal Pub Pvt. Ltd., p. 98–99.

114 Here, *śakti* does not denote the later tantric idea of 'divine feminine power', but simply means 'power'.

115 Saraswati, Satyananda, Swami. (2013). *Four Chapters on Freedom*. (reprint). Munger: Yoga Publication Trust, p. 147.

trapped in the cycle of identification trapped within the dichotomy of success and failure. This feeds emotions such as pride and despair as well as the image of a pretend personality with its attachment to a consciously or unconsciously underlying self-image. The means of escaping this cycle is to surrender one's Self (*samarpaṇa*).[116]

3. ***rāga*** — Desire/attraction. Desire is not only directed towards things, but also towards the attainment of satisfaction, e.g. through power, affection, recognition, etc. The identification of the senses with the object of desire prevents free and conscious action.[117] According to Vācaspati, one significant form of attachment is the perpetual attraction to pleasure.[118]

4. ***dveṣa*** — According to the *Yoga-sūtras* (2.6), *dveṣa* is both the avoidance of pain and the source of pain.[119] It is closely related to *rāga* and expresses aversion to or avoidance of experiences which do not give us pleasure. Aversion may derive from previous, unpleasant experiences, even though our situation may have changed since the time of the inciting incident. Or, we may feel aversion to things/situations which used to attract us — but, as the mind becomes bored with time and soon starts taking these things/situations for granted, it seeks new stimuli. This desire for renewed attraction leads to attachment to everything which attracts us (*parigraha*).[120]

   Svāmī Satyānanda says the following about this: '[*Rāga* and *dveṣa*] are the twofold expressions of an inner *rāga*. Liking for one thing involves repulsion for something else, so they are not the opposite of each other, but are the two sides of the mind. *Dveṣa* should be removed first and then *rāga* will also go. Even the spiritual aspirant is found to be subject to the influence of *rāga* and *dveṣa*. It is

116 Saraswati, Niranjanananda, Swami. (2002). *Yoga Darshan*. (1st edition, reprinted with corrections). Munger: Yoga Publication Trust, p. 282.

117 Ibid., p. 282–283.

118 Patañjali. (1998). *Patanjali's Yoga Sutras – with the Commentary of Vyāsa and the gloss of Vāchaspati Miśra, Prasāda, Rāma* (translation). New Delhi: Munshirm Manoharlal Pub Pvt. Ltd., p. 100.

119 Saraswati, Niranjanananda, Swami. (2002). *Yoga Darshan*. (1st edition, reprinted with corrections). Munger: Yoga Publication Trust, p. 100.

120 Ibid., p. 283.

dveṣa which is a more powerful binding force. It is a great hindrance. When *dveṣa* is removed, [deep immersion] becomes deeper and then *rāga* can be given up. It is said that man is affected more by *dveṣa* than by *rāga*, therefore, one should get rid of hate.'[121]

5. ***abhiniveśa***—the love of life and the fear of death. *Abiniveśa* is the survival drive, which expresses itself in the body-bound instinct for self-preservation and the striving for safety. According to Vyāsa, the desire to live cannot exist if the nature of death has not been experienced. This is inferred from the experience of previous lives.[122]

According to Svāmī Nirañjanānanda there is an opposing positive quality to each *kleśa*[123]:

avidyā	↔	Expansion of perception and correct discernment (*viveka*)
asmitā	↔	Self-surrender (*samarpaṇa*)
rāga	↔	A positive stance toward life
dveṣa	↔	Non-grasping (*aparigraha*)
abhiniveśa	↔	Acceptance of present circumstances.

The *kleśas* shape our unconscious reactions, thoughts and behaviour patterns. In our everyday lives, the *draṣṭā* attitude and action with awareness help us to recognise the influence of the *kleśas*, distance ourselves from it and consciously deal with it. This confrontation is not so easy, as the *kleśas* are naturally closely interwoven with suffering and emotional entanglements, which usually make it difficult to detach ourselves from identification with them or their causes.

In daily life, we may adopt the '*kleśa* lens', look closely at where the *kleśas* appear and tracing them back to their roots—the psychic seeds (*vāsanās*). This attitude can be practised as an actively aware stance in everyday life, as a meditation practice at the end of the day, and/or as a note in a spiritual diary.

---

121 Saraswati, Satyananda, Swami. (2013). *Four Chapters on Freedom*. (reprint). Munger: Yoga Publication Trust, p. 150–151.

122 Patañjali. (1998). *Patanjali's Yoga Sutras – with the Commentary of Vyāsa and the gloss of Vāchaspati Miśra, Prasāda, Rāma* (translation). New Delhi: Munshirm Manoharlal Pub Pvt. Ltd., p. 100.

123 Saraswati, Niranjanananda, Swami. (2002). *Yoga Darshan*. (1st edition, reprinted with corrections). Munger: Yoga Publication Trust, p. 284.

Contemplation of the aspects of *avidyā* on a daily basis is an excellent exercise. We can ask ourselves questions such as: 'When was I unhappy today and why?'—'What did I like today and what made me happy?'—'When did I feel insecure today?'—'What would help me to feel more secure?' With the help of such questions, we can recognise more clearly where we can strengthen ourselves in order to find our way out of dissatisfaction and insecurity. If we also accept the challenge of actively and consciously practising aspects we lack in everyday life—precisely in order to feel satisfied or secure—we sensitise ourselves to the perception of small things in our own lives. We should try to shift our perspective when interacting with others, engage with their viewpoint, and strive for understanding. This helps to reframe *asmitā*-driven identifications. As soon as the *asmitā* influence is released, we can recognise much more clearly when we are driven by the *raga-dveṣa* dyad and can control these tendencies better and more consciously.

It is very difficult to deal with fears of death (*abhiniveśa*). Overcoming the instinct for self-preservation can border on the impossible. Our striving for security and our instincts for self-preservation are deeply rooted in us and cannot be overcome by everyday awareness alone.

The exploration of the *kleśas* can become a fundamental basis for a successful self-study (*svādhyāya*) and self-development.

Attaining *Vidyā* through *Viveka*

Viveka, meaning 'discernment' or 'discrimination'—and sometimes referred to as *prajñā*, 'true knowledge'—is perhaps one of the most essential tools for the attainment of *vidyā*. It is the opposite of the limiting power of *avidyā*—distorted perception or lack of awareness.

In the *Yoga-sūtras* 2.27–28, Patañjali speaks of the seven stages of *viveka*. This does not refer to the knowledge arising from sense perception, memories, or the mind, but to a process of developing discriminating knowledge (*viveka-khyāti*) leading to higher awareness, which arises as a result of the constant practice of self-study.[124] Svāmī Satyānanda states: 'it appears that

124 Saraswati, Satyananda, Swami. (2013). *Four Chapters on Freedom*. (reprint). Munger: Yoga Publication Trust, p. 180.

during the process of *viveka-khyāti* the [individual] *purusa* or [individual] consciousness goes through different stages of experience. Those experiences are contemplative.'[125] In their commentaries, Vyāsa and Vācaspati explain these successive stages in detail.[126] The stages of *viveka-khyāti* are divided into two groups: four types of knowledge which liberate the individual from the causes of action, and three types of knowledge which liberate the mind.

The 'four kinds of knowledge which liberate from [bondage by] the causes of action (*catuṣṭayī kāryamuktiḥ prajñāyāḥ*)' are:

6. The pain to be removed is completely recognised without any residue (without any leftovers).
7. The cause of the pain to be removed is removed.
8. The destruction of the pain itself becomes the direct object of *nirodha-saṃādhi* (the transcendental state of dissolution).
9. The tools of cognition are actualised in the form of discriminating knowledge (*viveka-khyāti*).

The three kinds of knowledge which liberate the mind ([*trayī*] *cittamiktiḥ* [*prajñāyāḥ*]) are:

1. The intellect (*buddhi*) is released;
2. The three fundamental properties (*tri-guṇa*) of Nature (*prakṛti*) are withdrawn into their origin so that their future expression is completely avoided.
3. Dissolution of the individual consciousness (*puruṣa*) which has, at this point, overcome the fetters of the three fundamental properties (*tri-guṇa*) of Nature. This state can occur within a single lifetime; such a person is liberated from the cycle of rebirth, and usually referred to as a *jīvanmukta*.

Philipp Maas offers an additional nuance on the term *viveka-khyāti*, describing it as a state beyond the recognition of the distinction between *puruṣa* and *prakṛti*. The ultimate aim is to disentangle these two entities, allowing

125 Ibid., p. 181.

126 Patañjali. (1998). *Patanjali's Yoga Sutras – with the Commentary of Vyāsa and the gloss of Vāchaspati Miśra, Prasāda, Rāma* (translation). New Delhi: Munshirm Manoharlal Pub Pvt. Ltd., p. 149–150.

the *puruṣa* to disidentify from *prakṛti* and discern its distinction from *sattva*. What must cease is the projection of conscious content within the *citta*[127]. Only when the *citta* is devoid of content can the *puruṣa* observe the reflection of its own consciousness, analogous to light mirrored in a surface. In this state, the *puruṣa* becomes fully aware of its own nature, effecting a transformation in the yogin. This culminates in liberation while living — referred to as dharma-megha-samādhi or *viveka-khyāti* — a state that transcends the apprehension of the difference between *puruṣa* and *prakṛti*.[128]

Svāmī Nirañjanānanda translates *viveka* into the context of everyday life thus: '*avidyā* is a negative quality, so there must also be a [corresponding] positive quality. This positive quality is *viveka*. *Viveka* is right knowledge and *avidyā* is misconception, limited realisation. So, if we are able to overcome *avidyā* with the help of *viveka*, it becomes enlightenment.'[129]

When *viveka* is applied in everyday life, the main focus is put on one's own strengths and, at the same time, the conflict with individual limitations and restrictions ceases when we accept them for what they are. *Avidyā* (or *māyā* in late Advaita-Vedāntic terms) impedes the realisation of the reason why you strive for something seemingly missing in your life. Surrendering to this process of realisation results in an open approach to life, and you can develop courage and spontaneity so that you face challenges instead of fleeing away from them.[130]

Dissolution of the *Kleśas* and *Vṛttis* through Prolonged Immersive Focused Awareness (*Dhyāna*)

The mental afflictions which cause suffering (*kleśa*) can be weakened within Patañjali's system with the help of the so-called *kriyā-yoga*, consisting of austerity (*tapas*), self-study (*svādhyāya*) and surrender to the Cosmic Will (*īśvara-praṇidhāna*). It destroys their root — the so-called 'psychic seeds'

127 As pointed out before, in Pātañjala Yoga, the *buddhi*, *manas*, and *ahaṃkāra* are conceptualised as integrated within a single entity, the *citta*. This represents a significant innovation introduced by Patañjali, who uses the terms *citta*, *buddhi*, and *manas* interchangeably to denote the mental faculty.

128 Maas, Philipp, Dr. (2022). *The Yoga Sutras in Depth*. [Keen on Yoga Podcast] https://www.youtube.com/watch?v=ZFkGCIhEmVw&t=265s (accessed on 30.10. 2022).

129 Saraswati, Niranjanananda, Swami. (2002). *Yoga Darshan*. (1st edition, reprinted with corrections). Munger: Yoga Publication Trust, p. 285.

130 Ibid., p. 285–286.

(*vāsanā*). If this does not succeed, the *vāsanās* remain in their subtle form as the patterns and modes of the mind (*vṛttis*). The *vṛttis* can then be inhibited by means of *dhyāna* — a deep immersion in which concentration remains continuously focussed on one point. While the attenuation of the *kleśas* requires considerable effort, this is not the case with the *vṛttis*.[131] However, it is essential to first attenuate the *kleśas* in order to effectively address the *vṛttis*. How this dynamic is handled within the *yoga-nidrā* method shall be explained in detail in Part II.

In *dhyāna*, or by dwelling in a state of deep prolonged focused awareness of the chosen object, we can become aware of the mechanisms on the various levels of the body-mind system. The aim is to focus the awareness on not only one experience, but to extend it to all levels and branches of that experience. A *kleśa* can be invalidated by becoming aware of its associated components: the desire, ideas, its driving force and execution.[132] By dissolving these elements through targeted awareness, one can effectively address the *kleśa*.

Viveka and *dhyāna* are the two yogic methods Patañjali expounds for overcoming the *kleśas* and the *vṛttis*. *Dhyāna*, the seventh stage of Patañjali's so-called *rāja-yoga*, empties the mind while stimulating alertness.[133] *Viveka* is the quality which is close to the Vedāntic *jñāna-yoga* — the yoga of knowledge — and which emerges when we embark on a search for the true Self.

With the integral yoga approach, we learn to direct our outwardly-orientated, gross, material focus inwards as awareness and to become aware of our inner life. This ultimately enables us to harmoniously deal with both the inner and outer dimensions of afflictions and their causes.

---

131 Pātañjali. (1998). *Patanjali's Yoga Sutras – with the Commentary of Vyāsa and the gloss of Vāchaspati Miśra, Prasāda, Rāma* (translation). New Delhi: Munshirm Manoharlal Pub Pvt. Ltd., pp. 100–103.

132 Saraswati, Niranjanananda, Swami. (2002). *Yoga Darshan*. (1st edition, reprinted with corrections). Munger: Yoga Publication Trust, p. 286–287.

133 Clark, John H. (1983). *A Map of Mental States*. London: Routledge & Kegan Paul, p. 29.

The Eightfold yoga-path of Patañjali

The *Yoga-sūtra* are also sometimes referred to as Patañjali's *aṣṭāṅga-yoga*[134] (the eightfold yoga-path), because *sūtras* 2.27–2.29 describe a clearly structured instruction across eight limbs. Patañjali thus presents an integral system of practice.

The eight limbs of Patañjali's yoga are often interpreted as being in a sequential order in which each limb is linked to the result of a disciplined practice of the previous one. In this way, awareness is systematically channelled from the gross (material) to the subtle (energetic and spiritual) layers.

The first five of the *rāja-yoga* limbs and instructions described by Patañjali (*yama, niyama, āsana, prāṇāyāma, pratyāhāra*) relate to techniques which deal with the outer waking consciousness. They are defined as 'outer yogas' (*bahiraṅga-yoga*)[135] because they change and transform the outer aspects of the personality, its behaviour and interaction with the world, the concepts of name, form and idea. These first five, outer limbs of *rāja-yoga* support practitioners in weakening the *vṛttis*—the movement patterns of the mind which are stimulated and influenced by the external world.[136]

The last three limbs (*dhāraṇā, dhyāna, samādhi*) deal with both the inner states of consciousness and the techniques of *dhāraṇā* required to achieve *dhyāna* and *samādhi*. These are referred to as 'inner yogas' (*antaraṅga-yoga*). In *antaraṅga-yoga*, one experiences and engages with all states of mind. These last three limbs not only stop existing ones, but prevent the further accumulation of new *vṛttis* in the mental field.

The eight limbs of yoga according to Patañjali are:

1. *yama*—what discipline must be observed—behavioural guidelines to harmonise relationships with the outside world;
2. *niyama*—what is to be avoided—fixed rules for personal discipline to harmonise the inner world;

134 Not to be confused with the modern *Aṣṭāṅga-Yoga* of the contemporary guru Krishna Pattabhi Jois.

135 Not to be confused with Svāmī Satyānanda's categorisation of the different yoga paths in the yoga-cakra of Bihar Yoga. See Part I., Chapter 2. *Introduction to the Integral Approach to Yoga*.

136 Saraswati, Niranjanananda, Swami. (2002). *Yoga Darshan*. (1st edition, reprinted with corrections). Munger: Yoga Publication Trust, p. 131.

3. *āsana*—postures in which it is possible to effortlessly remain stable (for long periods of time);
4. *prāṇāyāma*—regulation of breath;
5. *pratyāhāra*—uncoupling of the sense perception from sense objects as prerequisite for focussing on the true nature of mind;
6. *dhāraṇā*—the practice of one-pointedness, focused awareness, binding the mind to a single object;
7. *dhyāna*—prolonged immersive focused awareness, whereby the mind remains constantly with the object of concentration while the subject is simultaneously aware of the individual self, the process and the object of absorption. It is the extension of one-pointedness over time with reference to the effort of understanding directed at the object of awareness, there being absence of desire to understand anything else at that time.
8. *samādhi*—transcendental state of absorption, where the mind dwells continuously on the object of concentration without being aware of the individual self and without discriminating between the object of absorption and the action of absorption.

Bahiraṅga-yoga—Outer yogas

Limb 1: *yama*—Yogic self-regulation, harmonisation of social and external interactions.

The five yogic behavioural guidelines for harmonising social and external interactions according to Patañjali are:

- non-violence (*ahiṃsā*),
- truthfulness/sincerity (*satya*),
- honesty (*asteya*),
- endurance/abstaining from sensual impressions (*brahmacarya*) and
- non-attachment (*aparigraha*).

Non-violence (*ahiṃsā*) is not the mere external act of eliminating violence from your actions, but the eradication of the violent nature in the personality.

According to Vyāsa, non-violence is both the cause and the goal of the other yamas.[137] Truthfulness (*satya*) is sincerity in word and thought. Honesty or literally 'non-stealing' (*asteya*) results from the absence of covetousness. Abstinence or abstaining from sensual impressions (*brahmacarya*) refers to worldly behaviour. Non-attachment (*aparigraha*) is the absence of greed.

Limb 2: *niyama* — Rules for personal discipline to harmonise the inner world.

Svāmī Satyānanda outlines the rules for personal discipline as purity (*śauca*)[138], contentment (*saṃtoṣa*), austerity (*tapas*), self-study (*svādhyāya*) and becoming established in/surrender to the Cosmic Will (*īśvara-praṇidhāna*). Purity (*śauca*) in this context refers to external purity such as bodily hygiene or eating 'pure' food; inner purity would be the removal of 'impurities' of the mind (e.g. the *vrittis*). Contentment (*saṃtoṣa*) is the absence of the desire to have possessions beyond the necessities of life. Austerity (*tapas*) consists of voluntarily enduring opposing sensations such as heat and cold, the desire for food or drink, standing and sitting, etc. According to Patañjali, self-study (*svādhyāya*) leads to connection with the chosen personal tutelary deity (*iṣṭadevatā*).

According to Svāmī Nirañjanānanda, self-study means analysing and knowing one's own personality or becoming aware of one's own qualities, strengths, weaknesses, ambitions and needs.[139] Becoming established in/surrender to the Cosmic Will (*īśvara-praṇidhāna*) means that the ability to enter into absorption (*samādhi*) becomes perfected in the one who surrenders completely to *īśvara*.[140] According to Svāmī Satyānanda, *īśvara-praṇidhāna* means 'placing your consciousness completely or fusing it completely in inner awareness'.[141] In some contexts *īśvara* or 'Lord' refers to Śiva, but Patañjali uses it

---

137 Patañjali. (1998). *Patanjali's Yoga Sutras – with the Commentary of Vyāsa and the gloss of Vāchaspati Miśra, Prasāda, Rāma* (translation). New Delhi: Munshirm Manoharlal Pub Pvt. Ltd., p. 155–156.

138 In this context, it is important to distinguish between the yogic and Christian meanings of the concept of purity. In Christianity, 'impurity' is associated with desire and lust of the flesh as well as with sin. The concept of sin does not exist as such in Indian thought. Here it is more about physical, ritual and especially spiritual purity (e.g. removing the *vrttis*), which is seen as a prerequisite for attaining higher states of consciousness.

139 Saraswati, Niranjanananda, Swami. (2002). *Yoga Darshan*. (1st edition, reprinted with corrections). Munger: Yoga Publication Trust, p. 135.

140 Patañjali. (1998). *Patanjali's Yoga Sutras – with the Commentary of Vyāsa and the gloss of Vāchaspati Miśra, Prasāda, Rāma* (translation). New Delhi: Munshirm Manoharlal Pub Pvt. Ltd., p. 168–169.

141 Saraswati, Satyananda, Swami. (2013). *Four Chapters on Freedom*. (reprint). Munger: Yoga Publication Trust, p. 138.

in a more impersonal way, which is taken slightly more theistically by some of his later commentators.

The external and internal transformation through the practices of *yama* and *niyama* should not come about through coercion and imposed rules, but through realisations that give the practitioner's lifestyle a new direction in a natural way.

In the process of becoming aware, it is essential to ask ourselves how we understand the *yamas* and *niyamas*, what they trigger in us and how we relate them to our own lives. We should observe our own behaviour, our interaction with others and our own thoughts, feelings and emotions in everyday life.

If we recognise patterns, we can learn to question them and understand when and why we function according to certain mechanisms. This enables us to consciously decide whether we want to maintain or change these patterns and mechanisms. It is essential to be honest with ourselves in order to find out whether these patterns are really necessary for our lives or whether we are impeding ourselves by maintaining them.

In this process of observation and self-study, inner transformations arise which allow us to not have to suppress destructive behaviour patterns, but to let go of them instead.

When disturbing thoughts arise during the practices of *yama* and *niyama*, the aim is to cultivate favourable qualities in order to enable a different perspective and shift the focus from negative aspects to constructive ones. This process is called *pratipakṣa-bhāvanā* (Yoga-sūtra 2.33).

Limb 3: *āsana* — Body posture

> Verse 2.46 states: *sthira-sukham āsanam*
>
> The posture should be stable and comfortable.[142]

In this context *āsana* refers to posture as a method of sitting. The posture should be effortlessly stable or, as Svāmī Satyānanda describes it, both stable and comfortable, allowing one to enter into immersion undisturbed. It must be underlined that this does not refer to the athletic-style exercises which are

---

142 Saraswati, Satyananda, Swami. (2013). *Four Chapters on Freedom*. (reprint). Munger: Yoga Publication Trust, p. 206; See the comments to the previous mention of this aphorism above.

usually associated with yoga in the West, but to *āsanas* such as *svastikāsana*, *siddhāsana*, *padmāsana*, *sukhāsana* and others.[143] Furthermore, it is not clear what Patañjali had in mind with regard to postures when he used these specific terms. In *sūtra* 2.48, he states that after mastering *āsana*, the opposites (e.g. cold and heat) can no longer have any effect.

Limb 4: *prāṇāyāma* — regulation of breath

According to Patañjali, *sūtra* 2.49: 'Being in that [*āsana*], regulation of breath (*prāṇāyāma*) is the [moment of] cessation in the movement of inhalation and exhalation' (*tasmin sati śvāsapraśvāsayor gativicchedaḥ prāṇāyāmaḥ*). Patañjali uses '*prāṇa*' to simply mean 'breath'. In the *Yoga-sūtras* and their commentaries, *prāṇāyāma* is the practice of non-breathing or cessation of the movements of breath. It is described as being of four types:

- *recaka* — (the stopping after exhalation; characterised by the impulse to inhale)
- *pūraka* — (the stopping after inhalation; characterised by the impulse to exhale)
- *kumbhaka* — (the stopping at any moment between inhalation and exhalation)
- *caturtha* — (lit.'the fourth'; when the other three have been surpassed)

In later parlance, however, the usage of the terms changed: *prāṇa* started to refer to *prāṇa-śakti* in the sense of 'vital energy' rather than to just 'breath'. Instead of referring to the cessation of breath under specific circumstances as in Pātañjala Yoga, the terms '*recaka*' and '*pūraka*' have come to be used in the sense of simply 'exhalation' and 'inhalation' respectively and then '*kumbhaka*' is used to refer to any type of 'breath retention'. Hence, nowadays *bahir-kumbhaka* or holding the breath after exhalation is what Patañjali refers to as *recaka*, which he characterises as 'external' (*bāhya*). Antar-kumbhaka or holding the breath after inhalation is what Patañjali refers to as *pūraka*, which he characterises as 'internal' (*ābhy-antara*). The third in Patañjali's system — *kumbhaka*, which he characterises as 'completely retrained' (*stambha*)

143 Ibid., p. 206.

i.e. when there is balance between the amount of air inside and outside the lungs—is not described by any term in modern yoga parlance. In this classical system, inhalation and exhalation are not the focus of regulation through timing repetition and control, but rather the intervals in-between.

In contemporary practice which has been influenced by later *haṭha-yoga* understanding and usage[144], however, the focus of *prāṇāyāmas* is more that inhalation and exhalation processes are regulated as well, and not just the standstill in between. Conscious and controlled breathing helps to achieve *kumbhaka* (i.e. what is to be achieved) in the contemporary sense. The techniques of *prāṇāyāma* change the normal pace of breathing, some more than others. In either case, *prāṇāyāma* increases the mind's ability to concentrate (*Yoga-sūtra* 2.53). While both approaches are aimed at achieving yoga, in Patañjali *prāṇāyāma* is aimed at removing the veil of ignorance (*Yoga-sūtra* 2.52), while in *haṭha-yoga* and some tantric traditions it is more aimed towards purifying *prāṇa* in the subtle channels of the body (*nāḍī-śuddhi*).[145] Vyāsa's *Yoga-sūtra-bhāṣya* (on the *Yoga-sūtra* 2.52):

> *prāṇāyāmānanuṣṭhānasya yoginaḥ kṣīyate vivekajñānāvaraṇīyaṃ karma yat tad āvaraṇam* |

> The *karman* of the yogin which veils or obscures discriminative knowledge is destroyed through the practice of *prāṇāyāma*.

Limb 5: *pratyāhāra*—Uncoupling the mind from sensory impressions

Yoga-sūtra 2.54–55 says:

> *svaviṣayāsaṃprayoge cittasya svarūpānukāra ivendriyāṇāṃ pratyāhāraḥ* || 2.54 ||
> *tataḥ paramāvaśyatendriyāṇām* || 2.55 ||

144 Mallinson, J. and Singleton, M. (2017). *Roots of Yoga*. London: Penguin Classics, p. 127–128.
145 Ibid., p. 130.

> 'Uncoupling from sense objects' is when the organs [of perception and knowledge][146] are disconnected from their own objects (spheres of perception) and they become like a resemblance of the mind's nature/form.
>
> Due to that, the organs [of perception and knowledge] are brought under full control.[147]

According to Mallinson and Singleton, *pratyāhāra* means the detachment of the senses from their objects, which leads to the senses beginning to imitate the mind. It is said that such withdrawal gives the yogin supreme mastery over the senses.[148]

If the mind can be consciously directed so that it succeeds in releasing its identification with the organs of knowledge (*jñānendriya*) and their impressions, it becomes possible for it to turn inwards. This is a particularly important point as *pratyāhāra* is often mistaken to be the process of turning inwards itself, rather than what makes it possible. The sensory perception then follows the mind spontaneously. Wherever the mind goes, the organs of knowledge and action naturally follow.[149] This allows the process of *saṃskāra* purification to be set in motion. The mind is thus prepared for the next stage: the practice of one-pointedness, focused awareness (*dhāraṇā*). Mastering the *pratyāhāra* state is a prerequisite for *dhāraṇā*. Through the daily practice of certain *pratyāhāra* techniques, this state can be achieved in a conscious and focussed manner.[150]

---

146 Patañjali does not explicitly distinguish here between the *karmendriya* – the organs of action (i.e. of perception) and the *jñānendriya* – the organs of knowledge. See Part I., Chapter 1. *Key Elements of Sāṃkhya*.

147 Translation from the Sanskrit: Georgi Krastev.

148 Mallinson, J. and Singleton, M. (2017). *Roots of Yoga*. London: Penguin Classics, p. 284.

149 As we will later see, this process is parallelled within the practice of *yoga-nidrā* described in the *Yoga-yajñavalkya* where the *prāṇa* also follows the mind, as awareness is circulated through the *marma* points of the physical body. See Part I. Chapter 5. *What is pratyāhāra*.

150 *Pratyāhāra* techniques of the Bihar Yoga tradition include *yoga-nidrā* (yogic sleep), *kāya-sthairyam* (body stillness), *ajapā-japa* (breath meditation with mantra), *antar-mauna* (inner silence) and *trāṭaka* (focussing the gaze on one point).

Antaraṅga-yoga — Inner yogas

Limb 6: *dhāraṇā* — Practice of one-pointedness, focused awareness

As soon as the sense perception turns inwards in *pratyāhāra*, the mind can enter a state of single-pointed focused awareness (*dhāraṇā*).[151] This is a complex process in which the mind is systemically guided through external, internal and intermediate states of focusing.[152] When the scattered mind is allowed to focus by means of a *pratyāhāra* practice, it calms down and, when focus is directed at a single point (object) over a longer period of time, deeper, prolonged focused awareness (*dhyāna*) can take place. Practicing '[...] fixation [*dhāraṇā*] sharpens perceptual clarity, as a result of which arises an effortless flow of concentrated awareness (or complete control of one's own ritually created reality), called meditation [*dhyāna*].'[153]

Limb 7: *dhyāna* — prolonged immersive focused awareness

After the mind has gone through *pratyāhāra* and *dhāraṇā*, it can enter the state of prolonged immersive focused awareness (*dhyāna*). Only then is this deeper immersive state achieved,[154] when awareness can be focussed on one point (one object) for a prolonged period of time with steadiness. The practitioner — the observer (*draṣṭā*) — is aware of himself, the object, and the process (*dhyāna*). Although immersive techniques can be learnt, for some — even a lifetime of practice may prove insufficient to reach the state of deep immersion.

> *Dhyāna* is often translated as 'meditation' or 'contemplation', but there is no word in Indian teachings which summarises all types of states of immersion. Various states of concentration, contemplation, visualisation, and immersion are named in yoga and tantric traditions in a very specific and nuanced way, which is why the word 'meditation' is deliberately avoided here as a direct translation as much as possible. The term *dhyāna* refers to a deeper, more refined process that goes beyond the general connotations of meditation in the modern, Western context.

151 *Dhāraṇā* techniques practised in the Bihar Yoga tradition include *cidākāśa-dhāraṇā*, hṛdayākāśa-dhāraṇā and *dharākāśa-dhāraṇā*.

152 Mallinson, J. and Singleton, M. (2017). *Roots of Yoga*. London: Penguin Classics, p. 283.

153 Ibid.

154 Ibid.

Limb 8: *samādhi*—a transcendental state of absorption

The *samādhi* state is the result and culmination of *dhyāna*. There is no awareness of the *draṣṭā* and of the absorption process of immersion as such. Only the awareness of the object of immersive concentration remains. Patañjali mentions several stages of *samādhi*.

The dissolution (*nirodha*) of the *vṛttis*, *pratyayas* and *saṃskāras*

Through the *antaraṅga-yogas*, the actual purification of the *vrittis* takes place. The *vṛttis pramāṇa* and *viparyaya* are weakened through the process of *pratyāhāra*. *Vikalpa*—conceptualisation—gradually fades away through increasingly deepened *dhyāna*. *Nidrā* is then the state of mind of predominant *tamas* and is overcome when awareness is maintained through *dhāraṇā* into *dhyāna*.[155] With practice, by maintaining this awareness the mind transitions from a state of unconsciousness and inactivity to one of focus and deeper immersion, moving away from the tāmasic influence.

According to Vācaspati's commentary on the *Yoga-sūtra* 1.10, deep sleep (*nidrā*) is neither the waking (*jāgrat*) nor the dreaming state (*svapna*). Its cause (*pratyaya*) is darkness (the quality of inertia; *tamas*), which obscures 'the light of the intellect' (*buddhi*). The resulting mental change is the deep state of sleep (*nidrā*). This means that the *tamas* property of the *tri-guṇa* predominates and *buddhi* is dominated by it. Thus, all knowledge and cognitive faculties are entranced (*saṃmohyate*) by that tāmasic *buddhi*. At this point, the individual *puruṣa*, is only aware of the quality of inertia (*tamas*), which means that it is asleep and its consciousness is directed inwards.[156]

Smṛti (memory and recollection) is the last to be dissolved, as it remains active even in *dhyāna* and stores completely new ideas in the form of *pratyayas*. Only in the highest *samādhi* is it completely transcended. The subconscious activating forces and deep memories (*saṃskāras*), which compulsively direct the awareness outwards, are uprooted. In this state, the yogin can consciously 'plant' positive behavioural tendencies (*śubha-vāsanā*) which can produce

155 Feuerstein, Georg. (2008). *The Yoga Tradition – Its History, Literature, Philosophy and Practice* (3rd edition). Arizona: Hohm Press, p. 413.

156 Patañjali. (1998). *Patanjali's Yoga Sutras – with the Commentary of Vyāsa and the gloss of Vāchaspati Miśra, Prasāda, Rāma* (translation). New Delhi: Munshirm Manoharlal Pub Pvt. Ltd. p. 23.

new mental activities—into his own consciousness. Memory and recollection have a coarse and a fine aspect. In *dhāraṇā* the coarse (gross) aspect is overridden, and in *samādhi*—in superconscious absorption—the fine (subtle) aspect is also neutralised.[157]

Patañjali and Vyāsa (2.11) explain that the *vṛttis* as produced by the *kleṣas* in their active state are attenuated by action, by continuous practice. Vācaspati explains (2.10) that when the *kleṣas* have thus been reduced to their potential state, their destruction is no longer something which can be achieved through human effort, but by the cessation of action and by the *manas* dissolving back into the *ahamkara*—its cause. This is since gross *vṛttis* are easy to remove, but potential ones require a more powerful contractive measure.

According to Vyāsa (1.41), the *pratyayas* are still present in samprajñāta-samādhi, but in their purified sattvic form. The mind concentrates on a single *pratyaya* which is clearly perceived, rather than the mind being scattered. Vyāsa outlines that (1.18) in *asamprajñāta-samādhi* the *pratyayas* are dissolved, and the subtle *vṛttis* remain only in their potential state, they are no longer active. Vācaspati elaborates, however, that the *vṛttis* can only then be fully suppressed when the support (focus) of the practice is not objective—i.e. one does not focus on an object belonging to the phenomenal world—real or imagined. This is because the state which transcends that, according to Vacaspati, cannot possibly have a worldly cause and must hence arise solely from pure spiritual insight. Hence, *asamprajñāta-samādhi*, where *saṃskāras* still remain, is considered a lower state than *nirbījā-samādhi*, which has no cause in any objective phenomenon.

---

157 Feuerstein, Georg. (2008). *The Yoga Tradition – Its History, Literature, Philosophy and Practice* (3rd edition). Arizona: Hohm Press, p. 952.

Preparing for *rāja-yoga*

haṭhaṃ vinā rājayogo rāja-yogaṃ vinā haṭhaḥ |
na sidhyati tato yugmamāniṣpatteḥ samabhyaset |
tasmātpravartate yogī haṭhe sadgurumārgataḥ ||[158]

Without *haṭha-*, *rāja-yoga* does not succeed, nor does *haṭha-* succeed without *rāja-yoga*. So the yogin should practice both until they are complete. Hence, he undertakes *haṭha-*, following the path of a good *guru*.[159]

Śiva-saṃhitā 5.222 / *Haṭha-yoga-pradīpikā* 2.76

There are various ancient scriptures which deal with *haṭha-yoga*. One of the *haṭha-yoga* manuals that is now considered a classic is the *Haṭha-yoga-pradīpikā* (for short: *Haṭha-pradīpikā*) by Svāmī Svātmarāma Yogīndra from the 15th century.[160] Svāmī Svātmarāma regarded *haṭha-yoga* as the path to *rāja-yoga*.[161]

Contents and structure of the *Haṭha-yoga-pradīpikā*

The *Haṭha-pradīpikā* of Svāmī Svātmarāma Yogīndra is divided into four chapters: 1. *āsana*, 2. *ṣaṭkarman* and *prāṇāyāma*, 3. *mudrā* and *bandha* and 4. *samādhi*. These chapters explain the techniques of *haṭha-yoga* and their effects.

The first chapter introduces *haṭha-yoga* and its origins as a preliminary stage for *rāja-yoga*. The basic principles and guidelines for *sādhana* and nutrition are given. *Āsanas* are described as specific postures which create stability of body and mind as well as health and flexibility of the limbs.

158 Mallinson, J. (2007). *The Shiva Samhita: A Critical Edition and an English Translation*. Woodstock: YogaVidya.com, p. 158.
159 Mallinson, J. and Singleton, M. (2017). *Roots of Yoga*. London: Penguin Classics, pp. 34–37.
160 Ibid., p. xl.
161 Ibid., p. 34.

Once the body is more stable in *āsana* and one has switched to a light diet, one can move on to the next stage, *prāṇāyāma*. Here, unlike in Patañjali, *prāṇāyāma* refers to the control of the breathing process or flow of subtle energy (*prāṇā*) and the cleansing of the energy channels in the body (*nāḍīs*). The secret cleansing techniques or *ṣaṭkarman* are also presented.

The concept of *kuṇḍalinī-śakti*—the dormant psychophysical life energy—and also the techniques of *mudrā* and *bandha*, which lead to the awakening of the *kuṇḍalinī*, are explained in the third chapter.

The fourth chapter describes the stages of *samādhi* and the path to liberation (*mokṣa*). The importance of *rāja-yoga* is emphasised. It is important to note here, that the *Haṭha-pradīpikā* 4.3 names *rāja-yoga* as a synonym of *samādhi*.[162]

Differences between the two paths of the *Yoga-sūtras* and the *Haṭha-pradīpikā*

The *Haṭha-pradīpikā* shows a path which starts with the physical instead of the mental, unlike in the Eightfold Path of Patañjali. The body is integrated into the spiritual conceptual framework and practice. Here, the classical philosophical concepts of *yama* and *niyama* of *rāja-yoga* are applied practically and directly to the body before moving on to the mental level. Beginning with purification through *ṣaṭkarmans*, continues with a discussion of discipline through *āsana*, followed by harmonisation of all body systems and energy in the two main subtle energy channels, *piṅgalā* and *iḍā*, achieved through *prāṇāyāma* (breath control), the *mudrās* (seals or gestures) and *bandhas* (body locks).

This is a process leading from the gross to the subtle, i.e. to the deeper states of *pratyāhāra*, *dhāraṇā*, *dhyāna* and *samādhi*. The basis for all higher states in the *Haṭha-pradīpikā* is a purified and balanced body, which is described by the author right at the beginning in verse 1 as a preliminary stage or prerequisite for *rāja-yoga*:

162 Ibid., p. 7.

śrī-ādi-nāthāya namo 'stu tasmai yenopadiṣṭā haṭha-yoga-vidyā |
vibhrājate pronnata-rāja-yogam āroḍhum icchor adhirohiṇīva ||

> Salutations to glorious Ādinātha, who taught the science (*vidyā*) of *haṭha-yoga*. It is resplendent as a stairway which leads those who wish to ascend to the lofty *rāja-yoga*. (1.1)[163]

Haṭha-yoga-pradīpikā propounds the attainment of *rāja-yoga* in the sense of *samādhi* through techniques which work with the anatomy of the subtle body, while the Eightfold Path of Patañjali[164]—through methods which work with the anatomy of the mind.

163 Ibid., p. 34.

164 As discussed above, Patañjali's system in its entirety is also later referred to as *rāja-yoga*, but it should not be confused with the *rāja-yoga* of the *Haṭha-pradīpikā*.

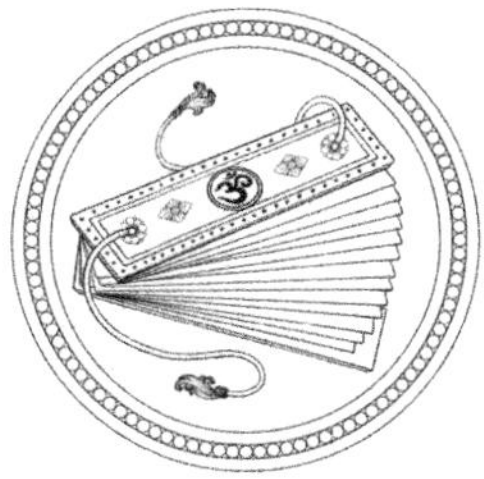

CHAPTER 4

History and Origins of *yoga-nidrā*

YOGA-NIDRĀ (F.) MAY REFER TO:

- a state: Viṣṇu's transcendental sleep, yogic sleep, psychic sleep, conscious deep sleep, the state between deep sleep and the waking state, a synonym for the fourth state of consciousness (*turiya*) and for the state of *samādhi*, etc.;
- a name: the goddess Yoganidrā from the *Mārkaṇḍeya-purāṇa*, the *Durgā-saptaśatī* (*Devīmāhātmya*), etc.;
- a process: how one goes about achieving or entering into the state of *yoga-nidrā*;
- a method: specifically Svāmī Satyānanda's method which incorporates either a *pratyāhāra* or a *dhāraṇā* focus, with the goal of attaining the state of *yoga-nidrā*.

The root √*drā́* means 'to sleep'. The prefix *ni-* has the meaning of 'down', 'back', 'into', 'within'. Thus ni√*drā́* is 'sleep', 'slumber', or 'sloth'.

The term *yoga-nidrā* rarely appears in traditional Yoga texts and refers to a state of *yoga-nidrā* rather than describing techniques for achieving that state. One possible explanation for this could be the oral transmission of yoga teaching, where knowledge was passed down from master to disciple, often in secrecy. As a result, modern research has encountered challenges in determining the precise age of the term *yoga-nidrā*. It is primarily through the surviving classical texts that we can trace the history of *yoga-nidrā* and discern its specific meanings in their historical context.

> In the West, *yoga nidrā* is often equated with relaxation and exercises involving 'mindfulness' or guided fantasy journeys.[165] This understanding does not correspond to either the intention or descriptions of *yoga-nidrā* discussed in traditional texts on yoga, or to the method developed by Svāmī Satyānanda in the 20th century.

The Goddess Yoganidrā and the Sleep of Viṣṇu

Yoga-nidrā as a state is mentioned in one of India's most famous epics, the *Mahābhārata* (ca. 400 BCE ~ 400 CE)[166], which is also one of the country's most significant philosophical works. This early reference highlights the historical foundations of the concept, suggesting its importance within the broader context of Indian spiritual and philosophical thought. There, the god Viṣṇu is described as being in a 'deep transcendental sleep'. He is depicted as resting in-between the creation cycles of the universe, lying on the eternal waters of the cosmic ocean and his state at that time is described in *MB* verse 1.19.13 as *adhyātma-yoga-nidrā* or 'sleep of union with the Supreme Self'. While he sleeps, a lotus flower grows out of Viṣṇu' s navel, symbolising the first manifestation of the material world and the seat of Brahmā—the creative power.[167] In later texts, where the term is used without the qualifier *adhyātma*, it becomes unclear what the yoga in '*yoga-nidrā*' refers to and opens

---

165 Feuerstein, Georg. (1990). *Encyclopedia Dictionary of Yoga*. Boston: Shambala Verlag.

166 Austin, Christopher, R. (2019). *Pradyumna: Lover, Magician, and Son of the Avatara*. Oxford: Oxford University Press, p. 21.

167 This interpretation can be encountered in textual sources such as the *Śrīmad-Bhāgavatam* (or *Bhāgavatapurāṇa*) 1.3.2. and the *Viṣṇupurāṇa* 6.4.6.

the compound to the possibility for relatively lax interpretation. Logically, one would expect yoga to be understood as qualified in some way, as when one speaks of 'union' or 'practice', that must be with or aimed at something. One cannot be in yoga with or practice yoga aimed at nothing in particular. However, in the context of the *Mahābhārata* it is very clearly identified as 'the deep immersion state', or 'the deep sleep' (*-nidrā*) 'of union with the Supreme Self' (*adhyātmayoga-*):

> *adhyātmayoganidrāṃ ca padmanābhasya sevataḥ* |
> *yugādi-kāla-śayanaṃ viṣṇor amitatejasaḥ* || 1.19.13 ||[168]

> And [it is the ocean which][169] serves as the repose of lotus-navelled Viṣṇu of splendour immeasurable,
> [for the] deep immersion state (lit.: 'the deep sleep') of union with the Supreme Self during the periods of time such as 'epoch' (*yuga*) and so on.[170]
>
> *Mahābhārata*, Book 1, Section XIX

The *Durgā-saptaśatī* (also known as the *Devīmāhātmya*) — a later adaptation of the latter part of one of the eighteen great *Purāṇas* — the *Mārkaṇḍeya-purāṇa* (ca. 7th–10th century CE[171]) as of its 81st chapter, describes the goddess Durgā as the supreme power and creatrix of the universe who has many forms. Even when reading the original, untouched by later, more explicit Śākta influence text of the *Mārkaṇḍeya-purāṇa*, however, we still encounter Yoganidrā personified as the goddess who overpowers Viṣṇu by inducing his cosmic sleep (*MP* 81.41–57; 66):

---

168 Mahabharata: *Adiparvan*. (1999). On the basis of the text entered by Muneo Tokunaga et al., revised by John Smith, Cambridge, et al. Electronic text. Pune: ©Bhandarkar Oriental Research Institute. http://gretil.sub.uni-goettingen.de/gretil/1_sanskr/2_epic/mbh/mbh_01_u.htm (accessed on 22.03.2022).

169 The square brackets [...] contain contextual additions which are not explicitly found in the source text, but which contribute to a better understanding of its contents in the target language. Furthermore, by these means, the translator's interpretation can be clearly distinguished from the content of the original source text.

170 Translation from the Sanskrit: Georgi Krastev.

171 Mallinson, J. and Singleton, M. (2017). *Roots of Yoga*. London: Penguin Classics, p. xxxix.

tan nātra vismayaḥ kāryo yoganidrā jagatpateḥ |
mahāmāyā hareś caiṣā tayā saṃmohyate jagat || 41 ||

It should not come as a surprise—the Yoganidrā of the Lord of the World—verily the Mahamaya of Hari—it is through Her that that world is entranced. (81.41)

jñāninām api cctāṃsi dcvī bhagavatī hi sā |
balād ākṛṣya mohāya mahāmāyā prayacchati || 42 ||

She, the Blessed Lady, the Goddess Mahāmāyā, draws by force the minds of even the wise and gives them over to entrancement! (81.42)

tayā visṛjyate viśvaṃ jagad etac carācaram |
saiṣā prasannā varadā nrṇāṃ bhavati muktaye || 43 ||

This whole world of moving and unmoving creatures is pushed out by Her—[and] when She is well-disposed, She becomes the bestower of boons for men, and finally produces their liberation. (81.43)

sā vidyā paramā mukter hetubhūtā sanātanī |
saṃsārabandhahetuś ca saiva sarveśvareśvarī || 44 ||

She is the supreme *vidyā* (female spell; knowledge)—Herself the eternal cause of liberation—and the cause of bondage in *saṃsāra*, verily She is the ruler all rulers! (81.44) [172]

According to purāṇic cosmology, the manifest universe returns to its causal or potential state at the end of a day of Brahmā (called a '*kalpa*') before the next cycle of creation begins. Traditional Vaiṣṇava symbolism depicts the supreme god Viṣṇu in transcendental sleep (*yoga-nidrā*) during this transitional period, stretched out on the thousand-headed serpent Śeṣa floating on the eternal ocean of the Cosmos.

172 Edition of and translation from the Sanskrit: Georgi Krastev.

One would presume that Viṣṇu enters the state of *yoga-nidrā* of his own free will. In the three verses which follow, however, he is under the power of the Goddess, who, as Yoganidrā, enters his eyes and body and forcefully overpowers him. Here, the Goddess is depicted in her supreme power as the ruler of the universe, both in its manifest and non-manifest states. Her power is confusion, attachment and entrancement—hence She is called 'She who is Great Entrancement' (*Mahāmāyā*). She is so powerful that She can conquer even Viṣṇu—the supreme *puruṣa*:

yoganidrāṃ yadā viṣṇur jagaty ekārṇavīkṛte |
āstīrya śeṣam abhajat kalpānte bhagavān prabhuḥ || 49 ||

tadā dvāv asurau ghorau vikhyātau madhukaiṭabhau |
viṣṇukarṇamalodbhūtau hantuṃ brahmāṇam udyatau || 50 ||

[For example:]

As Illustrious Lord Viṣṇu came unto the deep immersion state of union (*yoganidrā*), the Worlds having submerged into the [Cosmic] Ocean at the end of an aeon, spreading [himself] over the [snake] Śeṣa, (81.49)

two terrifying *asuras* called Madhu and Kaiṭabha arose from Viṣṇu's earwax with the aim of killing Brahmā! (81.50)

sa nābhikamale viṣṇoḥ sthito brahmā prajāpatiḥ |
dṛṣṭvā tāv asurau cograu prasuptaṃ ca janārdanam || 51 ||

tuṣṭāva yoganidrāṃ tām ekāgra-hṛdayasthitaḥ |
vibodhanārthāya harer harinetrakṛtālayām || 52 ||

Brahma—the Lord of Progenation—abiding in the navel-lotus of Viṣṇu—seeing these two terrible *asuras* and Janārdana (Viṣṇu) asleep, (81.51), with [his] heart one-pointedly concentrated on the goal of awakening Hari, praised that Yoganidrā, who had made the eyes of Hari into her abode. (81.52)

brahmovāca

viśveśvarīṃ jagaddhātrīṃ sthiti-saṃhāra-kāriṇīm . staumi nidrāṃ bhagavatīṃ viṣṇor atula tejasaḥ || 53 ||

Brahmā appealed [to Her] thus:

I praise the Venerable Sleep of Viṣṇu—the Lord whose energy is incomparable—Sleep who is the Ruler of the Universe, the Mother of the World, performing maintenance and destruction! (81.53) [...]

yayā tvayā jagat-sraṣṭā jagat pāty atti yo jagat |
so 'pi nidrāvaśaṃ nītaḥ kas tvāṃ stotum iheśvaraḥ || 64 ||

Who would be able to praise You who made even the creator of the world (*jagatsraṣṭā*) fall asleep, [the god] who (yo) protects (*pāti*) the world and who eats (*atti*) the world (81.64).

viṣṇuḥ śarīragrahaṇam aham īśāna eva ca . kāritās te yato 'tas tvāṃ kaḥ stotuṃ śaktimān bhavet || 65 ||

Since Viṣṇu, I (Brahmā) and Īśāna (Śiva) also have been forced to take bodily form by You, who among these is henceforth left with sufficient power to praise you [properly]? (81.65)[173]

According to Thomas Coburn, the personified *yoga-nidrā* is meant to suggest that entering a certain state brings about a certain dependence on that state.[174] In the narrative of the *Mārkaṇḍeya-purāṇa*, Yoganidrā, although an aspect of

173 Edition of and translation from the Sanskrit: Georgi Krastev.

174 Coburn, Thomas, B. (2002). *Devī Māhātmya, The Crystallization of the Goddess Tradition*. Delhi: Motilal Banarsidass Publications, p. 194.

Viṣṇu's consciousness is still a force which exerts an external influence on him, rather than it being actively initiated by him.

There, the Goddess Mahāmāyā, in her cosmic aspect as the creatrix of the Universe, is equated with Yoganidrā and is regarded as the ruler, sustainer and dissolver of the universe. She entrances all creatures by limiting their consciousness and maintaining cyclical existence (*saṃsāra*). It has to be noted, however, that even though this is an extreme Śākta view, in both Vaiṣṇavism and Śaivism, the Goddess is always construed as the power of the Supreme God and never as a standalone supreme feminine divinity.

It is obvious that the metaphor of deep sleep is used to express the duality of knowledge (*vidyā*) and non-knowledge (*avidyā*) — or, of absolute and individual consciousness. On the one hand, this perceived duality is represented as the transcendental sleeping state of the god (*yoga-nidrā*). On the other hand, Yoganidrā is the Goddess who simultaneously embodies Viṣṇu's transcendental sleep as a process and, in that capacity of hers, serves as the form of his consciousness while in that state.

The *Durgā-saptaśatī* is regarded as an attempt to reconcile the patriarchal Brahmanical pantheon and the Śākta traditions centring on the worship of female divinities, which were already widespread throughout the Indian subcontinent and still exist today. The text of the *Durgā-saptaśatī* synthesises a number of pre-existing mother goddess myths of Indo-Aryan and non-Indo-Aryan origin, which are skilfully integrated into a single narrative.[175]

Rather than embodying the state of 'deep sleep of union with the Supreme Self' (*adhyātma-yoga-nidrā*), some sources speak of the Goddess as the embodiment of the Supreme Deity's power, who is perceived as a luminous manifestation precisely in the intermediate state between wakefulness and deep sleep proper. For example, the Śaiva tantric text called the Vijñāna-bhairava-*tantra* (ca. 7th–8th century CE[176]) speaks of a goddess called Parā ('The Supreme') who 'shines forth' in the neutral state on the threshold between wakefulness and sleep. In verse 75, a particular stage in immersive practice is described with the help of which focused awareness (*dhāraṇā*) is to be aimed at and established while in this intermediate state, so that the Goddess would spontaneously appear:

175 Kumar, Kamakhya. (2013). *A Handbook of Yoga-Nidrā*. New Delhi: D. K. Printworld Ltd., p. 7.
176 Singh, Jaideva. (1991). *The Yoga of Delight, Wonder, and Astonishment: A Translation of the* Vijnana-bhairava *with an Introduction and Notes*. New York: SUNY Publishers.

anāgatāyāṃ nidrāyāṃ praṇaṣṭe bāhyagocare |
sāvasthā manasā gamyā parā-devī prakāśate || 75 ||

Within not-yet[-full] deep sleep (*nidrāyāṃ*), [yet] beyond the range of external [perception] (*bāhyagocare*),
it is by the mind having reached and become established in that state, that the Supreme Goddess/the Goddess Parā shines forth (*prakāśate*) [by herself].[177]

Patañjali also says that the apparition seen in a dream is a suitable object for practice (*Yoga-sūtra* 1.38).

According to Svāmī Satyasaṅgānanda, between each of the four states of consciousness (that is: wakefulness, the dreaming state, deep sleep and 'the fourth') there is a neutral state which must be crossed in order to reach the next state. These threshold states, which we unconsciously pass through every day, are not one of these four states themselves and are therefore 'unqualified and void-like'. In the *dhāraṇā* referred to above in verse 75, the mind focuses on the neutral state just before deep sleep—a liminal phase where consciousness disconnects from the external world but has not yet descended into deep sleep. If the practitioner is able to grasp this fleeting moment and enter this neutral space of the mind, they can experience this void[178], which is illuminated by Parā—the goddess who represents the supreme power of Bhairava—a wrathful form of Śiva. This moment of awareness in the transition between wakefulness and deep sleep allows the experience of the subtle energy of the highest divine power, as represented by Parā, within the void.[179] An important point is that this process is witnessed and that the image of the goddess is self-manifest and luminous and not willfully visualised, since deliberate imaginative visualisation is characterised by *vikalpa*.

---

177 Translation from the Sanskrit: Georgi Krastev.

178 Void here refers to it being empty of cognitive thought (*vikalpa*), not that nothing occurs.

179 Sarawati, Satyasangananda, Swami. (2004). *Sri Vijnana Bhairava Tantra – The Ascent*. Munger: Yoga Publication Trust, p. 262–263.

Yoga-nidrā in Contemporary Mythological Interpretation

Contemporary understanding of these texts and myths has, however, changed considerably. For example, Indian bestselling author Devdutt Pattanaik provides a socio-cultural interpretation of the application of myths in contemporary Indian society. It has to be noted, however, that, like many contemporary authors, his writing blends Śrīvaiṣṇavism, modern Śāktism and contemporary Indian views on religion and spirituality among others, which often superimposes new interpretations on the reading of ancient textual sources.

Pattanaik gives the following interpretation of the narrative of the *Mārkaṇḍeya-purāṇa*: Brahmā, who had observed all the events surrounding the emergence of the *asuras* (anti-gods, titans) threatening him while Viṣṇu was abiding in *yoga-nidrā*, addressed the Goddess in his hymn of praise as Yoganidrā, on the one hand, and as Mahāmāyā on the other. According to Pattanaik's interpretation, Nārāyaṇa (Viṣṇu sleeping) can be said to embody our sleeping mind, Viṣṇu our awakened mind and Brahmā our partially awakened mind. The *asuras* Madhu and Kaiṭabha are said to symbolise our negative thoughts arising from the partially awakened mind, while our positive thoughts are referred to as *devas* (luminous beings). The Goddess is construed as representing Nature ever-present, even when no human consciousness is present to perceive it.

According to this interpretation, the Goddess is said to manifest herself as Yoga-nidrā — the reality which is not observed by anyone — and she is also understood as Mahāmāyā[180] — the perceived reality which is observed by a partially awakened mind. 'Eventually, the mind will discover that she does not need him but he surely needs her', says Pattanaik. This perceived reality has many names, e.g. Śakti, the energy from which everything arises, Māyā — everything which the human vision defines and evaluates, Kālī — one of the forms revered as the Supreme Goddess, etc.[181]

Another interpretation by Pattanaik is that the male deity archetypes are mostly associated with verbs — their roles are to create (Brahmā), sustain

180 Mārkaṇḍeya-purāṇa uses the name Yogamāyā and has no mention of Mahāmāyā.

181 Pattanaik, Devdutt. (2014). 7 *Secrets of the Goddess*. New Delhi: Westland Ltd., p. 87.

(Viṣṇu) or destroy (Śiva). They therefore represent what can be actively done with what already exists. The female deity archetypes, on the other hand, are usually associated with nouns — inspiration (Sarasvatī), wealth (Lakṣmī) or power (Durgā) or with what is, regardless of what can be done with it or what happens to it. The female deity archetypes are paired with the male archetypes. Pattanaik surmises that in these myths, the male archetypes shape, preserve or destroy nature, which in turn is self-created and independent. These various ephemeral forms of the goddess are the perceived reality. His interpretative summary goes as follows: Brahmā tries to control Nature and creates culture to tame and domesticate the Goddess. Śiva is the ascetic who completely withdraws from Nature — his mind is pure and unclouded by thought. This makes him the destroyer of culture. He is so deeply embedded in our consciousness that we ourselves are not aware of it.[182] Our purpose in life would be to awaken this hidden and undiscovered potential. When Śiva awakens and realises Śakti, Viṣṇu is born. Viṣṇu is our wise mind, which should be able to understand the perceived nature, appreciate its autonomy and the mind's dependence on it. It should understand Brahmā's uncertainties and Śiva's significance and be able to balance both, which makes it the sustainer of culture.[183]

Contemporary understanding, however, moves away from the historical sources by accommodating modern themes and cultural and social currents, as we clearly see in the interpretation of authors such as Pattanaik, who attempt to break social stereotypes by reinterpreting old myths, but whose approach is visibly influenced by Western models and approaches, and Neo-Hindu thought.

---

182 Ibid., p. 89.

183 Ibid., p. 91.

Yoga-nidrā as a Synonym for the Fourth State of Lucidity (*turīya*)

> *That pure and equanimous state which is devoid of ego-sense and non-ego-sense, of the real and the [un]real, and which is free, is known as turīya (the fourth state). It is the state of the liberated sage. It is the unbroken witness consciousness (sākṣyavasthā vyavahṛtau sā turyakalanocyate). It is different from the waking and the dreaming states, which are characterized by movement of thought; it is different from the deep sleep state, which is characterised by inertia and ignorance. When the ego-sense is abandoned, there arises the state of perfect equilibrium in which the turīya manifests itself.*
>
> Words of Sage Vasiṣṭha from The Story of Ikṣvāku within the *Yogavāsiṣṭha* (6.132.14–33)[184]

According to Svāmī Satyānanda, *nidrā*—deep sleep—is one of the three possible states of embodied consciousness. These three states of consciousness (also sometimes referred to as 'states of lucidity') correspond to the gross, subtle and causal levels of existence: *jāgrat*—the waking state in which the mind experiences the physical world, *svapna*—the dream state in which the mind acts independently of the body and the external world, and *suṣupti* (also *nidrā*)—dreamless, unconscious sleep—a state in which there is no awareness of the world, the body, the mind or the ego, and which is characterised by the complete cessation of thought. They exist as transient forms of consciousness, distinct from the Ultimate (which in a Brahmanical framework would be the *brahman*—the infinite, transcendental Reality), the unobstructed perception of which is equated with the term *turīya*, 'the fourth'.[185] The fourth state of consciousness is said to go beyond waking consciousness, dream consciousness and deep sleep. *Turīya* is the experience of perfect unity with perfect awareness and the cancellation of all duality.

184 Adapted from Chapple, Christopher, Key and Venkatesananda. (1984). *The Concise Yoga Vāsiṣṭha*. New York: SUNY Publishers, p. 413.

185 Pattanaik, Devdutt. (2014). *7 Secrets of the Goddess*. New Delhi: Westland Ltd., p. 273.

The *Māṇḍūkya-upaniṣad* (ca. 100–200 CE[186]) one of the ten classical and most important Upaniṣads—also discusses the fourth state (there called *caturtha* instead of *turīya*). The Upaniṣad discusses as its main topic the significance of the mystical syllable and the primordial sound OṂ (ॐ)[187] as an expression of the four states of consciousness: A—the waking state (corresponding to the perceptions of the gross material body), U—the dreaming state (corresponding to those of the prāṇic body), and Ṃ—deep sleep (corresponding to those of the causal body), and finally the 'inaudible' fourth state of consciousness—*caturtha*, the primordial experience which both transcends and includes all multiplicity[188]—a conception very similar to the description we saw of the nature of the Goddess in the *Mārkaṇḍeya-purāṇa*, only in a strictly monistic context. The causal, prāṇic body, etc. will be discussed in more detail in Part I., Chapter 8. *Pañcakośa—The Five Sheaths of Being*.

The *Māṇḍūkya-upaniṣad* describes the three states of waking, dreaming and deep sleep as increasingly undesirable. Among the three, the waking state is considered most beneficial. The 'fourth' state (*caturtha*) is described as transcendental (*avyavahārya*). The totality of the four states as OṂ is then described the pure experience of the Self through the Self, in which knowledge is not gained through the mind, but through the experience of the *ātman*, as stated in the 7th verse of the *Māṇḍūkya-upaniṣad*:

nāntaḥprajñaṃ na bahiḥprajñaṃ nobhayataḥprajñaṃ na prajñānaghanaṃ na prajñaṃ nāprajñam | adṛṣṭam avyavahāryam agrāhyam alakṣaṇam acintyam avyapadeśyam ekātmapratyayasāraṃ prapañcopaśamaṃ śāntaṃ śivam advaitaṃ caturthaṃ manyante | sa ātmā sa vijñeyaḥ || 7 ||[189]

They consider the fourth quarter as perceiving neither what is inside nor what is outside, nor even both together; not as a mass of perception, neither as perceiving nor as not perceiving; as unseen; as beyond the reach of ordinary transaction; as ungraspable; as

186 Nakamura, Hajime. (2004). *A History of Early Vedānta Philosophy*, Part 2. Delhi: Motilal Banarsidass Publications, p. 268.

187 'O' consists of 'A' and 'U' according to Sanskrit grammar.

188 Wolz-Gottwald, Eckard. (2016). *Yoga Philosophie-Atlas*. (5th edition). Petersberg: Verlag Via Nova, p. 64–65.

189 The Sanskrit Project. (2020). *Göttingen Register of Electronic Texts in Indian Languages* (GRETIL). SUB Göttingen. https://gretil.sub.uni-goettingen.de/gretil.html (accessed 14.10.2024).

> without distinguishing marks; as unthinkable; as indescribable; as one whose essence is the perception of itself alone; as the cessation of the visible world; as tranquil; as auspicious; as without a second. That is the self (*ātman*), and it is that which should be perceived.[190]

Which Svāmī Rāma Bhāratī alternatively translates as follows:

> *Turīya* is the fourth state. In this state, consciousness is not turned inward nor outward nor both. It is undifferentiated; it is beyond the spheres of cognition and non-cognition. This state cannot be experienced through the senses or known by comparison or inference; it is incomprehensible, unthinkable, and indescribable. This is Pure Consciousness. This is the real Self. It is the cessation of all phenomena; it is tranquil, all-blissful, and one without second. Thus, real Self is to be realized.[191]

The ultimate goal of the *yoga-nidrā* method could be said to be the achievement of a superconscious state or *turīya*.[192] The yoga-master and scholar Svāmī Rāma Bhāratī (1925–1996, hereafter Svāmī Rāma) uses the term *yoga-nidrā* as a synonym for *turīya* in his commentary on the *Māṇḍūkya-upaniṣad*. However, he refers to the state of *yoga-nidrā* and not to the technique named after the state. He defines the *yoga-nidrā* technique as 'sleep with awareness, which aims to consciously shift awareness from one state of consciousness to another'—from waking—*jāgrat* (which he linked to the *ājñā-cakra*, regarded as being associated with the eyebrow centre) to dreaming—*svapna* (linking it to the *viśuddhi-cakra*, associated with the throat centre), and then to deep sleep—*suṣupti* (linking it to the *anāhata-cakra*, associated with the heart centre) in order to be aware of all three at the same time. While we work with the body, the senses, and then with our own state of consciousness, a deepening of sleep in the presence of awareness is achievable through guided practice: although the mind is turned inwards, one remains fully aware of oneself and also of one's surroundings. In some yoga traditions, the transition from

190 Olivelle, Patrick. (1998). *The Early Upaniṣads: Annotated Text and Translation*. New York/Oxford: Oxford University Press., p. 475.

191 Translation into English: Rama, Swami. (1982). *Enlightenment without God – Mandukya Upanishad*. Honesdale: Himalayan Institute Press, p. 55.

192 Saraswati, Satyanana, Swami. (2006). *Yoga Nidra*. (12th reprint). Munger: Yoga Publications Trust, p. 58; 177.

waking to dreaming to sleeping is sometimes also depicted as a passage through the subtle energy centres (*cakras*) along the spine. Discussing the *cakras* and the complex mechanics of subtle yogic physiology is a long and complex matter. As utilised in *yoga-nidrā* these elements are only subject to advanced forms of the practice, which must be integrated into a comprehensive *sādhana*, accompanied by *āsana*, *prāṇāyāma*, *mudrā*, and *bandha* in order to achieve its intended objectives. Therefore they are not discussed in this volume.

According to Svāmī Rāma, a serious practitioner should learn to master conscious sleep and understand the relationship between consciousness, mind and body, while the mind is being drawn inwards and consciously placed in deep rest. The practitioner should be able to gain self-assured, conscious access to all three states, be aware of them simultaneously and also experience their unity on an individual and a universal level simultaneously—a view shared by Svāmī Satyānanda[193]. Yogins describe this *turīya* or *yoga-nidrā* experience as a state of emptiness (of cognitive conceptual thinking) or bliss.

In the course of practice, we can attain wisdom in the form of knowledge about ourselves by recalling our *saṃskāras* (impressions), observing and understanding them, discarding unhelpful and disturbing thought patterns and strengthening helpful ones. In this way, the practitioner gradually 'enters' the 'hollow of the heart centre'—the *anāhata-cakra*, entering a state of 'absence of all impressions' and stillness of the mind. In this state, the clarity of mind is more profound than in the waking state. In the *Māṇḍūkya-upaniṣad*, the *turīya* state is described as being beyond all other states of the mind, and the state of bliss attained therein is the same bliss as experienced in deep sleep. Therefore, in some texts *turīya* is also used synonymously for the highest state of absorption—*samādhi*.

193 Ibid., p. 177.

Yoga-nidrā as a Synonym for the Highest State of Absorption — *samādhi*

In the *Yogatārāvālī*, (one of the later texts dating to 13th-14th century CE[194]) in which *haṭha-yoga* and *rāja-yoga* are integrated, the process of attaining *yoga-nidrā* is described in its quintessence, but is also used as a synonym for the attainment of *turīya*. In verses 17–19, entering into a state called 'mindful-less active state' (*unmanī*) is explained. There, the mind and senses are under volitional control in such a way that the breathing can be halted — in this text a synonym for *samādhi*. Verses 21 and 22 are dedicated to the *amanaskatā* state, in which the activities of the *manas* (thinking mind) are spontaneously halted and the breath transcends the mind. Then, as explained in verses 24–26, the state of *yoga-nidrā* is attained, and the practitioner is then encouraged to dwell in the *turīya* state, which three, in the system of Patañjali, could be said to roughly correspond to the states of formless absorption called *nirvikalpa-*, *nirbīja-* and then *asaṃprajñāta-samādhi*:

> *pratyagvimarśātiśayena puṃsā prācīnasaṃgeṣu palāyiteṣu* |
> *prādurbhavet kācid ajāḍyanidrā prapañca-cintāṃ parivarjayantī* || 24 ||

Preexisting attachments having been defeated by the Spirit[195] by means of considerable inner examination, [it is then that] non-torpid deep sleep (*ajāḍyanidrā*) manifests (lit: 'shines forth'), completely devoid of the multiplicity of conceptual thought. (24)

194 Nakamura, Hajime. (2004). *A History of Early Vedānta Philosophy*, Part 2. Delhi: Motilal Banarsidass Publications, p. 308.

195 Also referring to *puruṣa* or the Supreme Spirit, Soul of the Universe, Viṣṇu (*MW* [ID=125018]).

vicchinnasaṃkalpavikalpamūle niḥśeṣanirmūlitakarmajāle ||
nirantarābyhāsa-nitānta-bhadrā sā jṛmbhate yoginī yoganidrā || 25 ||

When the root of determination and indetermination (or: variegated ideation[196]) has been completely severed, the net of actions completely uprooted without a trace,

She, who is particularly pleased by uninterrupted practice, the *yoginī* who unfolds [then], is Yoganidrā. (25)
viśrāntimāsādya turīyatattve viśvādyavasthātritatayopariṣṭhe |
saṃvinmayīṃ kām api sarvakālaṃ nidrāṃ sakhe nirviśa nirvikalpām || 26 ||

Having come to repose (*viśrāntim āsādya*) in the realm of the Fourth [state], which is characterised by that condition of the Universe and so on of being situated above the triad [of the other states], it is that very deep state of non-conceptual (*nirvikalpām*) immersion (*nidrā*) which is characterised by understanding (*saṃvin-mayīṃ*), which you should enter, Oh friend! (26)[197]

These verses provide perhaps a most essential and important explanation of the subtle difference between *nidrā* and *yoga-nidrā*. In Vācaspati's commentary on Patañjali's *Yoga-sūtra* 2.41 it is explained that *nidrā* is that of the three states of waking, dreaming and deep sleep in which the mind (*citta*) is dominated by the quality of *tamas* (inertia, torpidity)—i.e. there is a lack of awareness or consciousness.

In another place (the commentary to *YS* 1.10) it is explained that sleep dominated by *tamas* results in a heavy body and a feeling of stupidity. The commentary further distinguishes that sleep in which *sattva* is present alongside *tamas* allows one to awaken feeling refreshed, whereas sleep in

196 It is possible (and possibly intended) to understand the compound *saṃkalpavikalpa* not only as consisting of two phenomena (determination and lack thereof) with a single root, but also as a single noun – 'variegated ideation'. The point here being that dualistic thinking is characterised by attraction and aversion, the need for limiting discrimination which brings along with it the unavoidable consequence of limited perception and focus, which result in a faulty perception and therefore also faulty understanding of Reality. Both ways of understanding convey the same idea.

197 Translation from the Sanskrit: Georgi Krastev.

> which *rajas* is present alongside *tamas* leads to awakening in a poorly rested state. The *Yogatārāvālī* explains how *yoga-nidrā* differs from the usual *tamas*-dominated state of just *nidrā* and how and why it is, in fact, identical to the Fourth State (*turīya*). While *nidrā* is the state in which awareness is normally inactive, *yoga-nidrā* is the state in which only the conceptual thinking apparatus (*vikalpa*) is inactive, while complete and full awareness is maintained. This is also the reason why *yoga-nidrā* is equated with *samādhi*, as this state presupposes the uncoupling of sense perception from the sense objects (*pratyāhāra*) and thus the absence of attraction (*rāga*) and aversion (*dveṣa*) towards these objects—that is to say the ability to be fully aware, impartially, of the nature of existence, or whatever one wishes to focus one's attention upon, without this nature being obscured by the abstractions of the intellectual mind. This, of course, is also a prerequisite for the Fourth State, as one learns in Patañjali's *Yoga-sūtra* 2.49, where *prāṇāyāma* ('breath control') is presented as the process by which the mind is prepared for further practices, which, in turn, is the prerequisite for the practice of focused awareness (*dhāraṇā*) (2.53). On the basis of this, it can be argued that the later *Yogatārāvālī* not only elaborates upon a system of yoga whose structure of practice seems uncannily similar to that described by Patañjali, but, in fact, clearly states that *yoga-nidrā* is a subtle yogic state which is demonstrably different from the unconsciousness of ordinary *nidrā*.

Georg Feuerstein (1947–2012) also equates *yoga-nidrā* with the state of *amanaskatā*, or, as he calls it—'transmentality'.[198] In this state, the conceptual mind dissolves and one becomes illuminated. *Yoga-nidrā* is one of the states in which being liberated whilst alive (*jīvanmukti*) is possible and which makes it possible to experience a feeling of universality. *Amanaskatā* is the *unmanī*-state which signifies a condition of exhilaration or elation, that is, of being out of one's mind, but in the above-mentioned positive sense of non-conceptual awareness. In the *unmanī*-state, the fullness of 'This is you' (*tat tvam asi*) becomes comprehensible.[199] 'The *unmanī* state is the product of prolonged abiding in *nirvikalpa-samādhi*. This leads to the dissolution of the mind (*mano-nāśa*), whereupon the transcendental Reality shines forth in its

198 Feuerstein, Georg. (2008). *The Yoga Tradition – Its History, Literature, Philosophy and Practice* (3rd edition). Arizona: Hohm Press, p. 520.

199 Ayyangar, Srinivasa. (1938). *The Yoga Upanishads*. Madras: Vasanta Press, p. 241–242.

solitary majesty.'[200] These states from *tāraka-yoga*—a yoga path on which the deep dimensions of consciousness and the Absolute can be experienced in various manifestations of light, are described in the eighth verse of the *Advayatāraka-upaniṣad*—ca. 100 BCE to 300 CE.[201]—and in the third book of the *Maṇḍala-brāhmaṇa-upaniṣad*.

In addition to the *Yogatārāvālī*, *yoga-nidrā* is used synonymously with *samādhi* in other texts: the *Śāṇḍilya-upaniṣad* (ca. 100 BCE to 300 CE[202]; verse 1.35), the *Amanaska* (11th or 12th centuries CE; verse 2.61), and the *Haṭha-yoga-pradīpikā* (14th century CE; verses 4.43–50). According to these texts, *yoga-nidrā* is achieved by means of *khecharī mudrā* (a tongue position in which the tongue is moved backwards into the throat and nose to touch the point between the eyebrows, *ājñā-cakra*). They explain that *khecharī* should be practised in order to reach the unmanī state and until *yoga-nidrā* occurs.

Yoga-nidrā vs. *nidrā-śakti*

In ordinary *nidrā* as explained above, both the body and the mind of animals (including humans) become motionless, whereas in the dreaming state, there is some degree of mental and occasionally even physical activity. This distinction may explain Patañjali's interpretation of *nidrā* as referring specifically to a state of deep unconscious sleep, where the intellect (*buddhi*) is dominated by torpor (*tamas*). In this state, awareness is entirely absent, as both mental clarity and physical activity are subdued by the inertia of *tamas*. However, Vācaspati explains in his commentary on the *Yoga-sūtra* 1.38 that sattvic *nidrā* is when the mind is naturally one-pointed (*ekāgra*) and it is, in fact, a form of experiencing *brahman*.

This is also visible in the narrative of the *Mārkaṇḍeya-purāṇa*, where Viṣṇu is completely under Yoganidrā's power. It is alluded, however, that Yoganidrā is herself an aspect of Viṣṇu's consciousness, which remains active, because

200 Feuerstein, Georg. (2008). *The Yoga Tradition – Its History, Literature, Philosophy and Practice* (3rd edition). Arizona: Hohm Press, p. 520.

201 Flood, Gavin, D. (1996). *An Introduction to Hinduism*. Cambridge: Cambridge University Press, p. 96.

202 Ibid., p. 96.

it is the embodiment of that very state — rather than portrayed as something negative, She is praised by Brahmā as the supreme power. In this context, coherent with the Śākta view, the existence of creation, sustenance and destruction is not refuted as the negative manifestation of Universal Illusion obscuring the Absolute as in later Advaita Vedānta, but as a natural aspect of existence. Furthermore, as we saw in the Śaiva *Vijñāna-bhairava-tantra*, it is precisely by entering a state close to deep sleep, maintaining awareness, but away from active waking consciousness, which can allow a yogin to behold by means of the special perception afforded by that very state, the luminous apparition of the power of the Supreme Divinity (in the particular case — the Goddess Parā).

Texts such as the *Pañcadaśī* — an Advaita Vedānta treatise by *Vidyāraṇya Mādhava* (1296–1386 CE), however, speak negatively of *nidrā* as the 'force which causes torpor' (*nidrā-śaktiḥ*). Unlike in Vācaspati's commentary on the *Yoga-sūtra* 1.38, however, in the *Pañcadaśī*, *nidrā* has an exclusively negative connotation, as Mādhava compares it to the power of Universal Illusion (*māyā*) as understood by Sureśvara, which in later Advaita is strongly synonymous with ignorance (*avidyā*). Hence, both dreams (*svapna*) and the power of torpidity which causes them (*nidrā-śaktiḥ*) are seen in this Advaita context as something entirely negative. The cause of the false perception one has in dreams and the false perception that there are such processes as creation, sustenance and destruction is taken to be the same. This is contrary to the views propounded in texts belonging to many Śaiva, Śākta and Yoga traditions. To exemplify this, in the third chapter of the *Pañcadaśī*[203], we read:

mṛcchaktir brahmaśaktir[204] *anekān anṛtān sṛjet* |
yad vā jīvagatā nidrā svapnaś cātra nidarśanam || 3.85 ||

The power of death — the power of creation, produces (lit.: 'excretes') many false things (lit.: things, which go against (*an-*) the Natural Order (*-ṛta*));
similarly, that [power] having entered a living being — it induces torpid sleep (*nidrā*) and dreams (*svapna*) in them.

203 Original text from: Acharya, Narayan, Ram. (1987). *The Pañcadaśi of Vidyāraṇya Muni*. Delhi: Chaukhamba Sanskrit Pratishtan, p. 576–577; Translation from the Sanskrit: Georgi Krastev.
204 The printed edition has *vahrahma-*.

nidrāśaktir yathā jīve durghaṭa svapnakāriṇī |
brahmaṇyeṣā sthitā māyā sṛṣṭisthityantakāriṇī || 3.86 ||

As She—as the force of torpor (*nidrāśaktiḥ*)—causes living beings to have variegated dreams,
So [it is also] She (*eṣā*)—as established (*sthitā*) in the brahman (*brahmaṇi*)—effecting the illusion (*māyā*) of creation, sustenance and destruction.
[...]

īdṛśo mahimā dṛṣṭo nidrāśakter yadā tadā |
māyāśakter acintyo 'yaṃ mahimeti kim adbhutam || 3.89 ||

If what is seen [in a dream] is endowed with the greatness of the power of torpor (*nidrāśaktiḥ*), then,
is it not strange to not think the same about the power of illusion (*māyāśaktiḥ*) [as the cause of the manifest world], since it is [equally] great?

śayāne puruṣe nidrā svapnaṃ bahuvidhaṃ sṛjet |
brahmaṇy evaṃ nirvikāre vikārān kalpayaty asau || 3.90 ||

As torpid sleep (*nidrā*) [and] multi-faceted dreams (*bahuvidhaṃ svapnaṃ*) within people (*puruṣe*) is produced when one lies down to rest (*śayāne*),
so, [also it/She] produces the changes of form in the unchanging [Nature of the] *brahman* (*brahmaṇi*).

Reading verses such as the above outside of their respective Advaita context, may lead a reader to draw parallels and connections solely on the basis of the use of the word *nidrā* (such as when it is used in compound terms such as *nidrāśakti*), oblivious to its different connotations when read in the context of works belonging to different religious and philosophical traditions. For example, *nidrāśakti* as a term appears to be specific to an Advaita context. Therefore, without acknowledging these distinctions, one risks misunderstanding the deeper meaning and implications of the term as it relates to its specific philosophical background.

Furthermore, adding a qualifier '*yoga-*' does not make the term *nidrā* more transparent, as we discussed above in the case of *adhyātma-yoga-nidrā*. Therefore, the term should always be looked at in its individual contexts. The compound *adhyātma-yoga-nidrā mentioned* in the *Mahābhārata* offers a clue as to the understanding of *nidrā* in that context. While *yoga-nidrā* on its own has an opaque etymology, adding *adhyātma-* permits two interpretations of the compound, namely: 'the *nidrā* of/relating to *adhyātma-yoga*' or 'the *yoga-nidrā* of/relating to *adhyātma*'. The former makes better sense both structurally and etymologically, as yoga on its own may have many and varied meanings, making the compound *yoga-nidrā* opaque in its semantic value. However, if yoga or 'Union' is understood in the sense of *adhyātma-yoga* or 'Union with the Supreme Self', then *nidrā* becomes not 'deep sleep', per se, but a word denoting a state of deep immersion or absorption, characterised by Union with the Supreme—be that Śiva, Viṣṇu, an impersonal form of the Divine, or a higher state of consciousness closer to the Ultimate, depending on the tradition. We also see its versatility by the fact it is used in precisely this way by many different traditions. Thus, we must carefully distinguish between contexts where *nidrā* is used in the sense of 'immersion', those, where it is used as a synonym for the normal dreaming state (*svapna*) and those, where it is seemingly treated as an entirely negative phenomenon (*nidrā-śakti*), a state of being afflicted by a form of ignorance (*avidyā*).

Yoga-nidrā and the *nidrā-vṛtti*

Patañjali describes sleep itself (*nidrā*) as a *vṛtti*—a fluctuation of the mind which should be overcome in order to achieve *samādhi*. In this state of deep, dreamless sleep, there is no flow of thoughts, but only the awareness of pure being, the state based upon 'defined by non-being' (*abhāva-pratyaya*), the stillness of the mind.

In this state of mind, which no longer has a focus, or 'support' (*ālambana*), the mind becomes particularly receptive and malleable. Some authors explain that, in this way, the power of the mental field can be influenced by your own intention and decision (*saṃkalpa*), which is particularly valuable in the process of learning and activating the self-healing powers of the body and mind.[205]

Patañjali's *Yoga-sūtra* 1.10 states:

abhāva-pratyaya-ālambanā-vṛtti-nidrā |

That fluctuation of the mind based upon being defined by non-being [is called] 'deep sleep'.

Or, according to Svāmī Satyānanda:

Sleep is the *vṛtti* of absence of mental contents for its support.[206]

In his commentaries on Patañjali's *Yoga-sūtras*, Svāmī Satyānanda states that, when we have a mental experience of an object, that experience is called 'content of mind' (*pratyaya*).[207] It can take the form of a vision or a dream, with or without contact of the senses with an object. When the manifest content of the mind is removed through a particular process, the mind is deprived of the support of awareness.

Patañjali explains 'what is known in a dream or deep sleep' can be a proper object for focus and immersion. However, Patañjali does not give any practical instructions, nor does he mention *yoga-nidrā*. In *Yoga-sūtra* 1.38 he states:

svapna-nidrā-jñāna-ālambanaṃ vā |

Or, [steadiness of the mind is achieved] by having the experience of a dream or deep sleep as one's object [of cultivation].[208]

205 Parker, S., Bharati, S. V. & Fernandez, M. (2013). Defining yoga-nidra: traditional accounts, physiological research, and future directions. *International journal of yoga therapy*, 23(1), p. 13.

206 Saraswati, Satyananda, Swami. (2000). *Four Chapters on Freedom*. Munger: Yoga Publication Trust, p. 54.

207 Ibid., p. 54–55.

208 Translation from the Sanskrit: Georgi Krastev.

Yoga-nidrā in the Buddhist Tradition

References to *yoga-nidrā* can also be found in the Buddhist tradition. Similar to the Yoga, Vedānta, and tantric traditions, *yoga-nidrā* (equated with a *samādhi-* and *turīya-*like state) is achieved in Mahāyāna Buddhism by allowing awareness to rest in the heart centre. The subtle heart centre is regarded as the centre of deep sleep.

In the Buddhist *Mahāmāyā-tantra* (ca. 10th century CE), *yoga-nidrā* is described as the freedom from mental distractions and a state in which secret knowledge can be realised.

> *yadi sarve buddhayanti jagatkrīḍā vinaśyati* |
> *tasmād guptam idaṃ jñānam aprakāśyam anakṣaram* || 18 ||
> *buddhayanti hi saṃbuddhā yoganidrāsamāgatāḥ* |
> *dhyāyanta ekarūpāṇi piṇḍaṃ tadgatamānasāḥ* || 19 ||[209]

> If all beings were to awaken, the play of the world would cease. Therefore, this knowledge is secret, unseen, and imperishable. (18)
> Since the completely awakened ones (the Buddhas) are awake to it, [the yogins] immersed in *yoganidrā*, dwell upon the singular nature of [all] forms in the form of a pill (*piṇḍa*) while in that state. (2.19)[210]

In Tibetan Buddhism and the Bön teachings, for example, a special area of conscious dreaming is recognised. 'Dream' yoga is a practice of immersion which has been known in Tibet since ancient times. The practitioner tries to remain conscious even when asleep in order to influence their own dreams. The ability to dream lucidly is not an end in itself, but provides an additional context in which to engage in advanced and effective practices to consciously traverse and explore the various states of consciousness and subsequently achieve liberation. The dream is significant in this tradition because it is one

---

209 Ratnākaraśānti. (1992). *Mahāmāyātantram with Guṇavatī* (Prof. Samdhong Rinpoche & Vrajavallabh Dwivedi, Eds.). Rare Buddhist Text Series (No. 10). Central Institute of Higher Tibetan Studies, Sarnath, Varanasi, India. p. 33.

210 *Śrī-mahāmāyā-tantrarājanāma Toh* 425; Degé Kangyur volume 80, F.169.a; Adapted from the translation by the Dharmachakra Translation Committee under the patronage and supervision of 84000: Translating the Words of the Buddha / First published 2013.

of the best ways to understand the deepest aspects of ourselves. Dreams are also considered the most important pathways to healing. This practice is not so much about what you do when you are asleep and dreaming, but rather how the mind is utilised when you are awake. In this way, the mind is trained to remain continuously in awareness around the clock.[211]

In this tradition, dream yoga (*rmi lam gyi rnal 'byor*) is followed by sleep yoga (*rnal 'byor gnyid 'thugs*), also known as the 'yoga of clear light' (*'od gsal gyi rnal 'byor*), which is an advanced practice. The aim is to remain conscious in deep sleep, when the gross conceptual mind and the activity of the senses come to a standstill.

This practice is understood as preparation for death (*pho ba*). In dying, we reach the borderline between *saṃsāra* and *nirvāṇa*—the intermediate state, the famous bar do.[212] The principles of the states and experiences of consciousness are very similar to those already mentioned with regard to tantric yoga texts.

211 Wangyal, Tenzin, Rinpoche. (1998). *The Tibetan Yogas Of Dream And Sleep*. New York: Snow Lion Publications, p. 4–5.
212 Ibid., pp. 15–19.

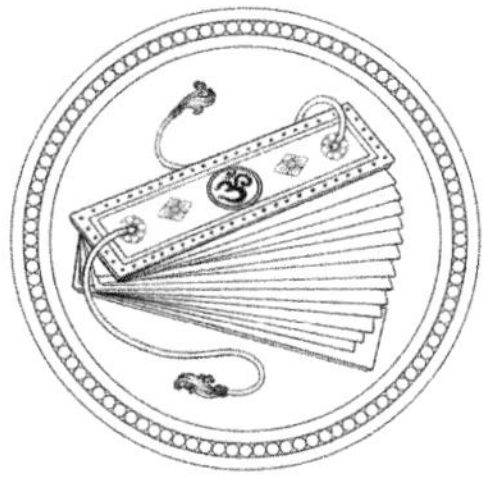

CHAPTER 5

Pratyāhāra as Foundation for *yoga-nidrā*

Svāmī Satyānanda's *yoga-nidrā* method is divided into progressively staged techniques, ranging from beginner to advanced, which, when practiced systematically, can lead to a specific desired state. Each technique always begins with stilling the body and mind. Then one starts by practicing a *pratyāhāra*-based technique suitable for everyone, subsequently moving onto *dhāraṇā*-based ones and finally becoming able to practice with techniques whose ultimate goal is achieving the state of *dhyana*,[213] the latter two of which necessitate direct instruction and supervision by a competent *guru*. An essential factor for the success of the practice is that you are aware of the respective focus of each technique, and that you proceed methodically in your own practice.

In order to grasp its full effects, *yoga-nidrā* should always be seen within the overarching yogic context, especially with regard to rāja-yoga[214] and Tantra[215]. Svāmī Satyānanda's *yoga-nidrā* technique which is available for general practice

213 Saraswati, Niranjanananda, Swami. (2002). *Yoga Darshan*. (1st edition, reprinted with corrections). Munger: Yoga Publication Trust, p. 170–17.

214 See Part I., Chapter 3. *Introduction to raja-yoga: the Path of the Souvereign*.

215 See Part I., Chapter 1. *Tantra*.

can be ascribed to the fifth limb of the eightfold yoga[216] — *pratyāhāra* — the process of purification from the layers of *saṃskāras*, *karmans* or archetypes of the personality, in which deep-seated tensions in the subconscious and unconscious are released. In *pratyāhāra*, the mind gradually detaches itself from identification with the sensory objects and perceptions, naturally assumes the attitude of an uninvolved observer, and is subsequently ready for further, more subtle immersions.

Svāmī Satyānanda's *Yoga-nidrā* Method with a *pratyāhāra*-focus

> *There are many kinds of pratyāhāra; [...] They are all meant for purifying the sense awareness and making it turn inward. [...] If you can master the technique of pratyāhāra, then concentration (dhāraṇā) becomes very easy. It is impossible to go on to dhāraṇā and dhyāna unless the field of pratyāhāra is crossed.*[217]
>
> Svāmī Satyānanda

With his *yoga-nidrā* method, Svāmī Satyānanda has made a systematic *pratyāhāra* practice available to the general public, based on tantric tecniques enabling the senses to be gradually turned inwards. This trains the mind to reach and remain in an actively inward-looking state. In this state of alertness, the senses are turned away from the perception of external stimuli, but the awareness within remains awake and active. The layers of impressions (*pratyayas*) accumulated in everyday life are dissolved at the level of the subconscious. Thus, the connection between the *pratyayas* and their source of power is weakened, limiting their range of influence.

> Through regular practice, we can learn to move between the different levels of consciousness. As this process facilitates the release of subconscious

216 See Part I., Chapter 3. *Role of the citta-vṛttis*.
217 Saraswati, Satyananda, Swami. (2002). *Yoga Darshan*. (1st edition, reprinted with corrections). Munger: Yoga Publication Trust, p. 219.

> tensions on the physical, energetic, and emotional-mental levels of being, it naturally gives rise to a state of profound relaxation, among other effects. Svāmī Satyānanda describes *yoga-nidrā* as 'yogic/psychic sleep' and also as 'unification of awareness during the state of relaxation'. 'This state in which we are aware, but not aware, that we are aware, is experienced in *yoga-nidrā*.'[218]

Patañjali defines yoga as the dissolution (*nirodhaḥ*) of the movement patterns (*vṛtti*) of the mind (*citta*) or *yogaś-citta-vṛtti-nirodhaḥ*. The term *citta* refers to the totality of the conscious, subconscious and unconscious fields. The simultaneous perception in the unified or complete awareness of these three fields is referred to by Svāmī Satyānanda as *turīya* or *aham asmi*—'I am'. This state, in which we are both conscious and unconscious of ourselves, is experienced in *yoga-nidrā*, in a process of imperceptible, inner sublimation.[219]

This powerful state of awareness can also be described as the threshold between the outer and inner worlds—between the waking and sleeping states, where we can achieve healing on all levels, connection with our inner being, inner strength and development of the creative potential of the mind.

From a yogic point of view, *yoga-nidrā* of Svāmī Satyānanda is, therefore, a powerful practice path where we can come closer to our true nature and reach a state of pure awareness free from the flow of thoughts and identifications.

The aims of Svāmī Satyānanda's *yoga-nidrā* method (from the *pratyāhāra* group) are:

- the cultivation of the *draṣṭā*—the observer attitude/stance;
- to bring body and mind into a unified state through deep relaxation;
- to withdraw the awareness from the body, the sensory and mental activities and to disidentify oneself from them by entering the subconscious with awareness in order to release the impressions (*saṃskāras*)—this is the process and, at the same time, one of the goals of *pratyāhāra*;

218 Saraswati, Satyananda, Swami. (2013). *Yoga Nidra – Water the Roots* 4. Munger: Yoga Publications Trust, 2013, p. 4–5.
219 Ibid., p. 5.

- to consciously experience and traverse the subtle sheaths of being (*kośas*);[220]
- to gradually immerse the awareness from the conscious via the subconscious into the unconscious in order to achieve unified awareness and to enable entry into the state of *dhāraṇā*;
- to go beyond all the above by illuminating the unconscious in the *dhyāna* state and thereby partaking in the experience of the superconscious state – *turīya* – or the union of outer and inner consciousness.

The individual stages of Svāmī Satyānanda's *yoga nidrā* method are presented in Part II. of this book.

What is *pratyāhāra*?

> *Many of us find that even after years of meditation practice, we have not achieved all that we expected. Trying to practice meditation without some degree of pratyāhāra is like trying to gather water in a leaky vessel. No matter how much water we bring in, it flows out again. The senses are like holes in the vessel of the mind. Unless they are sealed the mind cannot hold the nectar of truth.*[221]
>
> David Frawley

David Frawley also quotes the statement by Svāmī Śivānanda[222], that *pratyāhāra* should itself be called 'yoga', as it is the most important link in the *yoga-sādhanā*.[223] *Pratyāhāra* is also a main element of the Bihar Yoga system, which continues the teachings of Svāmī Śivānanda. An important factor here — just as in the teachings of Tantra — is the process of the expansion of individual awareness.

220 See Part I., Chapter 8. *Pañcakoṣa – The Five Sheaths of Being*.

221 Frawley, David. (n.d.). Pratyahara, Yoga's Forgotten Limb. *Yoga International*. https://yogainternational.com/article/view/pratyahara-yogas-forgotten-limb/ (accessed on 27.06.2020).

222 Svāmī Śivānanda is Svāmī Satyānanda's *guru*.

223 Ibid.

In modern, Western yoga, the aspect of *pratyāhāra* is largely neglected, presumably because it is not really understood. In the context of Patañjali's yoga system, it forms the threshold between the outer yoga stages (*yama, niyama, āsana, prāṇāyāma*), called *bahiraṅga-yoga*, and the inwardly-focused yoga limbs (*dhāraṇā, dhyāna, samādhi*)—*antaraṅga-yoga*. While *pratyāhāra* in Patañjali's *Yoga-sūtras*, belongs to *bahiraṅga*, in the *Yoga-yājñavalkya*[224] it belongs to *antaraṅga-yoga*. In the later yoga text *Gheranda-saṃhitā*, *pratyāhāra* is ranked before *prāṇāyāma*.

Within the integral approach to yoga, *pratyāhāra* can be a stage on the path, a state or a practice at the same time. After preparation through *yama, niyama, āsana* and *prāṇāyāma*, perception is diverted away from the external sense objects and the flow of *prāṇa* (here meaning 'vital energy' rather than 'breath')—originally focussed on the outside—is interrupted. This frees the senses from their external attachment and enables them to follow the mind inwards. In order to collect the mind and prepare it for the practice of focused awareness, continuously focusing the mind on a single object (*dhāraṇā*) and prolonged immersive focused awareness (*dhyāna*), *pratyāhāra* is an important step, indeed a prerequisite.

To think that *dhyāna* can be achieved without having mastered *pratyāhāra* is illusory. A holistic approach which addresses the individual in their entirety is essential in this process and on this path. It is not possible to jump from the physical to the spiritual level straight away. For example, in *haṭha-yoga*, these two levels can be connected by gaining control over one's vital energies, which is first done with the help of *prāṇāyāma*, then by controlling sensory perceptions and, finally, by dissolving the associated identifications on the mental level.

224 The text *Yoga-yājñavalkya* (between 900 and 1350 CE), written by an unknown author, describes the teachings of the seer Yājñavalkya. This text stands out from the other yoga texts of the same period and refers to Vedāntic and Tantric concepts.

The Process of *pratyāhāra*

It may be concluded that human consciousness operates within a limited range. Our mind is already conditioned by society in childhood to operate within a certain rational framework. The activities of the mind and its abilities are initially connected and identified with the senses, the 'sense objects' and physical sensory experiences. We cannot hear frequencies which our hearing cannot pick up, and we can only see as far as our visual system allows us to see. The barriers of personal perception do not allow us, for example, to see the nanoparticles of the universe with the naked eye or to hear ultrasonic waves. It is the mind which processes the information from the sensory organs, categorises it, stores it and thus creates our logically comprehensible world view in the context of social conditioning. In this way, the sensory object (*viṣaya*) is not merely the object itself, but arises from the combination of its various components, into which name, form, and time perception flow. The sense object is associated with identity, bodily structure, and the mental, emotional, and physical forces that shape the personality. From this form of conditioning arises duality, manifesting as *rāga* (attachment) and *dveṣa* (aversion).

One of the aims of *pratyāhāra* is to break these very links of sense perception associated with the three levels of name, form of the sense object, and the perception of it, which lead to physical (external), subtle (self-created) and causal (intrinsic) experiences. By withdrawing awareness from the external sense objects, we can redirect our focus to an internal focal point, allowing the mind to sink further unhindered into the *dhāraṇā* state.[225]

In order to experience the subtle boundlessness of consciousness, it is essential to overcome restrictive barriers and behavioural patterns, freeing the mind from its narrow confines. This requires cultivating a new inner attitude that interrupts our everyday habitual perception and opens our awareness to more subtle experiences, thereby expanding it. Consequently, we train our mind to detach from the flood of external impulses and to reduce identification with sensory perceptions.[226]

---

225 Feuerstein, Georg. (2008). *The Yoga Tradition – Its History, Literature, Philosophy and Practice* (3rd edition). Arizona: Hohm Press, p. 169.

226 Ibid., p. 164.

In the context of integral yoga, when the mind is withdrawn from the mechanical activities of the senses—seeing, tasting, smelling, feeling and hearing—the sense organs do not cease to function, but sense perception breaks its connection to the external sense impulses and can spontaneously follow the mind inward. Simultaneously, we strengthen the inner observer (*draṣṭā*) and achieve a certain distance from the material world (*prakṛti*). This does not imply a separation from real life; rather, the goal is to cultivate an aware and conscious approach to our sensory impressions. This awareness provides us with the opportunity to understand ourselves better, thereby enabling us to shape our lives more consciously. By looking inward, we become more attuned to the workings of our minds, which allows us to develop the ability to comprehend and direct the inner movements and patterns of the mind.

The mind possesses a life of its own, much like the body. Typically, we focus on the physical level, on the outside, and remain unaware of our mental processes. Just as we care for our bodies through *āsana* and *prāṇāyāma*, we must also learn to engage with the mind. In *pratyāhāra*, our perception should be directed inward to cultivate awareness and understand our mental processes—thoughts, memories and inner sense impressions—along with their associated connections. In this way, the perception of the inner and outer worlds is balanced.

The Stages of *pratyāhāra*

The term and the state of *pratyāhāra* have been interpreted in various ways. Throughout history, different authors and traditions have offered varied perspectives, levels, aspects, and approaches to understanding this state. Some of these interpretations are explained in more detail below.

In Patanjali's *Yoga-sutras* (2.54–55), *pratyahara* is introduced as the last link of external yoga, following *prāṇāyāma*. While Patañjali does not provide explicit instructions for the practice of *pratyāhāra*, Vācaspati's commentary clarifies that control of the senses is achieved through control of the mind. He explains that if each sense were to be restrained individually, additional effort would be required to manage the others. However, by controlling the mind, the senses are automatically controlled as well. Therefore, no further effort is needed to restrain the senses individually, making *pratyāhāra* the highest form of control over them.[227]

In his commentary on the *Yoga-sūtras*, Svāmī Satyānanda explains that *pratyāhāra* is a state in which one withdraws the mind from the sense objects: 'The capacities of smell, taste, sight, touch and hearing are withdrawn from their objects and the senses begin to follow the mind inward and not outward. This is withdrawal of the mind from the sense activities so that the sense perceptions also become introverted with the mind; they imitate the mind and follow it inside'.[228]

In the *Bhagavād-gītā* (2.58), the image of a tortoise withdrawing into its shell is used for the process of mastering sense perception — the tortoise's shell would be the mind, and the tortoise's limbs would be the senses. The scholar Vyāsa (ca. 5th or 6th century CE), however, compares the mind in his *Yoga-sūtra* commentary *Yoga-sūtra-bhāṣya* (on the *Yoga-sūtra* 2.54) with the queen bee: 'When the queen bee flies up, the bees swarm after her; when the queen bee settles down, the bees also settle down. Likewise, when the mind is mastered, the senses are mastered.' This approach is also reflected in the foundational texts of *haṭha-yoga* and in the *Gheraṇḍa-saṃhitā* (ca. 17th century CE).

In the *Kaṭha-upaniṣad*, the control of the senses is compared to a charioteer who reins in the horses:

ātmānaṃ rathinaṃ viddhi śarīraṃ ratham eva tu |
buddhiṃ tu sārathiṃ viddhi manaḥ pragraham eva ca || 3.3 ||

Understand the Self (*ātmān*) as a chariot driver,
with the body (*śarīra*) as the chariot.
Understand the intellect (*buddhi*) as the charioteer
and as the reins — the mind (*manas*). (3.3)

227 Patañjali. (1998). *Patanjali's Yoga Sutras – with the Commentary of Vyāsa and the gloss of Vāchaspati Miśra, Prasāda, Rāma* (translation). New Delhi: Munshirm Manoharlal Pub Pvt. Ltd., p. 177–178.

228 Saraswati, Satyananda, Swami. (2000). *Four Chapters on Freedom*. Munger: Yoga Publication Trust, p. 217.

indriyāṇi hayān āhur viṣayām˙s teṣu gocarān |
ātmendriya-mano-yuktaṃ bhoktety āhur manīṣiṇaḥ || 3.4 ||

The senses are called 'horses' by those with understanding,
the objects of the senses — 'the pasture for them'.
The one who is connected with the Self, the senses (*indriya*), and the mind, they call 'the enjoyer' (*bhokta*). (3.4)

yas tv avijñānavān bhavaty ayuktena manasā sadā |
tasyendriyāṇy avaśyāni duṣṭāśvā iva sāratheḥ || 3.5. ||

But he who due to an ever-untamed mind
is not a partaker of knowledge,
the senses do not obey him,
just as bad horses [disobey] a charioteer. (3.5)

yas tu vijñānavān bhavati yuktena manasā sadā |
tasyendriyāṇi vaśyāni sadaśvā iva sāratheḥ || 3.6 ||

But he who, through an ever-restrained mind,
partakes of knowledge –
the senses obey him,
just as good horses [obey] a charioteer. (3.6)

yas tv avijñānavān bhavaty amanaskaḥ sadāśuciḥ |
na sa tat padam āpnoti sam˙ṡāraṃ cādhigacchati || 3.7 ||

But he who is not a partaker of knowledge,
without a [restrained] mind, and is always impure –
he will not reach that place (state)
and enters into *saṃsāra*. (3.7)

yas tu vijñānavān bhavati samanaskaḥ sadā śuciḥ |
sa tu tat padam āpnoti yasmād bhūyo na jāyate || 3.8 ||

But he who is a partaker of knowledge,

has a [tamed] spirit and is always pure,
He reaches the place
from which he will not be born again. (3.8)[229]

In chapter 10, verse 6.1 of the *Haṭha-yoga-pradıpikā* (14th century)[230], a gradual and systematic withdrawal of the senses is described. In the *Yoga-darśana-upaniṣad* and the *Śāṇḍilya-upaniṣad* (both presumably 100 BCE–300 CE.[231]), in the *Vasiṣṭha saṃhitā* (pre 1250[232]) and in the *Yoga yājñavalkya* (between 900 and 1350 CE[233]), *pratyāhāra* is an active process. The *Yoga-yājñavalkya* explains the methodology for practising *pratyāhāra* as follows:

indriyāṇāṃ vicaratāṃ viṣayeṣu svabhāvataḥ |
balād āharaṇaṃ teṣāṃ pratyāhāraḥ sa ucyate || 7.2 || [234]

'One must direct [the mind] to the objects of the organs [of perception and action] in its natural state.
The retrieval (*āharaṇa*) of these [organs] due to force, that [process] is called 'drawing back in' (*praty-āhāra*).

yad yat paśyasi tat sarvaṃ paśyed ātmavad ātmani |
pratyāhāraḥ sa ca prokto yogavidbhir mahātmabhiḥ || 7.3 ||

[Then,] whatever you see is seen as being of the Self, within the Self.
This [state] is proclaimed by the great knowers of yoga to be *pratyāhāra*!

---

229 Translation into English after the German of Haas, Dominik. (2018). Die Kaṭha-Upaniṣad (translation). In Master's Thesis: *Vom Feueraltar zum Yoga. Kohärenz und Konzept der Kaṭha-Upaniṣad*. https://doi.org/10.1007/S10781–019-09408-Y (accessed on 22.02.2022), p. 13.

230 The lesser-known recension of the *Haṭha-yoga-pradīpikā* with ten chapters.

231 Flood, Gavin, D. (1996). *An Introduction to Hinduism*. Cambridge: Cambridge University Press, p. 96.

232 Wujastyk, D. (2017). *The Yoga Texts Attributed to Yājñavalkya and their Remarks on Posture*. Asian Literature and Translation, 4(1), p. 162.

233 Ibid., 159–186.

234 Divanji, Prahlad, C. (1954). *Yoga-Yājñavalkya. A Treatise on Yoga as Taught by Yogī Yājñavalkya*. Vol. 3. B.B.R.A. Society Mongraph. Bombay: Bombay Branch of the Royal Asiatic Society, p. 63–64.

karmāṇi yāni nityāni vihitāni śarīriṇām |
teṣām ātmany anuṣṭhānaṃ manasā yad bahir vinā || 7.4 ||

Those [ritual] actions, which are [are considered] indispensable and compulsory by embodied beings –
the practice (*anuṣṭhāna*) of these, [which takes place] within the Self [and is carried out] by the mind — this is [*pratyāhāra*] without [the need for] external [ritual practice].

pratyāhāro bhavet so 'pi yogasādhanam uttamam |
pratyāhāraḥ praśasto 'yaṃ sevito yogibhiḥ sadā || 7.5 ||

That, which is a *pratyāhāra* [practice], is truly the most excellent yogic practice!
This marvellous *pratyāhāra* [practice] is always practised by the yogins!

aṣṭādaśasu yad vāyor marmasthāneṣu dhāraṇam |
sthānāt sthānāt samākṛṣya pratyāhāro nigadyate || 7.6 ||

That [which consists of] the fixation of '[vital] wind' in the eighteen *marma* points
[and then] withdrawing [it] from those point by point, is referred to as 'drawing away' (*pratyāhāra*).'

aśvinau ca tathā brūtāṃ gārgi devabhiṣagvarau |
marmasthānāni siddhyarthaṃ śarīre yogamokṣayoḥ || 7.7 ||

Thus spake, Oh Gargī, the two Aśvins — the two excellent physicians of the *devas* –
about the *marma*-points for the sake of achieving the accomplishment of yogic liberation while in the living body![235]

235 Translation from the Sanskrit: Georgi Krastev.

Yoga-yājñavalkya is quoted in many of the later texts and can certainly be regarded as one of the main sources of *rāja-yoga*.[236] Yājñavalkya's teaching shows another complex path of 'yogic liberation', in which one learns to control the senses at will (*balāt*) and ultimately identifies both external and internal sense objects as the Self through perception (7.3). This could also mean that the prescribed daily ritual acts of the Vedic and Brahmanical traditions (in this case: *nyāsa*—the 'placing' of mantras on specific parts of the body of the priest, practitioner or image of the deity) are no longer performed externally but take place exclusively internally. In this way, yoga is detached from ritual. More recently, Mircea Eliade coined the term 'ritual interiorisation' in this context.[237]

In *Yoga-yājñavalkya* 7.6, special emphasis is placed on *pratyāhāra* utilising of the *prāṇa* or 'vital energy', which refers to the successive stopping and release of that *prāṇa* at the eighteen specific vital points of the body (*marmasthāna*)—very much akin to the principle described by Patañjali as to how the breath should be controlled during *prāṇāyāma*.

To achieve *pratyāhāra*, an additional carrier of consciousness is utilised in this practice: the *prāṇa-vāyus*, the 'vital energy winds', which are considered to flow outwards through the senses, dissipating and wasting energy in everyday life. Since it is challenging to individually and constantly restrain sense perception, the mind must first be purified and brought under control, allowing it to direct the senses and maintain this state. Once the mind is prepared, awareness is wilfully directed through the eighteen marma-sthāna (vital points). In this process, the *prāṇa* condenses through concentration at these points. This practice is similar to tantric *nyāsa*, in which the body is incorporated as an object of attention during immersion. In the 7th section of the *Jābāla-darśana-upaniṣad* (a late, probably post-classical text), the seer Dattātreya elaborates on the same process, but he introduces different focal points for the practice. In verses 7.5–13, for example, he describes a variation in which the focus is drawn down the central line of the body and fixed, with inhalation, at specific points: at the basis of the teeth, pit of the throat, the

236 Mohan, AG. (translation). (2000). *Yoga-Yājñavalkya*. Chennai: Ganesh & Co., p. 135.

237 Eliade, Mircea. (2009). *Yoga – Immortality and Freedom*. Princeton: Princeton University Press, pp. 111–114.

heart in the chest, the belly button in the navel, the tail bone, the knees, the shanks, and the toes of the feet. Then, with exhalation the focus moves back up to the forehead.

The *Yoga-yājñavalkya* (8.15–25) explains that the different regions of the body are each associated with one of the five elements and their respective deities. Practicing focused awareness (*dhāraṇā*) on each of these regions in a specific way is said to produce different supernatural yogic abilities (*siddhi*). According to Svāmī Nirañjanānanda, this practice results in *dhāraṇā* as a process of merging one element (*tattva*) with the next until nothing manifest exists. In *Jabala-darśana-upaniṣad* 8.1–6, too, the *dhāraṇā* reaches into the five *tattvas* of the body or the Self, leading on the path of yogic liberation. In this context, Svāmī Nirañjanānanda also makes a connection to the tantric scriptures.

In *Vijñāna-bhairava-tantra* verse 89, it is stated that through the mastery of a single sense perception, the emptiness in which the Self (*ātman*) becomes enlightened can be attained. By mastering the senses, the practitioner can transcend dualistic consciousness and enter a non-dual state. When control over the sense perceptions (*pratyāhāra*) is achieved, focussed awareness (*dhāraṇā*) follows. As soon as the mental focus is directed toward one point, enlightenment occurs effortlessly.[238] Verse 136 makes it clear that all perception — through contact with the senses — is what generates pain and pleasure. When you abandon the objects of the senses and direct your sense perception inwards (*indriya-pratyāhāra*), you dwell in the individual Self.[239]

There are therefore many paths to *pratyāhāra*, which some contemporary teachers also engage with. David Frawley discusses four main forms of *pratyāhāra* which he derives from his understanding: *indriya-pratyāhāra* — control of the senses, *karma-pratyāhāra* — control of action, *prāṇa-pratyāhāra* — control of the *prāṇa* and *mana-pratyāhāra* — withdrawal of the mind from the senses.[240]

238 Sarawati, Satyasangananda, Swami. (2007). *Awakening the Vijnānamayakośa*. Munger: Yoga Publication Trust, p. 294–295.

239 Ibid., p. 392–393.

240 Frawley, David. (n.d.). Pratyahara, Yoga's Forgotten Limb. *Yoga International*. https://yogainternational.com/article/view/pratyahara-yogas-forgotten-limb/ (accessed 27.06.2020).

Svāmī Nirañjanānanda points out two different approaches to *pratyāhāra*. On the one hand, he presents Patañjali's dualistic system, which has a Sāṃkhya background, where *pratyāhāra* is understood as the alignment of the mind, where the observer (*draṣṭā*) plays a central role. He emphasises the approach of what he terms 'pre-Patañjali *rāja-yoga*', which has a non-dualistic background and focuses on the alignment of the energies of the mind (*prāṇa-pratyāhāra*) and not with the functions of the mind (*vṛtti*) directly.[241]

Svāmī Nirañjanānanda thus proposes the following stages and definitions of *pratyāhāra*.

1. *indriya-pratyāhāra* — sense-perception-*pratyāhāra*

Two definitions of the word *pratyāhāra* have been handed down. If the word is understood as *prati-* (towards) and *-āhāra* (food intake), then according to the Sāṃkhya school of thought, it means the reciprocal reception of food — what is given to you, you give back.[242] But *pratyāhāra* literally also means: 'control over *āhāra*' or 'gaining mastery over external influences'. In Patañjali's rāja-yoga context, the term is usually translated as 'restraint of the senses'.

> *To penetrate into the depths of the mind, the contact with the object must be cut off. When the mind is in contact with the external world, it is not aware of the deeper facets of consciousness. When one is aware of these deeper facets, one does not know the world of the senses.*[243]
>
> Svāmī Satyānanda

In the Bihar Yoga system, most *pratyāhāra* and immersive techniques begin with an introductory period dedicated to withdrawal from sensory perception. This applies, for example, to *yoga-nidrā* Stage 1 and especially to the

241 Saraswati, Niranjanananda, Swami. (2019). *Yoga Chakrodaya* – Book 2/3. Bihar: Yoga Publications Trust, p. 231.
242 Ibid, p. 191.
243 Saraswati, Satyananda, Swami. (2000). *Four Chapters on Freedom*. Munger: Yoga Publication Trust, p. 218.

antar-mauna[244] (inner silence) practice. Advanced stages of *kāya-sthairyam* [245] (stillness of the body) further focus on this withdrawal. When the body has entered the state of stillness, sense perceptions are brought to a halt: one sense perception after another must be calmed and balanced. For, while the body is nourished by physical food, which includes the five gross elements (*pañca-mahābhūta*), the organs of knowledge and action (*indriya*) constantly 'feed' the mind through the five subtle sense experiences (the five *tan-mātras*: smell, taste, sight, touch and sound) with impressions which we store in the form of identifications and associations, in our subconscious. In a state of body stillness, this process is interrupted and reversed — the inwardly directed sensory perception is 'fed' in its subtle form with the mental content, which would otherwise remain unnoticed and thus active. This allows for the direction of perception toward a more subtle spiritual level, specifically to the stored memories and associations of the unconscious. Since our sense perception is the gateway to the organs of knowledge and action, silencing the senses, one sense at a time, is a powerful practice. The stillness of all outwardly directed senses leads to *indriya-pratyāhāra*. Only when this state has been perfected and there are no more disturbances in the practice of focused awareness (*dhāraṇā*) and prolonged immersive focused awareness (*dhyāna*), can the transition to deeper states of superconscious absorption (*samādhi*) take place.

2. *prāṇa-pratyāhāra*

According to Svāmī Nirañjanānanda, *prāṇa-pratyāhāra* is the second stage of *pratyāhāra* from the 'pre-Patañjali *rāja-yoga*' perspective. Unlike in Patañjali's Yoga, the focus here is on the interplay of the various energies, energy flows and energy levels in the body — and not on the mind. As described in the context of the *Yoga-yājñavalkya*, the awareness directs *prāṇa* to specific points in the body, redirecting the flow of *prāṇa* inwards. However, this prāṇic connection is also tied to identifications with people, objects and impressions.

---

244 The tantric technique *antar-mauna* is described in detail in the Saraswati, Satyananda, Swami. (2001). *Meditations from the Tantras*. (2nd edition). Munger: Yoga Publication Trust, pp. 211–224.

245 The higher stages of the tantric technique *kāya-sthairyam* with *indriya-pratyāhāra* are described in detail in Saraswati, Niranjanananda, Swami. (2018). *Progression of Pratyahara* 1. Munger: Yoga Publication Trust.

It exerts an emotional gravitational force, binding individuals and keeping them tethered. By reversing the *prāṇas* and breaking these connections, one can attain a greater and more conscious freedom of choice in daily life. Once the *prāṇas* have been removed from the objects of identification, they can merge with the mind.[246]

An advanced stage of *yoga-nidrā* leads to *prāṇa-pratyāhāra*. This particular technique is called *prāṇa-yoga-nidrā*, and involves becoming aware of the five vital energies, or *pañca prāṇa*.[247] The five are: situated in the lungs and heart inward- and upward-flowing (*prāṇa*), situated in the lower abdomen downward-flowing (*apāna*), situated in the throat and head upward flowing (*udāna*), situated in the navel sideways-flowing (*samāna*), all-pervasive outward-flowing (*vyāna*). Svāmī Nirañjanānanda defines *prāṇa-yoga-nidrā* as follows: when only a single *prāṇa* remains active, the third stage, called *prāṇa*[-*yoga*]-*nidrā* starts. Now you have to withdraw the intensity of *prāṇa-śakti* from all parts of the body, from all *marma* points, and concentrate on the *cakras*. This is *prāṇa*[-*yoga*]-*nidrā*.[248] *Prāṇa-yoga-nidrā* is similar in its principles to the technique for achieving *pratyāhāra* described in the *Jābāla-darśana-upaniṣad*.

3. *mana-pratyāhāra*

Svāmī Nirañjanānanda shows another meaning of *pratyāhāra* from the 'pre-Patañjali *rāja-yoga*', where the prefix *prati-* is also understood as related to *pratyaya* (in the sense of 'impressions', 'archetypes') and the latter part of the compound as *hāra* ('that which can be taken away or removed'). '*Pratyāhāra*' then is interpreted as 'to remove the impression, to dissolve it, to put an end to it—to not have it, to move forward'. *Pratyayas* are connected to desires, where everything in life revolves around fulfilment. The desires for fulfilment are threefold: the desire for wealth, comfort, prosperity, resources; the desire for offspring; the desire to be popular, recognised, valued and credible. These three desires guide the actions in life—the *karmans*.[249] *Mana-pratyāhāra*

246 Ibid., p. 35.

247 An example for the *prāṇa-(yoga)-nidrā* technique ibid., p. 101–112; See Part I., Chapter 8. *Pañcakośa – The Five Sheaths of Being*.

248 Saraswati, Niranjanananda, Swami. (2018). *Progression of Pratyahara* 1. Munger: Yoga Publication Trust, p. 88.

249 Ibid., p. 31.

refers to a process of purification of the mind in all its aspects such as *citta*, *buddhi*, *manas*, *ahaṃkāra* (cumulatively sometimes referred to as the *antaḥ-karaṇa*, see below) in order to allow the more gross mind to merge into the subtle mind.

4. *śūnya-pratyāhāra*

When the previous stages of *pratyāhāra* have been mastered on the physical, energetic and spiritual levels, the state of *śūnyatā*—'being in the void'—arises spontaneously. In this state, all attachment to the material world is overcome and one is ready to connect with the transcendent. However, the practitioner's task is to go even beyond this. The state of *śūnya* here can be said to be comparable to the state of *turīya*.

5. *prakāśatva-pratyāhāra*

After experiencing the *śūnya*, one transitions to *prakāśatva* (luminosity), wherein the *ātman* (Supreme Self) reveals itself. In this state, when all ties to the material world dissolve, one can connect with the Higher Self, leading to infusion of light. It is at this juncture that true *dhāraṇā* (one-pointedness) begins.[250]

The process of *pratyāhāra* thus also follows the basic direction of the 'pre-Patañjali *rāja-yoga*' approach with tantric elements—from the gross to the subtle. The immersion of the mind begins with the *tan-mātras*—the gross aspects of the sense perception (*indriya-pratyāhāra*)—and is directed towards the subtle aspects (*antaḥkaraṇa*) of the organs of knowledge and action (*indriya*) via the reversal of the *prāṇa-vāyus* (*prāṇa-pratyāhāra*). The stilling of all these aspects spontaneously leads to the even more subtle level of the *śūnya* (void) state and then to the *prakāśatva* state. In this way, a higher level of consciousness is achieved and the desired state, *dhāraṇā*, can be reached.

---

250 Ibid., p. 36.

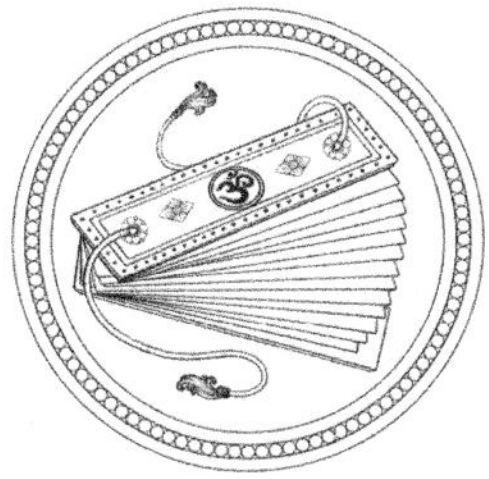

CHAPTER 6

Antaḥkaraṇa — Structure of the Mind According to Yoga Psychology

What is Yoga Psychology?

Yoga psychology is a contemporary approach which applies the principles of Yoga's subtle anatomy with the understanding and the management of the psyche and mind. This subtle anatomy encompasses the structure of the mind, various levels of consciousness and their interplay—a concept which has a long and complex history in yoga, spanning more than 1500 years. Although specifics of this anatomy differ across various texts and traditions, the foundational features and components generally adhere to consistent principles. In this chapter we will look at the principles of yoga psychology as applied in Bihar Yoga and their direct connection to the *yoga-nidrā* method of Svāmī Satyānanda.

Yoga psychology focuses on the mental, emotional, and subtle aspects of the mind, addressing both theoretical and practical elements of yoga aimed at enhancing these qualities. It seeks to provide tools and techniques for individuals to explore their inner landscape, fostering self-awareness and promoting mental well-being by effectively navigating life's challenges through the practices of yoga.

The primary aim of yoga psychology, as well as all traditional yoga disciplines, is to liberate limited perception and the deluded mind from its attachment and identification with the world of objects and from its ignorance of the Highest Reality in order to achieve liberation and knowledge of the Self. In the course of this process, the practitioner goes through various stages of inner purification, systematically removing the existing limitations and delusions afflicting the individual mind in all its aspects, allowing for an increasingly deeper experience of the more subtle aspects of reality. These afflictions are the product of the activities of the rational and cognitive aspects of the mind—*buddhi* (intellect) and *manas* (thinking principle)—when they operate without awareness. By cultivating the attitude of an impartial observer and conscious engagement with these aspects, practitioners can gradually transform these obstacles, leading to a clearer perception of reality and a deeper understanding of the Self.

The ultimate, highest goal of yoga is to find our way back to the source—or to gain yogic understanding of the evolution of individual consciousness. In other words, we are born out of an unmanifest origin into the manifest world (involution) in order to experience the gross planes of existence and to realise our Self through interaction with them so that we can eventually find our way back to the origin from here (evolution).

The Highest Awareness and the Manifestation of the Individual Consciousness

The concept of consciousness and the different levels of consciousness in yoga is similar to the concepts of the universe and the evolution of existence as we know them from the Vedānta, Tantra and Sāṃkhya schools of thought. However, it is essential to understand these parallels within the framework of each tradition and keep in mind the respective context and system. What is presented here is largely based on a Sāṃkhya-Vedānta synthesis elaborated with certain tantric elements, whereby the different evolutes of existence are characterised by aspects of both consciousness and energy.

Non-manifest (*avyakta*) consciousness (*brahman*) is associated with the primordial sound A—omniscience (nameless), U—omnipotence (formless) and M̊ —omnipresence (timeless) and stands for the *brahman*[251]. In this dimension, nothing is manifest, but there is only pure potentiality. From this consciousness and its aspect of omniscience arises *mahat*[252]—what Svāmī Nirañjanānanda also refers to as 'the supreme intelligence'. There we find the source which underlies every kind of life force, energy and expression.[253]

From the supreme intelligence (*mahat*) emerges the causal[254] ego (*ahaṃkāra*)—the principle of individuation, which had already begun to manifest in the supreme intelligence. *Ahaṃkāra* is not yet fully manifested and expresses the desire and will for multiplicity—this is when the first division of the mind takes place.[255] Then, from *ahaṃkāra* develops *manas*—the interactive faculty of mind.

Gross manifestation then begins when the subtle elements, the *indriyas* (the organs of knowledge and action), the *tanmātras* (the perceptual experiences of sound, contact, form, taste, smell) and *mahābhūta* (the gross elements of ether, air, fire, water, earth), arise from *ahaṃkāra*. The *tanmātras* develop from the causal, through the subtle to the gross forms of manifestation.[256]

Although not part of the classical Sāṃkhya system, Svāmī Niranjanananda introduces a particularly useful grouping of the 3rd, 4th and 5th manifestations of *prakṛti* combined with the notion of *citta* as 'storehouse/memory' used in Vedānta and Śaivism. This so-called composite 'inner organ' (*antaḥkaraṇa*) consists of the functions of the mind and is thus used to represent the inner functional structure of the psyche:[257]

---

251 See Part I., Chapter 1. *Indian Schools of Thought*.

252 We must note that in classical Sāṃkhya consciousness does not evolve and *mahat* (*buddhi*) is an evolute of *prakṛti*.

253 Saraswati, Niranjanananda, Swami. (2002). *Yoga Darshan*. (1st edition, reprinted with corrections). Munger: Yoga Publication Trust, p. 34–35.

254 'Causal' here refers to the most subtle of the three levels of existence, the productive foundational level.

255 Saraswati, Niranjanananda, Swami. (2002). *Yoga Darshan*. (1st edition, reprinted with corrections). Munger: Yoga Publication Trust, p. 35.

256 Ibid., p. 35–36.

257 Saraswati, Niranjanananda, Swami. (2008). *Samkhya Darshan*. Munger: Yoga Publication Trust, p. 5.

- *ahaṃkāra*: individuation, I-consciousness, I-thought—identifies
- *buddhi*: reason, intellect, will—analyses and determines
- *manas*: mind, thinking principle—processes impressions and experiences
- *citta*: the mechanism of memory, which compares new impressions with previously stored experiences.

These concepts are found in both the Sāṃkhya and Vedānta systems, with the exclusion of *citta*. In the Bihar Yoga view, *citta* can either represent the entire mind, including *ahaṃkāra*, *manas* and *buddhi*, or, based on the Vedāntic understanding, it can refer specifically to one part of the mind: memory and the subconscious. It has to be pointed out, that in the Vedāntic conception, *antaḥkaraṇa* is active only in the waking and dreaming states of consciousness, and not during deep sleep—a relationship we will explore further below.

Mahat is the aspect of *prakṛti* which pervades the entire structure of the human being. Its special dynamic can be more easily understood with the help of the concept of *antaḥkaraṇa*—the so-called inner organ, which encompasses all forms of mentation.[258] *Antaḥ-* means 'internal' and *-karaṇa* means 'cause'. *Antaḥ-karaṇa* is, therefore, an inner tool or organ, a way to conceptualise the inner functional structure of the mind.[259] The functions of the mind are as follows: to feel, to remember, to distinguish and to think.

Within the Bihar Yoga system, these correspond to the four components:

- *manas*—the interactive mind, the thinking principle (conducts awareness of the present, words, images, feelings, desires, impressions);
- *citta*—memory and recollection (provides a basis for the comparison of current experiences with stored experiences);

258 It has to be noted, that *antaḥkaraṇa* is a concept found mainly in Vedānta and certain streams of Śaiva philosophy and does not traditionally relate directly to the Sāṃkhya conception of the stages of manifestation of *prakṛti*.

259 'The psychic body [the psyche] is [in yoga unlike the western psychology] a deeper aspect of the subtle body and the causal body, or the subconscious and the unconscious. The subconscious area is known as the subtle body and the unconscious as the causal body. The approximate borderline zone between the subconscious and unconscious is known as the psychic body. The psychic body is the zone where both the inner and outer experiences are visualised and experienced.' From Saraswati, Niranjanananda, Swami. (2002). *Yoga Darshan*. (1st edition, reprinted with corrections). Munger: Yoga Publication Trust, p. 228.

- *ahaṃkāra*—I-consciousness, ego, ego-thought (identifies);
- *buddhi*—reason, intellect, will (analyses and determines);

Antaḥkaraṇa is in dialogue with the world of the senses, with name, form, idea, time, space, and object.[260]

Antaḥkaraṇa—The Mental Apparatus, The Mental Faculty; Yogic Anatomy of the Mind

Higher, or more actively manifest *antaḥkaraṇa* distinguishes humans from plants, animals and non-living matter. In these 'lower' life forms, *antaḥkaraṇa* exists in a dormant and tāmasic state. Human consciousness, which manifests its functions through the aspects of the *antaḥkaraṇa*, thus has the ability to think, plan, remember, categorise, interpret, classify, make assumptions, perceive and recognise information relating to past, present and future experiences. However, we do not utilise it to its full capacity. The reason for this is our limited perception. A rock lacks awareness. Humans have limited awareness. The full potential of the *antaḥkaraṇa* remains dormant and imperceptible until we begin to refine it. This refinement occurs when we begin to tune it to higher frequencies of energy and realise that *antaḥkaraṇa* is one with the Cosmic Will.[261]

260 Ibid.

261 Saraswati, Satyasangananda, Swami. (2005). *Tattwa Shuddhi*. Munger: Yoga Publication Trust, p. 48–49.

> *Like a musical instrument, the antaḥkaraṇa is sensitive enough to pick up the subtlest vibrations, which it continues to do irrespective of our conscious knowledge. [...] What is recorded there is a part which may never reveal itself to you, unless the clarity of cosmic awareness and the inner ear and eye, which can comprehend the subtle vibrations of cosmic sound and vision, are attained. Therefore, we have not only to discover what is stored in the antaḥkaraṇa, but also learn how to control it.*[262]
>
> Svāmī Satyasaṅgānanda

Although consciousness is available to each of us, its expression depends on how each individual's perception operates, which is determined by the mental 'gears'. Our conditioning reflects how we live, as we often find ourselves at the mercy of the mind. An idea or thought is interpreted and actualised differently by each of us. The result depends entirely on our own intellect, mind, memory and ego. The activity of the *antaḥkaraṇa* is the basis of our inner personality and identity. It is additionally subject to the influence of the *tri-guṇa*—*tamas, rajas, sattva*—the three qualities of primordial matter which shape the perception of the inner personality.

Buddhi—The Agent of Awareness, Capacity for Reasoning, Capacity for Logical Understanding, Capacity for Recognition, Capacity for Discrimination

Buddhi means 'to be conscious', 'to have the experience of something' or to recognise something experienced. This aspect of *antaḥkaraṇa* is closest to pure consciousness. *Buddhi* enables one to gain understanding and knowledge, it analyses, questions and compares in order to make a decision about new information.

Svāmī Nirañjanānanda makes a precise distinction between the meaning of *buddhi* and the translation of the term as 'intellect' and 'reason'. Reason is a faculty of the manifesting mind, while *buddhi* is a quality of consciousness.

---

262 Ibid., p. 50.

The intellect is only an analytical and comparative part of the mind, while *buddhi* means the ability to be aware.[263]

The influence of the *tri-guṇa* on the *buddhi* expresses itself in the following ways:

- *mahat*—the highest intelligence, is beyond the *guṇas*.
- The qualities of sattvic *buddhi* are wisdom, dispassion, reason, serenity, self-control, discernment, contemplation and equanimity. Through them, we can adopt the perspective of the *draṣṭā*—'I am aware'—the uninvolved observer stance (without *rāga* and *dveṣa*).
- Due to the influence of *rajas* (dynamism, activity), *buddhi* is contaminated by false knowledge (*viparyaya*) and ignorance (*avidyā*).
- tāmasic *buddhi* reacts to the incoming information with needs, instincts and desires and becomes the 'slave' of the perceptual information supplied to it by the *manas*, or it comes under the rule of the ego (*ahaṃkāra*) and is clouded by false judgements.

According to Svāmī Nirañjanānanda, *buddhi* encompasses three further aspects: firstly, the ability to focus awareness on a particular sensory stimulus like a filter and block out all others (*ekāgra*). Secondly, it involves the subtle awareness of the instincts of self-preservation (*abhiniveṣa*)—for example, when we keep our distance from fire. The third aspect comes into play when we consciously and deliberately detach our perception from the sensory stimuli (*pratyāhāra*). It is only by developing this latter ability to intentionally detach the mind from sensory inputs that the *buddhi* can actualise its true nature.

In Svāmī Satyānanda's *yoga-nidrā* method, every practitioner has the experience of having become aware of a part of the body according to a certain instruction—such as 'left thumb'—but only a moment later, the instruction is, seemingly suddenly, 'the whole body'. Despite the fact that you have not been asleep, you have not been aware of the series of instructions between 'thumb' and 'whole body'. There has been a detachment from the auditory sensory experience, even though we have heard the instructions. With time,

263 Saraswati, Niranjanananda, Swami. (2002). *Yoga Darshan*. (1st edition, reprinted with corrections). Munger: Yoga Publication Trust, p. 26–27.

the awareness is cultivated and sustained throughout the practice. As a consequence, *buddhi* becomes expressed as awareness in everyday life when directed outwards, and as self-awareness when directed inwards. When directed towards the higher levels of consciousness, *buddhi* strengthens our intuition and leads us to knowledge of the true Self.

Svāmī Nirañjanānanda goes on to say that consciousness and the experience of consciousness are different from the experience of the senses and their connection with the mind. This difference is not only difficult to articulate, but also hard to translate adequately. The presence of consciousness in its various forms can ultimately only be experienced in the way these forms express themselves, for example while we are sleeping or practising yoga-nidrā and techniques of immersion.[264]

Ahaṃkāra — Individuation, I-consciousness

Ahaṃkāra is the principle of individuation, the ability to identify, to entitify, to differentiate between entities. This, in turn, is the prerequisite for identification, because as soon as existence is perceived as differentiated into entities, these entities automatically have an identity — the *ahaṃkāra*. This identity can be active (*rajas*), passive (*tamas*) or balanced (*sattva*). According to Svāmī Satyasaṅgānanda, this is how the various evolutes of *manas* (the *indriyas*) arise from the sattvic *ahaṃkāra*. Since they have emerged from *ahaṃkāra* as their foundation, *ahaṃkāra* manifests in them in different ways. When we interact with the world, it is this manifest *ahaṃkāra* which we experience. In this respect, *ahaṃkāra* is related to the material world, is most clearly experienced in the form of 'I-ness' or 'ego' and the concept of possession, and results in attachment. This sense of possession is directed towards external objects as well as our own body, which is bound to sensory and intellectual experiences and thus experiences 'I-ness' — 'I know that I exist'. The seed of individuality is in the ego, and so the process of identification and attachment also begins there. The ego relates to the things around it and creates the sense of ownership, of 'mine' and 'yours'. *Ahaṃkāra* monitors physical, emotional, intellectual and psychological experiences and motivates, directs and guides

264 Ibid., p. 29–30.

the individual. In its pursuit of happiness and avoidance of pain, it reveals the paradox of creation: the ego both anchors us to objective experience and must be overcome to awaken the state of yoga.[265] *Ahaṃkāra* transforms the sensory impressions into a personal experience. As the mechanism of self-identification, it transforms the impersonal sensory impression 'A cake is seen' (*manas*) into the subjective experience 'I see a cake' (*ahaṃkāra*). Furthermore, it creates a feeling of separation from the world and of uniqueness and individuality.

According to Svāmī Satyasaṅgānanda, the influence of the *tri-guṇa* on *ahaṃkāra* is expressed as follows:

- Sattvic *ahaṃkāra* is responsible for the idea of 'I am' and acts as a catalyst in the process of coming to know the Self. It has the ability to lift latent impressions from the subconscious (*saṃskāras*) into consciousness, but temporarily withdraws under the influence of *sattva*.
- Rajasic *ahaṃkāra* is a dynamic force which ignites ego-possession in the individual, causes intense activity and restlessness and eventually leads to the dispersion of thought.
- tāmasic *ahaṃkāra* intensifies the painful and negative *saṃskāras* and causes doubt, apprehension and procrastination.[266]

Manas — The Interactive Mind, Capacity for Thinking, Capacity for Feeling

Manas is an aspect of the individual mind which has direct contact with incoming information and sensory impressions and coordinating them with various responses, including motor reactions. It is the individual aspect of consciousness, the outer level of the mind and the window of consciousness which opens to the outside world. As sensory impressions change from moment to moment, the mind is volatile and in constant flux. *Manas* does not operate independently and is guided by the logical conclusions of *buddhi* and the decisions of the *ahaṃkāra*. *Manas* plans or ponders, brings forth thoughts and their contradictions or doubts, idea and counter-argument, or opposing

265 Ibid., p. 37–38.
266 Saraswai, Satyasangananda, Swami. (2005). *Tattwa Shuddhi*. Munger: Yoga Publication Trust, p. 52–53.

thought, and connects the finer intuition to the outer, obvious and 'gross' awareness. The thoughts and feelings which arise from *manas* are not always appropriate and not always correct. We should learn to observe it, control it and detach ourselves from it.

Manas functions like an interface between the *buddhi*, the *ahaṃkāra* and the senses. It is the thinking mind which sees, perceives and scrutinises something, and has the following mechanisms:

- Capacity for Recognition — the process of giving meaning to information gained from the transmissions of our senses;
- Emotions — perceptions which are important to us and arise primarily in the form of strong instincts trigger an emotion. The emotion appears in a form appropriate to the stimulus and the memories (citta), e.g. love, joy, desire, anger, fear, sadness;
- Cognition — the mental processing of the information gained from sensory perception. *Manas* processes the impressions with the help of *citta*, *ahaṃkāra* and *buddhi* and sometimes reacts to situations appropriately, but also inappropriately.

Manas is in constant motion and is naturally under the sway of *rajas* and is therefore always distracted and scattered by its nature. Nevertheless, its quality changes under the influence of the other two *guṇas*:

- Under the influence of *sattva*, *manas* becomes steady, focussed and concentrated.
- *Manas* influenced by *rajas* activates the senses and unbalances the intellect (*buddhi*).
- tāmasic *manas* makes the intellect (*buddhi*) and the senses inert and inactive.[267]

267 Ibid., p. 54.

This rajasic tendency is altered when manas comes under the sway of ahaṃkāra to a state of tamas, and transformed when it comes under the sway of buddhi to a state of equilibrium or sattva. Thus ahaṃkāra and buddhi operate through manas, drawing upon the contents of past impressions stored in the citta to create an experience of happiness or unhappiness, pain and pleasure.[268]

Svāmī Satyasaṅgānanda

Citta —'Mind' vs.'Memory'

At this stage, it is necessary to recall that the term *citta* is used differently depending on the tradition. In the classical Sāṃkhya of the *Sāṃkhya-kārikā* of Īśvarakṛṣṇa, *buddhi*, *ahamkāra* and *manas* are distinct successive evolutes of *prakṛti* which also produce faculties (*indriya*) of the individual mind. In the *Yoga-sūtras* of Patañjali *buddhi* and *manas*, together with citta are used interchangeably as terms to refer to the totality of the individual mind, whose *vṛttis* are to be blocked. This is how Patañjali begins his *Yoga-sūtras* and shows the aim of Yoga.

In Advaita Vedānta, however, the *citta* is seen as the mental organ of memory and recollection, one of the four aspects of the 'internal organ' — *antaḥkaraṇa*. The corresponding element of Patañjali's system to the Advaita Vedānta idea of *citta* as 'memory' is *smṛti*, which, however, he considers a *vṛtti*.

In the context of Bihar Yoga, *citta* is a partial aspect of the experiencing mind, *antaḥkaraṇa*, as well as the seat of all experiences stored in the subconscious in the form of *pratyayas*, *saṃskāras*, archetypes and memories. Together with *manas*, *citta* represents the outer mind that can be experienced in the waking and dreaming state. As a repository of memory, *citta* reflects the external world and blends what is reflected with its own contents in the subconscious. Consequently, everything we think, feel and perceive is subjective and embedded in our own idea and interpretation of the world.

Memories overlay the canvas of *manas*, colouring perceptions. If the original experience that gave rise to these memories was tinted by emotions, those memories carry an emotional charge. Subsequent events that are subconsciously interpreted as sufficiently similar to the emotionally charged

268 Ibid.

experiences or memories can trigger latent *saṃskāras* from the sub- and unconscious level of the *citta*, provoking corresponding reactions.

Both *citta* and *manas* are not active independently; rather they are guided by *buddhi* and *ahaṃkāra*. When memories (*saṃskāras*) arise from the *citta*, they can be met with equanimity by a witnessing and awakened *buddhi*, causing them to lose their emotional power over our behaviour. This process frees us from our attachment to the instinctive modes of functioning. Furthermore, according to Svāmī Satyasaṅgānanda, *citta* is influenced by the *tri-guṇa* as follows:

- Under the influence of *sattva*, the sensory impressions stored in *citta* withdraw so that consciousness remains undisturbed.
- In *rajasic citta*, *saṃskāras* are awakened in the form of *vṛttis* as *vikalpa* (imagination) or as *viparyaya* (false knowledge). In this state, *citta* contains both knowledge and ignorance.

When *tamas* influences the *citta*, unwanted *saṃskāras* arise, the individual becomes clouded by *vāsanās* (deep-rooted desires, behavioural tendencies) that push all good *saṃskāras* into darkness. The *vāsanās* can only be removed by *dhāraṇā* and *dhyāna*.[269]

Using a simple example, the following mechanisms of *antaḥkaraṇa* can be illustrated as soon as we perceive something. Imagine we see a cake—the reactions will be as follows: *manas*: 'Something (a cake) is seen' (sense impressions, thoughts and feelings arise); *citta*: 'There is a stored impression: this is a cake, cake tastes good, hmmmmm… I remember the cake from my birthday.' (memories and experiences from the subconscious arise); *ahaṃkāra*: 'I see and smell a cake, I love cake and I want to eat this cake!' (identification); *buddhi*: 'Do I really need it? How much of it is good for me?' (intellect and discrimination).

If we compare the mind, once again simplified, with a computer, we could also say that *manas* functions like an interface operating with a computer's working memory which records temporary information, while *citta* resembles the hard drive which contains what has already been saved; in this metaphor, *buddhi* would correspond to the logic of a processor which can

269 Ibid.

evaluate information and execute tasks, while *ahaṃkāra* represents the dedicated application programme. Although a machine itself does not have an ego, it is the servant of a human ego which does pursue its own purposes. The comparison may seem inappropriate in this form, too technical and reduced, but it may also serve to clarify the point.

An Important Goal of Yoga: Developing *buddhi*

As practitioners and spiritual seekers, we can progress further on our path by engaging consciously with the *antaḥkaraṇa*. It is essential to strive not only to release the muscular and nervous tension of the body, but also to let go of mental tension — not merely for our everyday well-being, but equally for the sake of our spiritual development. In doing so, we can dissolve the unnecessary mental patterns that create unrest and tension in our lives, transforming the conditioning of the mind while purifying and harmonising its expression.

The *antaḥkaraṇa* has two primary forms of expression: awareness, on the one hand, and identification, on the other. Attention is an aspect of *manas*, which penetrates through the 'window of consciousness' and radiates outwards — simultaneously extending outwards towards sensory perception or sensory objects, and then inwards, into the space of *buddhi*, *ahaṃkāra* and *citta*. The manifestations of *ahaṃkāra* in the form of 'I-ness', self-importance, self-preservation and identity influence *manas*, *citta* and *buddhi*. As all these energies are in motion, the interaction between *ahaṃkāra* and *manas* gives rise to what we call emotion. The entire spectrum of ego-related emotions comes from the *ahaṃkāra*, and, when they are active, attention shifts from *manas* towards *ahaṃkāra*.[270]

We should learn to observe the mind with the *vṛtti*s and the emotions neutrally and not identify with them. By harnessing awareness through the faculty of *buddhi*, we can direct the mind and consciously take control of *manas*. This is how we develop and cultivate our inner awareness:

- inner clarity and being aware;
- the ability to take a step back and watch (*draṣṭā*);

270 Sarasvatī, Niranjanānanda, Svāmī. (2021). Shavasana-3. [Online-lecture] *Yoga-Chakra-Series*. May.

- an observer's attitude towards sensory impressions and mental concepts;
- awareness of the outside as well as the inside;
- the ability to make contact with (our) higher consciousness (intuition, direct knowledge).

Yoga provides us with the necessary tools to develop those skills that refine our *antaḥkaraṇa* through the stimulation of the sattvic aspects of *buddhi*. We should realise that we are not *manas*, not *ahaṃkāra* and not *citta*.

By training to develop the *draṣṭā* stance we learn to observe through awareness rather than merely reacting mechanically. By cultivating the quality of discrimination (*viveka*), we aim to support the expression of sattvic *buddhi* and the ability to make right decisions. The practice of non-attachment and letting go (*vairāgya*) aids in reducing our attachment to cravings through contentment (*santoṣa*), allowing us to increasingly embody a state that is beyond craving and obsession, as well as beyond attraction and aversion (*rāga* and *dveṣa*).

Towards this purpose, a resolve (*saṃkalpa*) can be made, preferably during a *pratyāhāra* practice, as in *yoga-nidrā* and integrated into daily life and practice. Through this tool, we can gradually transform our habits and attitudes, achieving goals with greater ease while gaining control and direction in our lives.

The *yamas* and *niyamas* help harmonise our relationships with others as well as with our inner attitudes and feelings. The cultivation of self-acceptance, self-awareness, and self-recognition through self-study (*svādhyāya*) forms an essential foundation in this process.

Antaḥkaraṇa and the Practice of *śavāsana* and *yoga-nidrā*[271]

The primary step towards purification and harmonisation of the *antaḥkaraṇa* is through *pratyāhāra*. It begins with achieving relaxation and stillness at the *manas* and *buddhi* levels.

The Satyananda Yoga Nidra method is practiced in the 'corpse' posture (*śavāsana*), so-named because the body is lying still, akin to that of a dead person — stretched out, lying on its back on the ground. We will address the details of the posture in the practice section of this book. If *śavāsana* is held for extended periods of time, it is referred to as a 'relaxation practice'. Now, relaxation is usually associated with sleep, tension — usually with wakefulness. However, the aim of *śavāsana* practice is to achieve a high state of relaxation while remaining fully awake and aware. That is why the *śavāsana* practice forms the foundation of and is the prerequisite for *yoga-nidrā*. Remaining conscious is essential when practising both *śavāsana* and yoga-nidrā, as falling asleep causes us to lose much of the effect and descend into the unconscious. In the state of deep sleep (*nidrā*), the mind consolidates its habitual patterns of worries and fears. However, by remaining conscious and attentive, awareness, engaged in the practice, is lured away from its entanglement with obsessive mental fears. The behaviour of the *antaḥkaraṇa* caused by that entanglement begins to weaken during *śavāsana* and begins dissolving during the *yoga-nidrā* practice.[272]

Our everyday life is also determined by the predefined impulses of our *prāṇa*, understood as 'vital energy,' and of our mind. The *prāṇa* controls our movements, while the mind perceives, thinks, shapes our feelings and acts without us being aware of what aspect of our conditioning is brought about by our nature and behaviour. Through the intention and desire to relax and turn inwards during *śavāsana*, all aspects of *antaḥkaraṇa* give a different kind of feedback. Mental preoccupation and identification play a significant role in the experience and can prove to be a hindrance during practice.

---

271 This section draws primarily on Sarasvatī, Niranjanānanda, Svāmī. (2021). Shavasana-3. [Online-lecture] *Yoga-Chakra-Series*. May.

272 Saraswati, Satyananda, Swami. (2006). *A Systematic Course in The Ancient Tantric Techniques of Yoga and Kriya*. (4th reprint). Munger: Yoga Publications Trust, p. 64–65.

- **Obstacles to practice at the level of *manas***

If the awareness is distracted by thoughts during *śavāsana* so that we do not hear the instructions of the facilitator, then — at that moment — the distracted state of *manas* is stronger than our attempt to let go and practise *śavāsana*. Whatever the forms of the predominant conditioning of the mind may be, it is those very thoughts which will come to the fore during *śavāsana*. When, during the practice of *śavāsana*, we experience such strong fluctuations and distractions at the *manas* level, we then tend to fall asleep and lapse into unconsciousness. As a result, we often make an effort during practice to focus our awareness on the instructions, even though there is a confrontation with our mental baggage. This in turn results in sensory and mental tension, defeating the purpose of *śavāsana* and preventing us from proceeding to *yoga-nidrā*. We should gradually learn to gently turn the awareness towards the instructions and guide it so that it is not drawn away by other stimuli.

- **Obstacles to practice at level of *buddhi***

If our practice is disturbed at the level of the *manas*, the expression of awareness at the level of the *buddhi* is also affected. The thought which comes to the fore in *manas* is analysed and intellectualised. This *vikalpa* prevents the experience and wisdom of the practice from taking effect. Conceptual thoughts then become the focus of awareness and reflective questioning may arise: 'Why am I doing this?', 'Have I learnt this and that before?', 'What is better?' etc. So, the *buddhi* being active in this way does not allow for direct experience, as we are preoccupied with weighing up which option might be the better for us. Yet another such negatively manifested aspect of the *buddhi* is self-doubt. Whatever the predominant conditioning of the *buddhi* (*rajas/tamas/sattva*),[273] it will manifest during *śavāsana*. We must gradually learn to mitigate it, in a manner analogous to how we deal with the distractions arising from the *manas*.

- **Obstacles to practice at level of *citta***

Dissolving identification with the elements of the *citta* is the main objective of *śavāsana* practice.

---

273 See Part I. Chapter 3. *Introduction to rāja-yoga: the Path of the Sovereign*.

The *Haṭhayoga-pradīpikā* gives the following definition of *śavāsana* in its Chapter 1, verse 32:

> *uttānaṃ śavavadbhūmau śayanaṃ tacchavāsanam* |
> *śavāsanam˙ śrānti-haraṃ citta-viśrānti-kārakam* || 32 ||[274]

> Lying stretched out on the floor like a corpse' is *śavāsana*.
> *Śavasana* dispels tiredness and brings calm to the mind.

Although we pass through the interactive mind (*manas*) and the capacity for reasoning (*buddhi*), we should ultimately reach the level of memory (*citta*). If *manas* and *buddhi* are not brought to a halt through the attitude of the observer (*draṣṭā-bhava*), we cannot consciously reach the *citta*. Our consciousness is usually concerned with the present only for short periods of time. During the rest of the time, we are preoccupied with the past—and for all intents and purposes, an endless source of material, which occupies the *manas* and the *buddhi*. When *śavāsana* is practiced properly, the material of the *citta* comes to the surface, where it needs to be purified, harmonised and regulated, which regulation can be done by means of *yoga-nidrā*.

- **Obstacles to practice at the level of *ahaṃkāra***

Awareness of the identification with the elements of the *ahaṃkāra* is connected with the *citta*. During the initial relaxation process which takes place in *śavāsana* practice, the aim is to dissolve the identification with the elements of the *ahaṃkāra* by detaching the awareness from their negative attraction and neutralise that attraction. It is the first conditioning which arises in the course of a *śavāsana* practice which becomes the object of identification. This is exactly what we need to work on and dissolve.

- **Purification of the *antaḥkaraṇa***

In yoga, mental tension is released through inner purification. This does not mean stopping the flow of thought. The mind is seen in the totality of its four aspects. The purpose of *śavāsana* practice is therefore to begin purifying,

274 Svatmarama. (2002). *The Hatha Yoga Pradipika*. Akers, Brian Dana. (translation). New York: Yoga Vidya Publications.

transmuting and 'reprogramming' the contents of the mind (*manas*) together with the capacity for reasoning (*buddhi*). This process is deepened in *yoga-nidrā* and provides the tools which enable us to consciously direct it.

The *manas* level is transmuted, sublimated and purified when we are able to turn sensory awareness into subtle awareness, connect body and breath and consciously and intentionally create the conditions for the different states to arise in our body, for example creating the feeling of lightness — such as in Stage 5 of *yoga-nidrā* — 'Pairs of Opposites'.[275] Can we manage to experience this feeling at any moment of the day without feeling the need to lie down? While we are sitting in a chair, travelling, enjoying ourselves or even when we feel pain?

In order to balance and harmonise awareness and identification at the *buddhi* level, the *draṣṭā* stance (objectivity) must be cultivated. We should be able to observe events in our everyday life neutrally at all times without being influenced by them. Only then will *buddhi* be balanced and purified.

Then, at the *citta* level of identification and awareness, it is a matter of experiencing and allowing opposites, whereby the disturbing components of our lives are transformed and neutralised by cultivating their positive counterparts. This is associated with the discipline of *pratipakṣa-bhāvanā* — 'cultivating the opposite view'.

At the *ahaṃkāra* level, the process of disidentification takes place through awareness and visualisation. Visualisation is seen by yogic and tantric traditions as a very powerful tool for transforming mental conditioning and identifications. For each type of identification, we should visualise it and subsequently gradually transform it into its positive opposite through directed attentive awareness, leading to peace, balance and harmony at the *ahaṃkāra* level. While visualisation is regarded as a type of *vikalpa* by some traditions, predominantly employed in practices related to the mundane and subtle levels of existence, rather than those aimed at liberation. For this reason, although visualisation is incorporated into the *yoga-nidrā* method, its use is strictly delineated, with clearly prescribed principles, and its purpose is directed towards cleansing the stored impressions in the sub- and unconscious.

Purification of the mind, transformation of mental states and the associated change in attitude towards life take place in *pratyāhāra*. Life is not seen

---

275 See Part II., Chapter 14. *Foundations of the Eight Stages; Pairs of Opposites in yoga-nidrā.*

as a collection of situations in which one is constantly confronted with reflections of the ego, but approached with a constructive and positive outlook. This is why the practice of *śavāsana* is so effective and powerful. *Savāsana* is the first step towards *yoga-nidrā* and is an essential tool on the path of *pratyāhāra*.

The Song of Self-Realisation

According to legend, Śaṅkara—the great Vedāntic saint of India—wandered in search of a true master who embodied the truth and had attained self-realisation. During this quest, he encountered *guru* Śrī Gauḍapāda, who is said to have asked him: 'Who are you?' In response, Śaṅkara, then only eight years old, is said to have spontaneously composed six verses, which have come to be known as the *Nirvāṇāṣṭakam*.[276]

Nirvāṇāṣṭakam ~ Eight Verses of Realisation

manobuddhyahaṅkāracittāni nāham |	Neither thinking, nor intellect, ego or mind
na ca śrotrajihve na ca ghrāṇanetre |	neither ear, nor tongue, nor nose, nor eyes,
na ca vyomabhūmir na tejo na vāyuḥ |	neither wind, nor earth, nor sun, nor sky:
cidānandarūpaḥ śivo 'ham śivo 'ham || 1 ||	Of the glory of consciousness bliss am I, bliss am I! (1)
na ca prāṇasañjño na vai pañcavāyuḥ |	I'm called neither 'the Breath', nor the winds am I five,
na vā saptadhātur na vā pañcakośaḥ |	nor the elements seven,[277] nor the sheaths am I five,
na vākpāṇipādaṃ na copasthapāyu |	neither tongue, nor hands, feet, anus or privates:
cidānandarūpaḥ śivo 'ham śivo 'ham || 2 ||	Of the glory of consciousness bliss am I, bliss am I! (2)

276 Translation into English adapted from the German of Dominik A. Haas.

277 These are the seven elements of the body according to the *Garbha-upaniṣad*: chyle, blood, flesh, fat, bone, marrow, and semen.

na me dveṣarāgau na me lobhamohau |
mado naiva me naiva mātsaryabhāvaḥ |
na dharmo na cārtho na kāmo na mokṣaḥ |
cidānandarūpaḥ śivo 'ham śivo 'ham || 3 ||

I harbour no hatred, no passion, no greed,
no delusion, no pride, nor envy I need,
nor charge or gain, no enjoyment or freedom:
Of the glory of consciousness bliss am I,
bliss am I! (3)

na puṇyaṃ na pāpaṃ na saukhyaṃ na duḥkham |
na mantro na tīrthaṃ na vedā na yajñaḥ |
ahaṃ bhojanaṃ naiva bhojyaṃ na bhoktā |
cidānandarūpaḥ śivo 'ham śivo 'ham || 4 ||

Neither merit nor sin, nor pleasure or pain,
Nor mantra, nor side, neither Veda, nor rite,
Neither eating, nor food, nor enjoyer am I:
Of the glory of consciousness bliss am I,
bliss am I! (4)

na me mṛtyuśaṅkā na me jātibhedaḥ |
pitā naiva me naiva mātā na janmaḥ |
na bandhur na mitraṃ gurur naiva śiṣyaḥ |
cidānandarūpaḥ śivo 'ham śivo 'ham || 5 ||

I fear no death, nor am I bound by blood,
I have no father, nor mother, nor birth,
no relatives, friends, no disciple or master:
Of the glory of consciousness bliss am I,
bliss am I! (5)

ahaṃ nirvikalpo nirākārarūpo |
vibhutvāc ca sarvatra sarvendriyāṇām |
na cāsaṅgataṃ naiva muktir na meyaḥ |
cidānandarūpaḥ śivo 'ham śivo 'ham || 6 ||

I am free of ideas, I am formless of being,
However, wherever you look — there I am,
I am neither division, nor whole or the measure:
Of the glory of consciousness bliss am I,
bliss am I! (6)

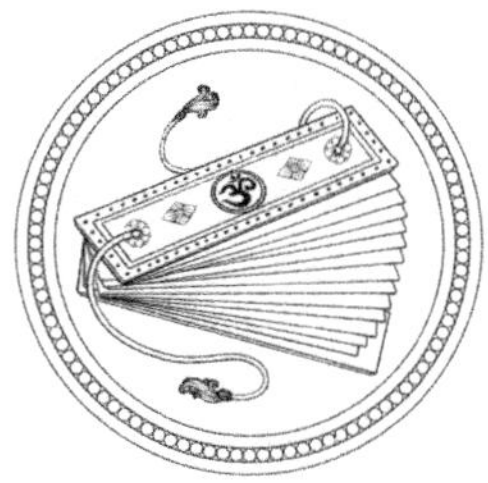

CHAPTER 7

Pratyāhāra — the Purification Process of the Impressions of the Subconscious Mind

As discussed above, it is the *antaḥkaraṇa*, the 'internal organ' with its four aspects, which we specifically address in *pratyāhāra* in order to initiate the purification process of the deeply rooted inner impressions in the subconscious and unconscious. *Pratyāhāra* in the Vedāntic sense means removing the superimposed layers of impressions (*pratyayas*) or archetypes from the *citta* and disidentifying from them.[278]

The countless impressions which are accumulated every day penetrate the various layers of consciousness and are stored in the *citta*, manifesting as conscious, subconscious and unconscious life experiences. The different impressions of these everyday experiences which constantly feed the mental flow are called *pratyayas*. They subsequently push outwards and unconsciously influence our attention and perception of life. These impressions manifest on the surface of waking consciousness in the form of gross

278 Saraswati, Niranjanananda, Swami. (2018). *Progression of Pratyahara* 1. Munger: Yoga Publication Trust, p. 30.

citta-vṛttis, mental obscurations and patterns of behaviour. We lose valuable mental energy through these mostly unconscious and uncontrolled mental activities. The *citta-vṛttis* are, in fact, the subject of Patañjali's first *yoga-sūtra*. Svāmī Nirañjanānanda, offers another perspective on Patañjali's concept of *citta-vṛttis* in the sense of 'storehouse of impressions'-*vṛttis*, rather than as 'modifications of the mind'. Although the terminology of the two systems is not directly compatible[279], Svāmī Nirañjanānanda emphasises that Patañjali does not refer to *manas vṛtti*, *ahaṃkāra vṛtti*, or *buddhi vṛtti*; instead, he specifically chose *citta-vṛtti* to indicate the 'location' of stored latent impressions and to highlight the significance of *citta pratyāhāra* practice.[280] He explains that *manas*, *buddhi*, and *ahaṃkāra* can be regulated through their respective *pratyāhāra* practices. Consequently, the *citta-vṛttis* constitute the primary focus of *rāja-yoga*, rather than the faculties of mind (*manas*), intellect (*buddhi*), or ego (*ahaṃkāra*).

We should endeavour to become aware of the *citta-vṛttis*—*pramāṇa*, *viparyaya*, *vikalpa*, *nidrā* and *smṛti* and the *pratyayas* which arise with them. Initially, we should recognise the most recent impressions by means of the *draṣṭā* stance, preparing ourselves for their release and purification. Only thereafter can the deeper layers of impressions be accessed. In this context, *smṛti* functions as the repository of conscious, subconscious, and unconscious memories, which must first be processed before higher immersive states can be attained.[281]

The imprints, *pratyayas*, cause *saṃskāras*—permanent marks or scars, conscious and unconscious impressions which have shaped us in the past and determine our way of thinking and actions in the present.

---

279 I.e., as we mentioned before, Patañjali uses *manas*, *citta*, and *buddhi* interchangeably to mean 'mind', whereas in the Advaita context, these three – along with *ahaṃkāra* – are considered as the four parts of the 'internal organ' (*antaḥkaraṇa*) and ultimately not of the nature of the Supreme Self.

280 Ibid., p. 31.

281 Ibid., p. 31–32.

> *Pratyatas are connected with desires (vasanas*[282]*). It is desires that make pratyatas. What you wish is what you do, so it is desires that build your life. [...] desires have been identified as threefold: vitteṣaṇā — desire for wealth, comfort, prosperity, resources, finances; putreṣaṇā — desire for progeny; lokeṣaṇā — desire to be popular, recognised, appreciated, thanked, believed in. These three desires guide the actions in life, the karmas. These karmas, fulfilled or unfulfilled, create pratyayas. The pratyayas are impressions that can emerge when the time is ripe: as nature, a trait, a quality, a behaviour, an attitude, an understanding.*[283]
>
> Svāmī Nirañjanānanda

A *pratyaya* is like the image of an impression received by consciousness. It is experienced in the form of memory, knowledge, *saṃskāra* and *karman*. On these different levels, the *pratyayas* form the gates of perception to our waking consciousness, the sub- and the unconscious. Opening these gates is the goal of *dhyāna*.[284] When we purify the *citta-vṛttis*, we also *purify* the *pratyayas*. According to Vyāsa (1.18; 1.41), the complete *pratyaya-nirodha* only takes place after *saṃprajñāta-samādhi*, that state of absorption in which one is aware of the difference between knowledge, the object of knowledge and the knower.

Buddhi plays an important role in filtering and classifying the sensory experiences which are stored as memories. When these memories are activated and flushed to the surface by the mind (*manas*) according to external circumstances and situations, it is important to recognise and reflect with the help of *buddhi* in what way an event is caused or influenced by them and what actions result from it.[285]

According to Svāmī Nirañjanānanda, the word *saṃskāra* consists of the word parts *saṃ* — 'with', 'together', and *ākāra* — 'form'. It indicates connection and continuity. It expresses continuity or the flow of transition from one

---

282 According to Feuerstein, the *vasanas* are whole chains of similar karmic driving forces; Georg Feuerstein. (2008). *The Yoga Tradition – Its History, Literature, Philosophy and Practice* (3rd edition). Arizona: Hohm Press, p. 911.

283 Saraswati, Niranjanananda, Swami. (2018). *Progression of Pratyahara* 1. Munger: Yoga Publication Trust, p. 31.

284 Saraswati, Niranjanananda, Swami. (2002). *Yoga Darshan*. (1st edition, reprinted with corrections). Munger: Yoga Publication Trust, p. 125.

285 Ibid., p. 126.

stage to the next.[286] The *saṃskāras* are memories which are difficult to understand rationally and are naturally stored in the unconscious. They are imprints, impressions or after-effects and are usually understood psychologically as patterns or psychological tendencies. Some *saṃskāras* are transformed into archetypes to be stored in the deepest layers of the unconscious. There they lie latent, some without appearing outwardly. They are carried with us from life to life and are seen as our karmic inheritance. Most memories from early childhood are also stored in the unconscious because rational thinking is not yet developed at this stage of life. A *saṃskāra* takes a long time to rise from the unconscious to the subconscious and from there to the waking consciousness, and again a long time to be recognised. When *saṃskāras* manifest, they emerge as our strongest *vṛtti*s with the greatest power of attraction. They are not easy to dissolve and become disturbingly noticeable in deeper states of immersion and absorption.[287] The *saṃskāra-nirodha* only takes place in the *asaṃprajñāta-samādhi*—the state of absorption in which one is no longer aware of the difference between knowledge, the object of knowledge and the knower.

As Svāmī Nirañjanānanda explains, our recallable memories or imprints can be distinguished from a *saṃskāra* as follows:

> *When an impression or an experience goes beyond every kind of rational perception, it becomes a saṃskāra. In the sphere of the rational we have thoughts, intellect, emotions, desires, ambitions, etc., everything that we can experience now in our life and manifest now in our own activity. If something does not fit into any of these categories, it becomes a saṃskāra.*[288]
>
> Svāmī Nirañjanānanda

He further clarifies that different types of experiences are imprinted on different levels across the five sheaths of being (*pañcakośa*).[289] Thus, emotionally charged experiences will remain in the mental-emotional sheath (manomaya-kośa), while the experience of chanting devotional songs (*kīrtana*) or reciting mantras will be stored in our bliss-sheath (*ānandamaya-kośa*).

---

286 Ibid., p. 210–211.
287 Ibid., p. 127–128.
288 Ibid., p. 128.
289 The different layers of being, the *kośas*, are explained in the next chapter: 08. *Pañcakośa*.

The *pañcakośa* will be discussed in some detail below. According to Svāmī Nirañjanānanda, if an experience does not fit into our current personality pattern, if it is outside our realisation and we cannot deal with it, it becomes a *saṃskāra*.[290] The *saṃskāras* have the property of being hard or soft. Experiences which are less emotionally charged are stored as soft *saṃskāras* and are barely felt when they come up. Experiences which have a strong emotional intensity, such as traumas, radically change our perception of life and become particularly powerful hard *saṃskāras* and are also stored as such. They strongly influence our entire personality as soon as they come to the surface and manifest themselves.[291]

All these impressions cause *karmans*, which means 'actions'. The top layer, the *citta-vṛttis*, cause our current immediate *karmans*, while '*pratyayas*' we call our past accumulated *karmans*, and the *saṃskāras* chart the consequences of those *karmans*. Svāmī Nirañjanānanda states that the aim of '*rāja-yoga*' as applied to the approach of Patañjali is not primarily to achieve *samādhi*, but to dissolve these imprints while in the *pratyāhāra* state. Once the citta-vṛttis are managed and the *pratyayas* are released through *pratyāhāra*, *dhāraṇā*, and *dhyāna*, then *samādhi* can be experienced in a natural and spontaneous way.[292] A certain multitude of *saṃskāras* will nevertheless remain because the body, the senses and the mind continue to exist as our tools in the interaction with matter and the external world.

Karman itself has various aspects which interact with with one another. *Karman* means, among other things:[293]

- a ritual action (which reflects its older Vedic meaning)[294];
- the principle of cause and effect which governs every aspect of creation;

290 Saraswati, Niranjanananda, Swami. (2002). *Yoga Darshan*. (1st edition, reprinted with corrections). Munger: Yoga Publication Trust, p. 128–129.

291 Ibid., p. 130.

292 Saraswati, Niranjanananda, Swami. (2018). *Progression of Pratyahara* 1. Munger: Yoga Publication Trust, p. 22.

293 It must be noted that *karman* (usually '*karma*' in English) does not mean 'fate' or 'destiny'.

294 While the root √*kṛ* from which *karman* is derived generally means simply 'to do', the notion of *karman* as fate, or destiny as a consequence of one's actions is a slightly later development. For example, in the context of the Vedic religion, the *pañca-karmans* were five special ritual actions, which every adult initiated *brahmin* was required to make daily. This is, in turn, connected with the Vedic idea that ritual actions maintain and rectify the order of the Universe (*ṛta*).

- the basic pattern of the personality of the individual with all his thinking and knowledge as experienced in life;
- an action performed by the intellect, mind and senses to enjoy the fruits of the material world;
- an action of the hidden dimension of life;
- the primordial seed of desire that guides the thoughts, actions and behaviour of every individual.

The *karman* should also be seen in connection with the identification aspect of the *ahaṃkāra*. Selfish actions arise from both interactions, and, subsequently, also from the impulse for further selfish *karmans*. To transform our *karmans*, we should try to become aware of our *saṃskāras*, for example, by reliving the aspect of pain or pleasure they contain.

Hence, the practice of *karma-yoga* within the integral yoga context—the conscious, selfless and expectation-free action of awareness—is a reliable method for consciously recognising *saṃskāras* as they mature. Subtle reactions are particularly observed, and efforts are made to transform selfish actions into selfless actions. *Karma-yoga* can be practised at any moment and anywhere. The aim is to remove the negative and disruptive influence of the *saṃskāras* from the mental level. *Saṃskāras* appear in the form of attraction and aversion, ideas or images. In *karma-yoga*, what matters is the inner attitude with which an action is performed, rather than the action itself. It is about cultivating awareness during the action and recognising how we can become aware and conscious of our inner attitudes and transform them. Through this realisation, restrictive and negative *karmans* can also be purified. In this context, the *karmans* are the roots of desire (*kleśas*).[295]

The *kleśas* are of a sensory nature and, according to Svāmī Nirañjanānanda, just like the *karmans*, pass through three stages: 'the latent form (the seed), the active form (a fully laden tree) and the 'burnt out' form (the dead tree), which no longer has the ability to produce blossoms or fruit'.[296] They therefore exist in a latent, active or 'burnt out' form, regardless of whether it is a thought, an idea or a physical action. In this respect, *karmans* and *kleśas* are linked in their course. In the *pratyāhāra* and *dhāraṇā* states, we become

---

295 Saraswati, Niranjanananda, Swami. (2018). *Progression of Pratyahara* I. Munger: Yoga Publication Trust, pp. 59–68.
296 Ibid., p. 284.

aware of their 'burnt out' and their active forms, with the active form coming to the foreground and the 'burnt out' form remaining in the background. Especially in the *dhyāna* state, we can become aware of the latent form of the *kleśas*. The *kleśas* can only be removed when we recognise them in their subtle form, and only then can the associated *karman* be overcome. Only in the *dhyāna* state can our awareness simultaneously expand to all four subtle levels—idea, desire, motivation, and realisation.

Awareness in the Process of Purifying the *pratyayas*

As Svāmī Nirañjanānanda points out, the first step in the process of purifying the *pratyayas* is very similar in both the *pratyāhāra* and *dhāraṇā* states. We are impartial observers, who look at what is happening in an uninvolved and non-judgemental way. We largely detach ourselves from identification, unless we become aware of a connection to the deeper areas of our personality. Thus, both aspects of perception are therefore active here: the perception of the object on which the awareness, concentration and observation are focussed, and at the same time the knowledge or awareness of the process of observation itself.[297]

In the *dhyāna* state, three types of awareness are present, leading to an uninterrupted flow of experience:

- continuous flow of awareness of an object;
- awareness of the self;
- the awareness of the process of prolonged immersion.

In this state, the *pratyayas* can manifest in various forms and dissolve in the course of *dhyāna* once we have recognised them.[298]

We can practise *pratyahara* and *dhāraṇā* purposefully. However, *dhyāna* has several stages of refinement of the awareness and can only be experienced

297 Ibid., p. 185–186.
298 Ibid., p. 187.

spontaneously. If we deal with the concept of *dhyāna* but have not yet experienced this state and try to understand it rationally with our functional mind, it remains an abstract and theoretical level of experience. At the levels of *pratyāhāra* and *dhāraṇā* we have enough material and opportunities to deal with our awareness and the patterns of the mind (*vṛttis*).

The Effect of Purification by *yoga-nidrā* in Everyday Life

The processes of purification become more tangible in everyday life as soon as we establish a *sādhana*—consistent, regular, disciplined practice. Given the inherently scattered nature of the mind (*manas*), the cultivation of *pratyāhāra* constitutes an essential foundation. The *pratyāhāra* techniques, and particularly the *yoga-nidrā* method of Svāmī Satyānanda, train the mind to enter an inwardly focused state of active awareness and to remain established therein. In the process, the layers of impressions in the *citta* (*pratyayas* and *samskaras*) accumulated in everyday life, are released in the subconscious. As already mentioned, if these tensions are not released, the awareness cannot engage with the more subtle layers of the mind.

After the first stage of *pratyāhāra*, when the sense perception is already directed inwards and the stance of 'being aware', the *draṣṭā* is established—it is then that the process of releasing the subconscious tensions on the physical, energetic and mental levels of being begins. This enables the practitioner to naturally enter a state conducive to the release of tension, as exemplified in *yoga-nidrā*.

> In *pratyāhāra*, we 'feed' the mind through the finer sense impressions stored at the inner and deeper levels of our consciousness (subconscious and unconscious) that are not of a physical nature, i.e. they do not originate from the outside. Once we succeed in integrating *yoga-nidrā* into our everyday life, we soon notice how the underlying layer of overstimulation of the senses and nervous system, which we could not dissolve in any other way, gradually diminishes. In our daily experiences, we find that by releasing energy through the alleviation of underlying tension in *yoga-nidrā*, fatigue

> disappears, revitalising the body, while mental tension also subsides and the elasticity of the brain is restored.

On a very practical and tangible level, this process is a kind of daily 'hygiene' for the mind. We engage in it to 'digest' everyday impressions. Most practitioners report a noticeable lightness of mind, body and spirit, allowing them to approach their daily tasks or activities in a relaxed state. Furthermore, the quality and depth of interactions with family, friends and the working environment increase. It is precisely in these interactions that we often find ourselves unconsciously caught in a cycle of pleasure and displeasure, where the mind reacts quickly and automatically, as many thought constructs and patterns are old and habitual. Becoming aware of this allows us to cultivate more loving and conscious relationships, enabling us to perceive others more truthfully.

The *yoga-nidrā* method of Svāmī Satyānanda can assist us in recognising our behavioural patterns, evaluations and beliefs more clearly, helping us filter out disturbing old burdens from our behaviour. This practice empowers us to dwell in the clarity of the moment, creating a sense of having more space for conscious action.

During *yoga-nidrā*, we also experience a connection with several layers of consciousness, depending on the depth of awareness. Relaxation, a pleasant experience, or even sleep can occur. When the subconscious is engaged, we experience an apparent suspension of gravity, as perception temporarily detaches from the body. This can also evoke other, quite different sensations. The detachment from sensory impressions is based on the subconscious' own language, in the form of symbols, colours and sounds. In the course of the practice, when the deeper layers of the subconscious and unconscious are accessed, latent *saṃskāras* are released, creating space within the storehouse of the *citta*. This process enhances mental energy and the capacity for further immersive states. Occasionally, yet profoundly, during *yoga-nidrā*, it is possible to penetrate to the core of the unconscious, where deep latent impressions, not linked to sensory perception, can be released.

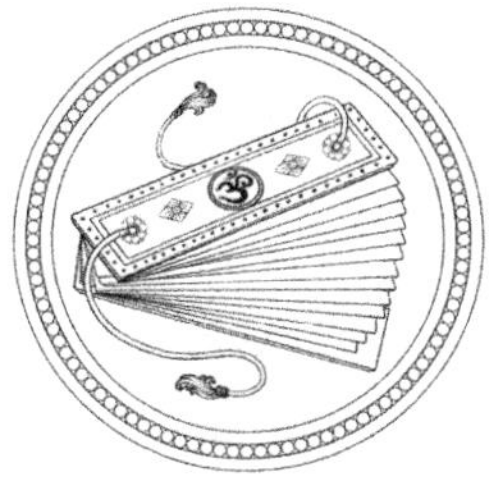

CHAPTER 8

Pañcakośa — The Five Sheaths of Being

ANOTHER RELEVANT CONCEPT WITH RESPECT to the individual comes from Vedāntic subtle physiology — the *pañcakośa* or 'the five sheaths' which cover the Self (*ātman*). They form a holistic system for understanding a being as composed of 'bodies' (*kāyas*) existing across different planes of subtlety, ranging from the gross to the nearly transcendental. Most of the five sheaths are very subtle and can be directly experienced in various immersive states.

Pañca means five, and *kośa*, among other meanings, refers to a 'layer', 'sheath', 'vessel', or 'dimension'. The Vedāntic doctrine of the three subtle bodies, the causal (*kāraṇa-śarīra*), the subtle (*sūkṣma-śarīra*), and the gross (*sthūla-śarīra*), and the five sheaths or *pañcakośa* is presented for the first time in the *Taittirīya-upaniṣad* (2.1–5)[299]. This text discusses ways and means of attaining *brahman* and describes in detail the dimensions of the Self.[300] Yogic theory of the subtle physiology mentions this concept only after the 17th century, which indicates that it is most likely a later adoption.[301]

299 *Taittirīya-upaniṣad* embedded as three chapters in the *Taittirīya-āraṇyaka* of the Kṛṣṇa *Yajur-veda*. It dates back to around the 6th century BCE and is one of the primary Upaniṣads.

300 Sharvananda, Swami. (1921). *Taittiriya-Upanishad*. Mylapore: The Ramakrishna Math, pp. 1–3.

301 Mallinson, J. and Singelton, M. (2017). *Roots of Yoga*. London: Penguin Classics, p. 469–470.

The concept of *kośas* functions like a map, illustrating our levels of experience from gross to subtle in order to recognize them and find our way into the more subtle layers of our being. These sheaths are in constant activity and influence one other, either in a balancing or disruptive way. The aim is to harmonise and balance the different levels as much as possible. Therefore, a holistic approach to yoga is essential.

> As a method which indirectly affects all levels of being by utilising their interconnectedness, Svāmī Satyānanda's *pratyāhāra-yoga-nidrā* technique is an ideal tool for addressing imbalance on any level in a safe and systematic manner, without the risks associated with advanced targeted practices, which work directly with subtle energies, energy centres or the sub- and unconscious afflictions of the mind. Attempting advanced practices without proper preparation or the supervision of a qualified master typically carries risks, offers minimal benefits, and is generally unsustainable as a *sādhana*. Reliable progress on the yoga path can only be achieved through consistent practice.

The five sheaths are:

annamaya-kośa—the food or body sheath: the sheath which we experience most directly on a daily basis. It is seen as the gross manifestation of energy and the elements (earth, water, fire, air, ether), i.e. what we are made of—matter in various states and quantities. It forms the gravitational centre of all other *kośas* and is the only sheath which can be seen by physical vision and which we can physically touch. According to Svāmī Nirañjanānanda[302] it occupies around 75% of our everyday awareness. Our daily rhythm and habits have a direct impact on the state of our *annamaya-kośa*.

The yoga techniques aimed at harmonising this 'physical body sheath' are primarily:

302 Saraswati, Niranjanananda, Swami. (2002). *Yoga Darshan*. (1st edition, reprinted with corrections). Munger: Yoga Publication Trust, p. 40–41.

- *ṣaṭkarman*—by cleansing the mucous membranes and the digestive tract;
- *āsana*—by strengthening, activation, flexibility, relaxation, detoxification, etc., and developing a heightened awareness of the physical body;
- *prāṇāyāma*—by increasing breathing capacity, vitality and relaxation and by learning to regulate the breath;
- *yoga-nidrā*—by relaxing all body systems and releasing muscular tension, activating the parasympathetic nervous system, resolving psychosomatic disorders of the organs, resolving *saṃskāras* which affect the body-mind complex, etc.

prāṇamaya-kośa—the sheath of vital energy. This sheath surrounds *annamaya-kośa* and is more subtle. *Prāṇa* is the essence of life, the microcosmic life energy, which is limited within us, but links all other *kośas* from the gross to the most subtle and vitalises them. It is indispensable for all physiological functions of the human organism. According to Svāmī Nirañjanānanda, this is the energy which manifests itself in various forms: as physical strength and vitality, mental willpower and *saṃkalpa*, as well as in its physio-electric aspect in the form of measurable electromagnetic oscillation frequencies in the brain—the alpha, beta, theta and delta waves.[303] Similarly, *prāṇamaya-kośa* is said to occupy only about 2% of our everyday consciousness because the experience of energy is linked to mental experience.[304]

In the tantric view of the subtle body, *prāṇa* flows through a network of thousands of *nāḍīs*[305] (energy pathways) which converge to form various energy plexuses (*cakras*) in the various joints and along the subtle channel of the spine (*suṣumṇā*). The two other main *nāḍīs*, through which the life energy flows together, are located on both sides of the *suṣumṇā*: *iḍā* is the left *nāḍī*, through which the mental force flows. It controls the subtle prāṇic experience and can be said to also control the *antaḥkaraṇa*. The one on the right is *piṅgalā*, in which the life force circulates and which controls the gross or material

303 Ibid., p. 38.

304 Ibid., p. 41–42.

305 Many sources speak of 72,000 *nāḍīs* of the *prāṇamaya-kośa*. This figure can vary depending on the source. It is significant that we generally assume a very large number of *nāḍīs*.

prāṇic experience. Through the central *nāḍī*—*suṣumṇā*, the *kuṇḍalinī-śakti* rises during its awakening. According to Svāmī Nirañjanānanda, *iḍā* extends through the two other, more subtle *kośas*—the *manomaya-* and vijnānamaya-kośa, with *piṅgalā* controlling both *annamaya-* and the most subtle—the *ānandamaya-kośa*.[306] One of the main goals in yoga is to harmonise *iḍā* and *piṅgalā* and activate the *suṣumṇā*. These three main energy channels run through the seven major *cakras* along the spine. There are five other prāṇic manifestations *prāṇa*, *apāna*, *udāna*, *samāna*, and *vyāna*;[307] each of them operates in its own area in the body, has its own direction of movement and function in the body, yet they are all interdependent and interconnected.

If the flow within the energy pathways (*nāḍīs*) in the body is disturbed, an imbalance occurs on both the physical and mental levels. This imbalance has a direct impact in the form of illness or mental disorders. The breath is our most direct connection with *prāṇamaya-kośa* and at the same time our tool for balancing *prāṇamaya-kośa* and expanding our life energy. Incorrect breathing patterns can be the cause of physical and mental disharmony and illness. Our mind and its flow of thought patterns (*citta-vṛtti*) have a strong connection with our breath, so these two forces mirror each other. If we learn to regulate our breath, we can therefore also influence our state of mind. Thus, *prāṇamaya-kośa* is the level where our physical and mental sheaths interface. Whereas Patañjali's terminology reflects a psycho-centric approach to inner purification, the integration of the *kośas* with *haṭha-yoga* concepts like *nāḍīs* and *cakras* offers a distinctly somato-centric framework for approaching the same objective. Consequently, in Bihar Yoga, the *kośas* are understood through a Tantra-influenced psycho-physiological lens.

Thus, the yoga techniques aimed at harmonising the energy sheath are mainly:

- *ṣaṭkarman*—by purifying the *prāṇa* flow in the body;
- *āsana*—performed with awareness, with inner focus and breath awareness, releases blockages and regulates the energy in the entire body;

306 Saraswati, Niranjanananda, Swami. (2002). *Yoga Darshan*. (1st edition, reprinted with corrections). Munger: Yoga Publication Trust, p. 43.

307 See Part I., Chapter 5. *Pratyāhāra as Foundation for yoga-nidrā*; *Stages of pratyāhāra, prāṇa-pratyāhāra*.

- *prāṇāyāma*—purifies, balances, directs and regulates *prāṇa* flow and increases vitality;
- *yoga-nidrā*—by directing awareness to different parts of the body and breath, both hemispheres of the brain are balanced and the *prāṇa* flow throughout the body is harmonised and energetic blockages and *saṃskāras* may be released. *Prāṇa* is affected indirectly, through the awareness of the physical body and the breath;
- *prāṇa-(yoga)-nidrā*—through this technique the prāṇic sheath can be worked with directly and in much greater depth and detail than during *pratyāhāra-yoga-nidrā*. However, this practice is intended solely for advanced practitioners and should only be undertaken under the guidance of a qualified master.[308] The technique's name is often shortened to *prāṇa-nidrā*;
- Immersive techniques such as *ajapā-japa* (breath meditation with mantra) or the recitation of mantras and the practice of *kīrtana*—singing hymns and repetitively intoning mantras.

manomaya-kośa—the emotional or mental sheath is even more subtle than the former two. This is where the *antaḥkaraṇa* (*manas*, *buddhi*, *ahaṃkāra* and *citta*) begins to perceive, function and permeate through all levels of existence as an 'inferior' mind by means of the senses. This is the level of our thoughts in the form of memories, projections and constructs as well as our emotions in the form of *prāṇa*. This 'inferior' mind is the tangible aspect of consciousness, the bridge between the individual and the universal. A different kind of mental energy is active in the mental sheath, it is called *citta-śakti*. *Manomaya-kośa* is thus considered to occupy about 20% of our everyday consciousness.[309]

Only a small part of our mental functions take place on the conscious level. The closer we look at the interaction between mind and body, the more their differences become blurred. The body-mind complex is in a continuous dialog in which information processing and exchange constantly take place at all levels of physical existence—from the cellular to the organ level. All body systems and sensory perceptions with their functions and reactions interact

---

308 See Ibid.

309 Saraswati, Niranjanananda, Swami. (2002). *Yoga Darshan*. (1st edition, reprinted with corrections). Munger: Yoga Publication Trust, p. 40–41.

with the mind in the background of our everyday perception, forming a complex interplay of requirements, subtle processes and adaptations of which we are not aware.

Techniques aimed at harmonising the mental sheath are primarily those directed towards attaining *pratyāhāra*. In this context, *pratyāhāra* is understood as a state in which awareness is directed, or more precisely, focused within a specific field of concentration or aspect of existence, such as the physical body. By narrowing the scope of awareness in this way, its depth and intensity are enhanced, while distractions and the dispersion of energy are reduced. Techniques for achieving this include:

- *āsana-pratyāhāra*—practicing *āsana* in full awareness, focusing on its different aspects in succession: for example, first focusing on the physical body, then proceeding with performing the *āsana* by adding focus on the breath/*prāṇa*, then on the energy centres (*kṣetras* and *cakras*), and finally on mantra;
- *antar-mauna*—(inner silence), which helps us to get to know and understand the workings of the mind and harmonise its function;
- (*pratyāhāra-*) *yoga-nidrā*—it helps us to disidentify from the outer world and turn inwards to discover the inner subtleties of the mind, as well as to release *pratyayas* and *saṃskāras*. This process works indirectly by creating a balanced inner environment, which stimulates the desired subtle effects.
- All *dhāraṇā*—practices used in Bihar Yoga, which also engage strongly with the *manomaya-kośa*. For example, as *pratyāhāra* in *yoga-nidrā* deepens with time and experience, it becomes possible to develop a *dhāraṇā*-oriented *yoga-nidrā* practice, enabling focused and direct engagement with the subtle elements of the mind. As with *prāṇa-(yoga)-nidrā*, this practice should only be undertaken under the guidance of a qualified master.

vijñānamaya-kośa—*vijñāna* means knowledge from cognition. This is the wisdom sheath and the gateway to the subtlest of the *kośas*, to ānandamaya-kośa—the bliss sheath. At this level, the intellect is transcended and our access to intuition is enabled. According to Svāmī Nirañjanānanda, when our awareness is raised to this level, the mind is focused and higher experiences become possible as well as the attainment of certain *siddhis* (extraordinary abilities). Here, alignment with the higher consciousness can unfold. It is, however, often refracted through the influence of *buddhi*, *ahaṃkāra* and *manas* and thus it becomes impossible to judge whether an intuitive insight is genuine and correct or if it is a product of delusion. This causes doubt. It is the obfuscations of the lower functions of the mind which are to be transcended at this level so that genuine intuition can be allowed to unfold without filter. *Vijnānamaya-kośa* is considered to make up about 2% of our consciousness.[310]

In yoga, the approach to the *vijnānamaya-kośa* is achieved by successively engaging with the lower three *kośas* as well as through all techniques which promote the development of the higher aspect of *buddhi* — knowledge and wisdom — such as the higher stages of *yoga-nidrā*, deep states of immersion, mantra recitation or chanting of certain hymns.

ānandamaya-kośa, the bliss sheath or the causal body, is the subtlest of the five sheaths and is only experienced in deep absorption. This *kośa* is in closest contact with the Self — the *ātman*. It is the purely spiritual level which we cannot describe and from which *buddhi* and subsequently all other individual aspects of the mind arise. *Ānanda* is not emotional bliss, it is the transcendental joy of contact and merging with the highest consciousness which cannot be described in words. However, *ānandamaya-kośa* is still a sheath and must eventually also be transcended in the course of our further development.[311]

The *kośas* form a model of the different dimensions of human experience — from the gross (*annamaya*) and subtle (*prāṇamaya*) through the more subtle (*manomaya* and *vijñānamaya*) to the causal (*ānandamaya*) level. All *kośas* are in constant interaction and cannot be separated from each other. The more we become aware of the subtler levels of our being, the more our awareness expands and the more our personality develops and is refined. The model shows the path for growth beyond the level of individual personality to awareness of the Self. To address the whole system, we should develop an integral approach to yoga.

---

310 Ibid., p. 48.
311 Ibid., p. 42–43.

Yoga-nidrā and the *pañcakośa*

> *To awaken vijnānamaya[kośa] you have to transcend the influence of the mind [(manas)] and intellect [(buddhi)]. The easiest and quickest way to influence the analytical mind and logical intellect is to provide it with a set of practices that defy [conceptual] logic. [...] Mystic practices, involving mantras, rituals, worship, music as well as dance as in the case of the whirling dervishes and Sufi traditions [...] have been utilized since time immemorial by [many peoples] through the world [...]. [...] And all mystic practices, all practices dealing with the esoteric, have some link with yoga. So, you can easily use the practices of yoga, such as āsana, prāṇāyāma, mudrā, bandha, pratyāhāra, dhāraṇā, dhyāna, to awaken vijnānamayakośa.*[312]
>
> Svāmī Satyasaṅgānanda

In the Satyananda Yoga Nidra method, the consistent and systematic guidance of awareness through the various layers of the human being is of central importance. This method guides the awareness specifically from the gross to the subtle or from *annamaya-kośa* to *vijnānamaya-kośa*. Only the systematic traversal of the various stages of practice enables deeper experiences in the subtler sheaths. The regularity of practice is of paramount importance, as continuous development is only possible through consistent practice; without it, one is likely to revert repeatedly to old patterns and states.

The focus of *yoga-nidrā* is on two of the more 'subtle' levels of existence—those of *manomaya-kośa* and *vijnānamaya-kośa*, although *prāṇa* is also used as an essential tool in the process. Awareness at these two *kośa* levels influences all and interacts with all other *kośas*, forming an interlocking, dynamic system.

Through the observer attitude, which becomes more refined and therefore more profound as the practice progresses, we shift our awareness experience from the gross level of *annamaya-kośa* to the more subtle level of vijnānamaya-kośa. This is viewed as a process of purification of the mind (*śodhana*), through which we can begin to loosen and release the mental conditionings,

312 Sarawati, Satyasangananda, Swami. (2007). *Awakening the Vijnānamayakośa*. Munger: Yoga Publication Trust, p. 19.

pratyayas, *saṃskāras* and *karmans* that bind us to the worldly plane. This process opens up the possibility of reaching the higher level of consciousness represented by *ānandamaya-kośa*. More importantly, it enables us to manage our personality, life and daily experiences more consciously and to engage with them more fully.

This purification process largely takes place at the level of *manomaya-kośa*. The first layer of the subconscious consists of *pratyayas* (mental impressions in their seed form) from the past which are stored in the *citta*. These impressions, as mentioned earlier, can be positive, neutral or associated with pain or trauma. When the present situation evokes memories of a past experience, these impressions resurface, become conflated, and distort our present experience by imposing a false view (*viparyaya*). This process can lead to a confrontation with our repressed experiences, disrupting our mental balance. Consequently, we often find ourselves unconsciously reliving our past instead of being in the present.

Vijnānamaya-kośa is the realm where the unconscious, vast, super-personal mind begins, while *manomaya-kośa* is the constructed, personal mind. Deep *saṃskāras* and *karmans* are stored at this level, forming a reservoir of encoded experiences or memories (*citta*) which enter the *manomaya-kośa* and manifest as our conditioned personality.

The aspects of our consciousness we suppress, because they are deemed unacceptable to our egocentric self-image form our 'personal unconscious'. *Yoga-nidrā* and other *pratyāhāra* techniques such as *antar-mauna* (inner silence) make it possible to bring these *pratyayas* to the surface and face them in a gentle way. Through practice, we develop the ability to engage in this process as a neutral and aware observer (*draṣṭā*).

Influence of the *tri-guṇa*

Our awareness will gradually deepen as we purify the *manomaya-kośa*, leading to a greater understanding of the inner functions of the mind. We will increasingly succeed in identifying with the higher and more balanced (sattvic) aspects of *buddhi*, *manas* and *ahaṃkāra*.

Again, *buddhi* is essential for this process. When *buddhi* under the predominant influence of *rajas* and *tamas*, its attention becomes focused on actions and desires in the external world, on fantasies, or even on nothing at all. As a result, our perception remains limited to the level of *manomaya-kośa*, and this is the experience we will also have during *yoga-nidrā*. However, when we experience *buddhi* in its sattvic aspect while practicing yoga-nidrā, the mind operates at the higher level of *vijnānamaya-kośa*. In this state, *buddhi* separates the 'real' from the 'unreal' and expresses discrimination (*viveka*) accurately.

By means of *yoga-nidrā*, the sattvic *buddhi* enables us to incorporate 'higher wisdom', intellect and intuition into our judgments. While it is not consciousness itself, its bright and clear sattvic quality allows it to reflect, accept, and express the nature of consciousness in our mental functioning.

CHAPTER 9

Levels of Experience of Consciousness and *yoga-nidrā*

Awareness is different to consciousness. According to yogic principles, there is just one continuous state of being, of perception, of knowledge, which is called cetanā. Cetanā is known as 'consciousness'. This consciousness never changes; it is changeless.[313]

Svāmī Nirañjanānanda

THE WESTERN TERM FOR '*CONSCIOUSNESS*' comes from the Latin *conscius* 'knowing', 'aware', from *con-scire* 'to know', 'to be privy to something', 'to be mutually aware'—and is used differently depending on the context. The terms 'spirit', 'mind', 'consciousness' and 'awareness' are often used both as

313 Saraswati, Niranjanananda, Swami. (2002). *Yoga Darshan*. (1st edition, reprinted with corrections). Munger: Yoga Publication Trust, p. 22.

synonyms and with different meanings. However, these definitions only partially approximate the yogic understanding.

Mind, Consciousness and Awareness in Yoga

Citta [...] evolves into cetanā, the state of consciousness, and you the individual — is known as citi. Citta is in you, but you are citi. Citi means the knower of consciousness. Citta here becomes the building block of experience (cetanā), [...] and you become the experiencer of that [citta/cetanā].[314]

Svāmī Nirañjanānanda

The three terms *citta, citi* and *cetanā* derive from the same root — √*cit* 'to think', 'to perceive', 'to observe'. However, they come from several different systems of thought. According to Patañjali, *citta* is the mind-complex where *vṛttis* occur and *saṃskāras* are stored (*Yoga-sūtras* 1.2–1.4). *Cetanā* means 'consciousness' in Sāṃkhya and Vedānta. *Citi* refers to pure consciousness, and even universal consciousness, especially in some tantric texts.

According to Svāmī Nirañjanānanda, however, *cetanā* — the highest consciousness — represents the unmanifest aspect of the Cosmic Will (*īśvara*), possessing the ability to know, create and manifest. Its reality lies beyond time, space and personal perception. The highest consciousness is a constant state of being, perception, and knowledge.[315]

Cetanā can be construed as the embodied uninterrupted, unconditioned, fully aware flow of conscious activity — the continuous field of illuminated mental activity. Its meaning is broad, encompassing sensory, intellectual and also psychological experiences. While it remains uninterrupted, it may appear otherwise, as its focus shifts between the various expressions of the different aspects of the mind.

---

314 Saraswati, Niranjanananda, Swami. (2018). *Raja Yoga Yatra* 2 – Understanding Pratyahara. Munger: Yoga Publication Trust, p. 43.

315 Saraswati, Niranjanananda, Swami. (2002). *Yoga Darshan*. (1st edition, reprinted with corrections). Munger: Yoga Publication Trust, p. 136.

In yoga teachings, in contrast to Western understanding, the mind is the expression and tool of consciousness. Patañjali states in *Yoga-sūtra* 4.19: *na tat-svābhāsaṃ dṛśyatvāt* that the mind cannot illuminate itself or be the source of consciousness because it is the subject of knowledge and perception and can itself be perceived as an object.[316] Yoga does not seek to understand rationally what the mind is, but instead to experience its essence directly. This is only possible because through yoga we learn to observe the mind (*draṣṭā*), which indicates that there is a state of consciousness beyond the mind that involves this observing capacity.

Functioning of the Human Mind

Mind (*citta*) in yoga is understood as an aspect of consciousness. A distinction is made between three modes in which the mind functions:

- inferior, 'impure' mind — is subject to desires, wishes, ambitions, follows sense objects and seeks fulfilment outside; it is subject to the influence of *tamas* and *rajas*;
- higher, 'pure' mind — is clear and does not seek external stimulation; it is under the influence of *sattva*;
- total mind — refers to the two principles of consciousness (*śiva*) and energy (*śakti*) as a whole. It stands above the *tri-guṇa*.[317]

Five Evolutionary States of the Human Mind

In the commentaries by Vyāsa and Vācaspati Miśra on Patañjali's *Yoga-sūtra* 1.1. five states of mind — from the tāmasic states to the total mind — are referred to as follows:[318]

---

316 Saraswati, Satyananda, Swami. (2000). *Four Chapters on Freedom*. Munger: Yoga Publication Trust, p. 334.
317 Saraswati, Niranjanananda, Swami. (2002). *Yoga Darshan*. (1st edition, reprinted with corrections). Munger: Yoga Publication Trust, p. 33.
318 Patañjali. (1998). *Patanjali's Yoga Sutras – with the Commentary of Vyāsa and the gloss of Vāchaspati Miśra, Prasāda, Rāma* (translation). New Delhi: Munshirm Manoharlal Pub Pvt. Ltd., p. 1–5.

- *mūḍha* (deluded) — *tamas*-dominated; the mind is cloudy, confused, dull and sluggish;
- *kṣipta* (scattered) — *rajas*-dominated; the mind is scattered and restless.

These first two stages represent the worldly expression of the mind. The state of yoga can only begin taking place when the third stage, beyond the *tri-guṇa*, is reached. The three further stages or states of the mind are:

- *vikṣipta* (partially distracted) — constantly oscillating between *rajas* and *sattva*, the mind moves between distraction and concentration. According to Svāmī Satyānanda[319], this is the state of all meditation practitioners. He recommends studying and learning the interplay of the *tri-guṇa* and its influence on oneself as well as consciously directing the *tri-guṇa* by practicing techniques which weaken the elements of *tamas* and *rajas*. However, Vācaspati Miśra's interpretation entails the danger of confusing *vikṣipta* with complete yoga, since during *vikṣipta* a temporary stability of mind can occur, which, in contrast to complete yoga, is immediately followed by an unstable state. This relates to *dhāraṇā*;
- *ekāgra* (constantly focused) — *sattva-guṇa* state; *tamas* and *rajas* are not present. This is the state of complete concentration, the concentration of the mind on one point. In yoga, the aim in all disciplines is to achieve 'one-pointedness' (*ekāgratā*) through regular practice. This relates to *dhyāna*;
- *niruddha* (suppressed)[320] — according to Svāmī Satyānanda[321] a state above the *tri-guṇa*, the mind is not influenced by any of the three qualities of nature (*tri-guṇa*). Constant, uninterrupted awareness beyond all fluctuations of the mind, or according to Patañjali's definition of yoga: *yogaś citta-vṛtti-nirodhaḥ* (*YS*: 1.2). This relates to *samādhi*.

---

319 Saraswati, Satyananda, Swami. (2000). *Four Chapters on Freedom*. Munger: Yoga Publication Trust, p. 38.

320 The term is derived from the root √*rudh* – 'to stop', 'to close', 'to shut' with the prefix *ni-*, meaning 'down', 'back into', or 'within'. Thus *ni-*√*rudh* means 'to surround', 'to catch' or 'to overtake'. However, the root √*rudh* can also be related to √*ruh* – 'to grow', 'to ascend', 'to climb', through which lens *niruddha* can be interpreted as 'suppressed' in the sense that 'in that state latent seeds are suppressed and not given the opportunity to sprout'.

321 Ibid., p. 38–39.

The Four Experiential Levels of Consciousness

> *In modern psychology, the dreaming and sleeping states are thought to be unconscious states, but Vedānta psychology explains that they are not actually unconscious for the yogis who can attain conscious access to the dreaming and sleeping states.* [322]
>
> Svāmī Rāma

In Western psychoanalysis, three levels of consciousness are generally distinguished: the conscious, the preconscious (or subconscious), and the unconscious. The unconscious contains repressed drives, impulses, and experiences that are not normally accessible to awareness and can only be brought into consciousness through reflection, analysis, or therapeutic techniques. In contrast, the yogic approach aims to cultivate awareness of increasingly subtle layers of the mind, including those analogous to the subconscious and unconscious, as part of a progressive ascent toward self-realisation or enlightenment.

In yoga, consciousness is described as operating on four experiential levels:

- *jāgrat*—the gross experience (*sthūla*); alertness, the 'conscious' level of mind, waking consciousness, acute external sensory experience, superficial thinking and perception of the external world;
- *svapna*—the subtle experience (*sūkṣma*); the sleep or dream state, the subconscious level of mind, e.g. the dream, in which the conscious experience is distorted or reduced; the subconscious comes forth more distinctly, the individual memory predominates, external sensory experience is dampened;
- *suṣupti* or *nidrā*—the causal experience (*kāraṇa*); deep sleep, the 'unconscious' level of mind; states in which consciousness is greatly reduced or absent;[323]

---

322 Rama, Swami. (1982). *Enlightenment without God – Mandukya Upanishad*. Honesdale: Himalayan Institute Press, p. 38.
323 Ibid., p. 19.

- *turīya*—also *caturtha* with the meaning (the) 'fourth' (from *catur*—'four'); denotes the fourth state of consciousness, the superconscious state, cosmic consciousness, the enlightened state.[324]

Our usual point of reference for other states of consciousness is the waking, decision-oriented state of consciousness. In this waking state, existence is perceived in the form of a separation of subject—identified with the ego—and object, i.e. dualistically. This state is also characterised by the illusion of being in control. In other words, the function of dualistic perception is to enable the 'normal' functioning of an independent entity in an ultimately boundless world. Without the separation of subject and object, a person would not be able to filter the information from their environment; such states can manifest in mental disorders such as schizophrenia. Inversely, a yogin consciously trains to release the shackles of dualistic perception in a controlled and targeted manner.

In contrast, our consciousness seems less clear during the dreaming state; the images and dreams which arise spontaneously are almost impossible to control voluntarily. We recognise that our experience of consciousness appears distorted in dreams or in dream-like states and entitification is less discrete.

Even though such a categorisation is usually made into four 'states of consciousness', it should be noted that the experience of consciousness is by no means divided into different, strictly distinguishable phenomena. Rather, the different states flow into each another—they form a continuum of experience which ranges from wakefulness to unconscious sleep. The fourth state goes beyond this distinction. Known as *turīya*—the fourth state—is not the fourth in a series, but represents a qualitatively different experience of consciousness compared to the three coloured by the three *guṇa*s.

Yoga recognises consciousness as a fundamental principle of existence, although our experience of it is often limited by our identification with the body. Due to our preoccupation with individual sensory perception, our ordinary waking experience of consciousness is only a faint shadow of what is possible to experience.

---

324 *Turīya* is found in various spellings and is a term for the highest state of consciousness in the *Haṭha-yoga-pradīpikā* (4th chapter, verses 3–4) and *Māṇḍukya-upaniṣad* (verse 7), a synonym for *samādhi* in *rāja-yoga* and other terms such as *amanaska*.

In the understanding and experience of Svāmī Satyānanda, in *yoga-nidrā*, our awareness can traverse all three levels of consciousness to move from the conscious to the subconscious and finally to the unconscious. Awareness is purposefully expanded. Practitioners are trained to perceive these three levels simultaneously in order to gradually aim at attaining the fourth state of consciousness, *turīya*—the superconscious. E.g., this is what early texts such as the *Māṇḍukya-upaniṣad* focus on.[325]

Māṇḍukya-upaniṣad and *Yoga-nidrā*

nāntaḥprajñaṃ na bahiḥprajñaṃ nobhayataḥprajñaṃ na prajñānaghanaṃ na prajñaṃ nāprajñam | adṛṣṭam avyavahāryam agrāhyam alakṣaṇam acintyam avyapadeśyam ekātmapratyayasāraṃ prapañcopaśamaṃ śāntaṃ śivam advaitaṃ caturthaṃ manyante | sa ātmā | sa vijñeyaḥ | || 7 ||

Of the fourth, they mean that it neither perceives inwardly, nor perceives outwardly, nor perceives in both directions, that it is neither wholly insight, nor insight nor non-insight, that it is invisible, intangible, ungraspable, imperceptible, unthinkable, unmarkable, that it is the core of the concept of the One Self, that it is the cessation of multiplicity and pacifies, happy and non-dual. It is the Self, it is to be recognised.[326]

The *Māṇḍukya-upaniṣad*, probably from the 1st or 2nd century CE[327], is the shortest *Upaniṣad*. However, it is considered more profound than any other. Its twelve verses discuss the nature of the material and spiritual world, the nature of consciousness and the meaning of causality.

325 From the 1st or 2nd century CE.

326 The *Māṇḍūkya-Upaniṣad*, after the Sanskrit text and German translation of Haas, Dominik, A. (2019). https://orcid.org/0000–0002-8505–6112 (accessed on 27.10.2022).

327 Vergl. Nakamura, Hajime. (2004). *A History of Early Vedānta Philosophy*, Part 2. Delhi: Motilal Banarsidass Publications.

Māṇḍukya-upaniṣad describes the three states of consciousness of the individual self and the state of consciousness which lies beyond them. It also explains how the eternal sound OṀ[328] exists beyond past, present and future, transcends time, space and causality, represents the entire universe and is connected to the four states of consciousness.

amātraś caturtho 'vyavahāryaḥ prapañcopaśamaḥ śivo 'dvaitaḥ |
evam oṃkāra ātmaiva | *saṃviśaty ātmanātmānaṃ ya evaṃ veda* || 12 ||

The fourth [state], the inconceivable, the cessation of multiplicity, the happy, non-dual, is moreless[329]. In this way, the sound '*oṃ*' is the Self. He who understands this enters into the Self by the Self.[330]

The terms used in the *Māṇḍukya-upaniṣad* for these three states of consciousness are synonyms for those already explained — *vaiśvānara* ('common', i.e. the waking state), *taijasa* ('shining', i.e. the dream state), *prajña* ('in-sight-ful', i.e. deep sleep) and the fourth state *turīya*.

Mantra AUṀ	Terms	Consciousness State	Mental Levels	Reality Levels
A	*jāgrat/ vaiśvānara*	Waking consciousness	Conscious	*sthūla* gross/material
U	*svapna/ taijasa*	Dream consciousness	Subconscious	*sūkṣma* subtle
Ṁ	*suṣupti/ nidrā/prajña*	Deep sleep	Unconscious	*kāraṇa* causal
Stillness	*turīya*	The fourth	Superconscious/ Self/*ātman*	absolute

TABLE 3: Overview and comparison of terms used in the *Māṇḍukya-upaniṣad*.

328 In Sanskrit, diphthongs (clusters of two consecutive vowels) are considered equivalent to long vowels (e.g. o and e) – in other words, o is considered to consist of a and u, e is considered to consist of a and i. This is why it is often explained that *oṃ* consists of three parts (a, u and ṃ). In the Māṇḍukya-upaniṣad, the meanings of the three sounds are interpreted.

329 *Mora* or more (from Latin *mora* 'period') is the smallest metrical unit of time in verse.

330 The *Māṇḍūkya-Upaniṣad*, after the Sanskrit text and German translation of Haas, Dominik, A. (2019). https://orcid.org/0000-0002-8505-6112 (accessed on 27.10.2022).

Svāmī Rāma (1925–1996), one of the greatest yoga adepts, masters and writers of the 20th century and founder of the Himalayan Institute in Rishikesh, India, in his commentary on the *Māṇḍukya-upaniṣad* from the 1980s, cites *yoga-nidrā* as a method for traversing the three conventional states of consciousness and gradually reaching *turīya* — the state in which the knower knows and knows that he knows[331]. He describes this as follows:

To accomplish this [*turīya*], yogis learn to go into a deep state of voluntary sleep, called *yoga-nidrā*, and yet remain fully aware of the environment. In this state, the clarity of mind is more profound than in the waking state.[332]

Svāmī Rāma, like Svāmī Satyānanda, emphasises that the Sanskrit term *yoga-nidrā* cannot be translated into any other language. Both masters emphasise that yogins use this technique both during sleep and for reaching deep states of immersion. Svāmī Rāma refers to *yoga-nidrā* as 'yogic sleep' or 'sleepless sleep'. According to his description, *yoga-nidrā* is an advanced practice in which the practitioners learn to immerse the mind in deep relaxation, allowing them to traverse all three levels of consciousness while remaining fully aware. The goal is to maintain awareness of all three levels simultaneously. After experiencing all states of consciousness, one's essential nature — pure consciousness — is consolidated and the practitioner can realise that these states or modes of consciousness arise from a single source and ultimately dissolve back into it.

> Svāmī Rāma elaborates that *yoga-nidrā* is different from ordinary sleep. Instead of entering a state of unconsciousness, as occurs in the dreaming state and deep sleep, the practitioner remains conscious. Similarly, yoga-nidrā differs from practices of seated 'meditation', as they do not involve an effort to consciously experience the state of deep sleep. In fact, falling asleep is a known obstacle to the proper practice of seated meditation. However, *yoga-nidrā* can support and enhance 'meditation' practice.

Yoga-nidrā is beneficial in addressing the greatest challenges faced by every practitioner — laziness and sluggishness. It has a revitalising effect, providing complete rest to the mind, brain, nervous system, senses and body.

331 Rama, Swami. (1982). *Enlightenment without God – Mandukya Upanishad*. Honesdale: Himalayan Institute Press, pp. 46–52.
332 Ibid., p. 47.

Through immersion techniques and *yoga-nidrā*, the entire mind, including the subconscious, can be quietened. Svāmī Rāma also emphasised that practitioners can cultivate their willpower by strengthening their determination (*saṃkalpa-śakti*), enabling them to voluntarily enter a state of deep sleep and return to a state of full consciousness at will. Consequently, the practitioner strengthens their practice of immersion and observation. They learn to analyse and dissolve all their desires, thoughts and feelings through the practice of *yoga nidrā*, allowing them to place their mind into deep rest as needed.

Antaḥkaraṇa and the Levels of Consciousness

> *The unconscious mind is used as a vehicle for the individual self, but when the individual self drops all attachments to the unconscious mind, the individual self establishes itself in its essential nature and realises that its self is the Self of all. Such a state of realization is called liberation, turīya, the very origin of pure consciousness.*[333]
>
> Svāmī Rāma

As already discussed, *antaḥkaraṇa* includes the *buddhi* aspect of the mind, through the quality of which we can learn to control our awareness. *Buddhi* means to recognise something experienced; it is an aspect of our 'higher' mind and the vehicle of awareness. With the development of *buddhi*, however, awareness can be trained and maintained in those states in which we normally experience a loss of awareness, i.e. in the dream state and in deep sleep, but also in our experience of being present.

- *jāgrat*

In *jāgrat*, the mind is focussed on the gross level of sensory experiences and their mental representation in the form of images, memories, thoughts, and emotions. It is thus influenced by *ahaṃkāra*.

---

333 Ibid., p. 35.

- *svapna*

In the dream state—*svapna*—the mind is disconnected from the sensory impressions and constructs its own action from the reflection of the interplay between the outer, gross, and the inner, subtle level. Here *citta* (the memory) is predominantly active and creates dreams. Awareness in the dream state can be maintained through specific practice in order to explore and transform the mind through conscious dreaming.

- *nidrā* or *suṣupti*

In deep dreamless sleep—*nidrā*—the mind is in contact with the causal state, which is beyond desire and interest in the outside world. This is a state in which there are neither thoughts nor familiar objects on which our awareness can focus. Here, *ahaṃkāra* is still present despite its inactivity.

- *turīya*

If awareness can be directed and maintained even in the causal state of *nidrā*, we can realise a 'higher consciousness'. *Turīya* is the fourth, absolute, enlightened state of consciousness which transcends the experiences of the other three levels of consciousness as separate. Through the cultivation of *buddhi*, we can attain expanded awareness and move beyond duality.

When awareness is directed with equal intensity at all three levels—*jāgrat*, *svapna* and *nidrā*—and can be sustained simultaneously, its full potential as a homogeneous experience is achieved. Thus, *turīya* is spontaneously attained and experienced as a state of superconsciousness or cosmic consciousness. This state of realisation transcends individual experience and personality, facilitating total awareness across all aspects of the mind and levels of consciousness simultaneously, ultimately bringing us closer to enlightenment.[334]

---

334 Saraswati, Niranjanananda, Swami. (2002). *Yoga Darshan*. (1st edition, reprinted with corrections). Munger: Yoga Publication Trust, p. 25.

The Definition of Awareness and the Meaning of Being Present

Buddhi is like a big searchlight that lights up an area. You just have to expand the area of the light. The more you expand the area of light, the clearer things become. Clarity of vision, knowledge and experience, and clarity in the situation and environment are some of the benefits of evolving awareness.[335]

Svāmī Nirañjanānanda

All yoga techniques aim to expand human awareness and perception. In the yogic understanding, consciousness itself is all-pervading and omnipresent and cannot be expanded beyond that. It is our awareness that we want to increase, and that means expanding the receptivity and analytical structure of *buddhi*.[336]

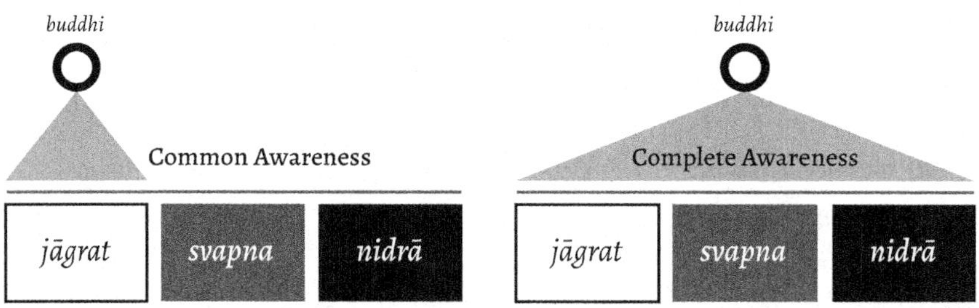

FIGURE 11: Awareness and *buddhi*[337]

The path to expanding awareness is characterised by the cultivation of the attitude of being present, or being established in awareness. This happens by means of cultivating alertness and awareness in every situation and action in everyday life, as well as through the practice of certain techniques such as *yoga-nidrā*, which immerse us in the *pratyāhāra* state and strengthen the *draṣṭā* stance.

335 Ibid., p. 26.
336 Ibid., p. 24.
337 Ibid., p. 23.

Awareness is our individual focal point in the endless field of consciousness (*cetanā*). It is the foreground and draws the light of consciousness into our experience. Thus, yoga techniques are designed to cultivate single-pointedness of mind. Our awareness is developed in two ways: by expanding, and by deepening the intensity of its focus. Expansion involves increasing the range of our awareness. This can initially involve sharpening the awareness of sensory impressions and lead to the ability to experience our life in all its facets much more consciously.

Another way to develop our awareness is to focus its intensity. In daily life, we are always surrounded by many stimuli and activities and only perceive a very limited part of them. Typically, what we perceive as meaningful or significant is at the forefront of our perception. By practising yoga, we can simultaneously expand and focus our awareness and direct it into states of experience beyond sensory perception. This intensification of our conscious experience occurs when we achieve a higher degree of clarity in our perception—a very high goal and a lifelong pursuit.

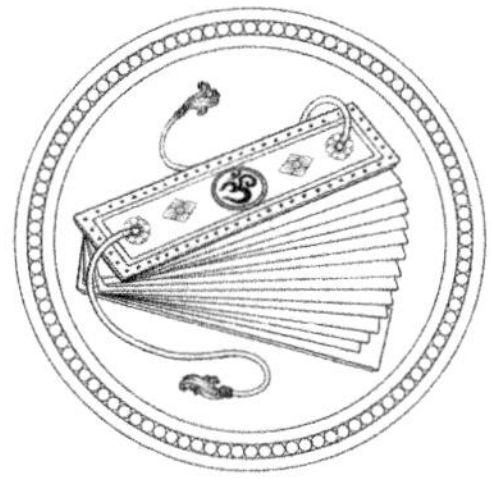

CHAPTER 10

Brain activity and states of consciousness during *yoga-nidrā*

Brain research is using ever more sophisticated examination equipment, such as brain scanners, but we are still no nearer to answering the crucial questions. [...] We can visualise which areas of the brain are switched on during certain tasks and how high their metabolism is, but nobody knows why this happens and what precise conclusions I can draw from these activities in my brain.[338]

Ulrich Warnke

DESPITE ALL THE TECHNOLOGICAL ADVANCES of our time, we remain unable to determine where the binding interface between consciousness and the material world is located, or even to measurably ascertain whether such an interface exists at all. This is largely because the human mind and consciousness are not objectively measurable phenomena. In 1930, the Czech

338 Warnke, Ulrich. (2017). *Quantenphilosophie und Spiritualität*. München: Goldmann Verlag, p. 93.

mathematician Kurt Gödel expressed a view aligned with many profound mystical traditions, asserting that 'the mind is not limited to the human brain but exists everywhere'.[339] The reduction of the body-mind complex to purely physical processes and the attempt by consciousness-orientated brain research and neuroscience to decipher and explain human consciousness through biological or physical phenomena has yet to yield definitive solutions. It remains undisputed that psychological phenomena — such as fear, joy, love, every train of thought and every surge of emotion — trigger and influence certain processes in the brain and body as well as in matter outside of them.[340] With the discovery of electroencephalography (EEG) in 1929[341], which allowed for the first time the measurement of electrical activity in the brain, neuroscience gradually gained a broader overview of the physiological processes within this organ. Today, electroencephalography (EEG), magnetoencephalography (MEG), measurement of electrodermal activity (EDA), functional MRI (fMRI) and positron emission tomography (PET) are the most important measurement methods in brain research and clinical diagnostics.

Most EEG devices are not designed to measure frequencies below 0.5 Hz. However, in recent years, increasingly sensitive, high-density measuring devices have been developed which can visualise previously unknown frequency spectra of brain activity. In certain measurement series, EEG and MEG devices are used in combination, as these methods are closely related and complementary. The same applies to the combination of EEG devices and PET scanners, through which a certain depth of measurement can also be achieved. Whenever possible, these methodological combinations should be analysed together in order to provide more accurate data.

Magnetoencephalography (MEG) records weak magnetic fields outside the human head, providing millisecond-precise information about neuronal currents which support human brain function. The small size of these neuromagnetic fields makes MEG recordings technically challenging. In addition to using low-noise sensors, it is essential to eliminate interference from external sources of electromagnetism, such as power lines, which

---

339 Schmieke, Marcus. (2009). Gödel's theorem and beyond. Cited in Ulrich, Warnke. (2017). [*Veden-Akademie*]. https://veden-akademie.de/bibliothek/naturwissenschaft/ (accessed on 27 October 2022).

340 Warnke, Ulrich. (2017). *Quantenphilosophie und Spiritualität*. München: Goldmann Verlag, p. 24.

341 The German neurologist and psychiatrist Hans Berger (1873–1941) is regarded as the inventor of electroencephalography (EEG) in 1929.

could contaminate the recordings. For instance, experiments are conducted in shielded rooms (Faraday cages) in order to block external sound sources and capture 'clean' data, or specialised filters are employed for data analysis.[342] Contemporary measuring devices are becoming increasingly sophisticated, making it exciting to anticipate the new findings which neuroscience will uncover.

Brainwave Frequencies in Summary

As previously mentioned, the states of consciousness in yoga — similar to those in Western psychology — are classified into three main categories: the waking state (conscious), the dreaming state (subconscious) and deep sleep (unconscious). With advancement in science, particularly in measuring brain activity, additional dimensions have been added in understanding these states.

The brain contains many billions of neurons organised in functional groups and interconnected by a complex network of connections between cortical regions and subcortical brain structures. These groups of cortical neurons undergo cycles of activity in which they are activated sequentially. This coordinated activity is represented by rhythmic waves in the EEG, which are registered at specific locations and can be recorded under certain conditions or after stimulation. The cyclical pattern of activity produces a distinct waxing and waning of the wave rhythms, showing fluctuations that occur over a timescale of several seconds and display considerable variability.[343]

By analysing the measured EEG voltage curves, the following general statements can be made about the different states of consciousness:

---

342 Hari, R, Baillet, et al. (2018). IFCN-endorsed practical guidelines for clinical magnetoencephalography (MEG), in *Clinical Neurophysiology*, Volume 129(8), 1720–1747. https://doi.org/10.1016/j.clinph.2018.03.042 (accessed on 27.10.2022).

343 Cascella, Marco; Bandyopadhyay, Susanta. (2023). Lambda Waves, 2022, in *Treasure Island* (FL): StatPearls Publishing LLC., 1. https://www.ncbi.nlm.nih.gov/books/NBK553088/ (accessed on 07.11.2022).

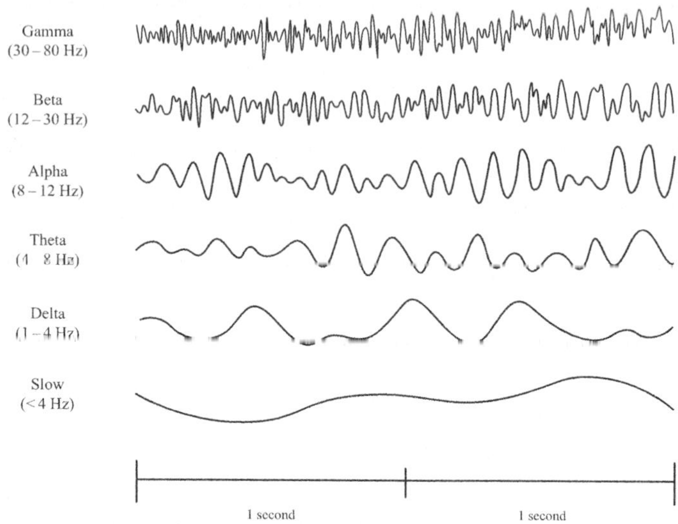

FIGURE 12: Brain activity frequency spectrum (EEG)[344]

- the gamma waves (from about 30 Hz) and hypergamma waves (from about 100 Hz) indicate the formation of a coherent, uniform perception; subjective state of transcendence;[345]
- the beta waves (12–30 Hz) indicate the waking state;
- alpha waves (8–12 Hz) indicate brain activity in a hypnagogic or hypnopompic state and in deep relaxation;
- the theta waves (4–8 Hz) indicate the subconscious state;
- the delta waves (0.5–4 Hz) indicate the unconscious state.

Gamma waves are fast beta waves which occur during peak (physical and mental) performance and deep concentration and are related to the ability to assemble a series of small fragments of information from different regions of the brain into a single, coordinated image. Hypergamma waves are extremely high-frequency waves which are associated with high-level cognitive abilities such as insight, psychic powers and out-of-body experiences.[346]

344 Image by © Immanuel Stürzebecher.

345 Nataraja, Shanida. (2008). *The Blissful Brain – Neuroscience and proof of the power of meditation*. London: Octopus Publishing Group Ltd., p. 100.

346 Ibid., p. 98.

Beta waves have a high frequency and indicate our waking state. They are associated with higher cognitive functions, such as active thinking, attention or problem-solving skills, while the brain is busy processing incoming sensory information.[347]

Alpha waves have a slightly lower frequency than beta waves. In general, alpha waves indicate a deeply relaxed, yet conscious state in which the parasympathetic neuronal functions and the integration of the right and left hemispheres of the brain are promoted and balanced. It is 'a state of wakefulness: the eyes might be closed and the mind and body relaxed, in a state of inner-directed attention and non-linear, holistic thinking'.[348] In this state, the brain is particularly receptive to new information. A significant increase in alpha wave activity in the frontal areas of the brain indicates creative thinking.[349]

Theta waves are even lower in frequency than alpha waves and are associated with the creative subconscious. They indicate the activity of large groups of neurons, which are associated with the ability to generate inner images and thus strengthen the power of imagination. Accordingly, their activity is particularly pronounced both in dream sleep and in deep immersion. They are also the predominant brainwave rhythms in children aged two to five years.[350]

Delta waves have a very low frequency and are associated with processes in the unconscious. They reflect the activity of the neurons which generate intuitive thinking, empathy and instinctive insight. Delta waves occur mainly in infants, sleeping adults and adults with brain tumours, patients during surgery in deep anaesthesia or in a coma.[351]

There is a whole range of other brain waves that can be recorded with modern equipment. The wave patterns are rarely pure, as the different waves occur in combination. Typically, different frequencies are recorded simultaneously, e.g. alpha waves predominate in a relaxed state, but depending on the depth of relaxation, some beta or theta activity may also be present.

---

347 Ibid., p. 97.

348 Lustenberger, C., Boyle, M. R., et al. (2015). Functional role of frontal alpha oscillations in creativity. In *Cortex Magazine*, 67, 74–82. https://doi.org/10.1016/j.cortex.2015.03.012 (accessed on 14.09.2023).

349 Ibid.

350 Nataraja, Shanida. (2008). *The Blissful Brain – Neuroscience and proof of the power of meditation*. London: Octopus Publishing Group Ltd., p. 97–98.

351 Ibid., p. 98.

If theta waves are measured in a person in a deeply relaxed but conscious state, a certain amount of alpha waves will also be present. This can be the case during deep immersion or lucid dreaming.[352]

Sometimes the parameters of the measured brainwaves differ slightly in the various studies, which is probably due to the current state of development of research. We can also look forward with curiosity to the rapid developments in science in this area.

Brain Waves and the Subjective Experience in a State of Immersion

Since the 1960s, research has expanded to include experiments on brain activity during various immersion practices or meditation methods. The EEG remains the most widely used method for this purpose, as it records the combined electrical activity of large groups of neurons in the brain, making it visible and measurable. Changes in the frequency spectrum of the EEG signals allow researchers to observe alterations in brain activity throughout the different phases of immersion.

However, typical EEG recordings are complex, making it challenging to establish definitive rules for the changes induced by immersion, especially when attempting to measure the subtleties of the different states. The results often represent a gross simplification of the intricate processes occurring in the brain during immersion. Based on these measurements, it is hypothesised that electromagnetic waves generated by the brain correspond to specific states of consciousness. As the brain becomes more active, nerve cells transmit more impulses per second, leading to more dynamic and denser voltage curves recorded by the EEG device.

As early as 1987, the British psychophysiologist and biophysicist Maxwell Cade published insightful findings on the relationship between various brain waves and immersion experiences, particularly the relaxation response. These results are very interesting with regard to *yoga-nidrā*, as they also documented intermediate states and subjective descriptions of the immersion experience.

---

352 Nilsson, Robert. *The relaxed State and Science*. Scandinavian Yoga and Meditation School. https://www.yogameditation.com/reading-room/the-relaxed-state-and-science/ (accessed on 07.11.2022).

Using a special multi-channel EEG system he developed, known as Mind Mirror EEG, Cade discovered that different levels of consciousness and even distinct psychological states encountered during immersion practice can be linked to specific brain wave patterns. He posited that the brainwave activity produced through regular meditative practice represents one of several possible brainwave patterns generated by the human brain. In fact, based on his measurements, he identified five observable states of consciousness/perception:

- dreaming sleep
- the hypnagogic and hypnopompic states
- the waking state
- the meditative state and the
- 'Awakened Mind' (lucid awareness).[353]

Although Cade took his measurements from a group of practitioners with different backgrounds and levels of experience, the results were very similar:[354]

Relaxation Response (% change)	EEG Readings Spectrum	Subjective Description of State of Relaxation
Below 25 %	Intermittent beta and alpha	Subjects begin to relax; may report difficulty in stilling the mind and/or restlessness.
25–35 %	Reduced beta and continuous alpha	May report feeling dizzy or having a fuzzy consciousness, as well as the frequent desire to fill the mind with everyday thoughts
35–45 %	No beta; continuous alpha, and intermittent theta	Sense of calmness and relaxation; intermittent attention; flashback memories of childhood or the past

353 Nataraja, Shanida. (2008). *The Blissful Brain – Neuroscience and proof of the power of meditation*. London: Octopus Publishing Group Ltd., p. 103.

354 See: Cade, Maxwell, C. & Coxhead, Nona. (2011). *The Awakened Mind: Biofeedback and the Development of Higher States of Awareness*. USA: Element Books Ltd.

Relaxation Response (% change)	EEG Readings Spectrum	Subjective Description of State of Relaxation
45–55 %	Continuous alpha of ever lower frequencies, with almost continuous theta	Sensation of floating, lightness, rocking and swaying. Attention becomes sustained and imagery clearer and more frequent
60–70 %	Continuous alpha and theta of ever lower frequencies	Extremely vivid awareness of breathing, heartbeat or other bodily sensations; effortless attention; fluctuation between external and internal awareness
70–80 %	Continuous theta and alpha of a frequency close to the alpha/theta border	Lucid impression of altered state of consciousness which is deeply satisfying and associated with intense alertness, calmness and detachment
Over 80 %	Very little electrical activity except occasional delta	Synthesis of opposites into a higher unity, combined with a new intuitive insight into old problems

TABLE 4: Relaxation response and states of consciousness according to Cade[355]

It is important to emphasise that the distinction here is not between different modes of consciousness which shift, but rather between states of perception which fluctuate and of which we become aware. While consciousness itself remains immeasurable, but we obtain physically measurable results which reflect the multidimensional interaction of the body-mind complex.

Most studies on consciousness and brain activity have been conducted in the English-speaking world, focusing on methods such as *transcendental meditation*[356] since the 1960s and *mindfulness meditation*[357] since the 1970s. These findings are of great interest and have contributed significantly to enhancing our understanding of states of consciousness during practice of these particular methods and their clinical and therapeutic applications. However, these results cannot be directly transferred to *yoga-nidrā*, despite the temptation many authors feel to do so. A comparative study between these methods

355 In Nataraja, Shanida. (2008). *The Blissful Brain – Neuroscience and proof of the power of meditation*. London: Octopus Publishing Group Ltd., pp. 104–105.

356 In 1960, the American physician Robert Keith Wallace submitted his doctoral thesis in which he presented meditation as the fourth major state of consciousness.

357 Harrington, Anne, and John D. Dunne. (2015). When Mindfulness Is Therapy: Ethical Qualms, Historical Perspectives. *American Psychologist*. 70(7), pp. 621–631.

and *yoga-nidrā* has yet to be undertaken, and any parameters for such a study should be selected with great care, explicitly specifying which *yoga-nidrā* technique is being applied.

Scientific Research on Satyananda Yoga Nidra and the Brain

Since the 1970s, *yoga-nidrā* has been studied extensively as a method of immersion through various EEG and PET scanner examinations. The results of these studies can differ considerably from one group to another, influenced by factors such as the participants' experience levels, the measurement methods employed, and the specific *yoga-nidrā* technique used. Given the broad definition of *yoga-nidrā* outside the context of integral yoga, the neurobiological studies conducted encompass a wide range of techniques, which explains the variation in findings. Nevertheless, despite the simplified settings and the different experiences of the practitioners, these studies appear to show several common, crucial elements inherent to this type of immersive experience.

For a professional study on *yoga-nidrā* to be conducted properly, at least three further parameters must be considered as essential prerequisites in addition to the biological characteristics of the test subjects, such as sex, age, state of health, etc. These include the specific technique practiced, the amount of experience each participant has with that technique, and also whether the individual practices other awareness-expanding methods in addition to *yoga-nidrā* in their daily life, such as those offered by integral yoga. That being said, many studies have indeed specifically been done on the Satyananda Yoga Nidra method.

Most studies that examined Svāmī Satyānanda's *yoga-nidrā* method[358] used EEG equipment and PET scanners. It has been demonstrated that states of consciousness during or after the practice of *yoga-nidrā* are associated with measurable changes in brain activity.[359] *Yoga-nidra* is a 'sleepless sleep' because

358 This refers to the *pratyāhāra* variant of the Satyananda Yoga Nidra method, which has been made available for general use. It consists of the classic eight stages of the exercise, which have also been described in this book. The higher stages of this method have not yet been clinically researched.

359 Kjær and Lou (1997, 1999 and 2002), Gosh (1988) and Immink (2012).

it induces a state of deep relaxation in a short period of time and the practitioner can learn to enter the state between waking and sleeping without loss of awareness.

During the various Stages of the *yoga-nidrā* technique, all subjects displayed definite and clearly visible changes of activity in various areas of the brain. Notably, improved communication between the two hemispheres was observed, indicating a greater level of integration in brain function. The subjects also displayed a high degree of relaxed, effortless concentration. Additionally, the measurements made it clear that the test subjects were able to be fully aware in such a deep and stable state of relaxation—i.e. the brain activity indicates that the mind remains conscious and controllable during *yoga-nidrā*, highlighting the technique's potential for enhancing mental clarity while promoting relaxation.[360]

A detailed summary of the studies listed below can be found in Part III, Chapter 20 of this book: *Clinical Studies and Scientific Findings on Satyananda Yoga Nidra* and Part V. Appendix 2. *Summary of Clinical Studies and Scientific Findings on Satyananda Yoga Nidra.*

In his study, Gosh (1988)[361] concluded that practice of Satyananda Yoga Nidra leads to an alpha-wave-dominance in the brain, which is associated with mental relaxation. As Roney-Dougal (2001) also found, the EEG of the subjects initially showed pronounced beta activity with intermittent alpha activity. As the session progressed, the beta activity was slowly replaced by alpha activity and then by a consistent, well-formed alpha activity of the so-called hypnagogic/hypnopompic state. After thirty *yoga-nidrā* sessions, improved alpha activity had set in, intermittently with theta wave activity as practice progressed, indicating a deep state of relaxation.

Gosh conducted his study in a Faraday cage to eliminate interference and took measurements using Brain Electrical Activity Mapping (BEAM) at 2.5 seconds per image. The results showed that on average, subjects showed increased alpha activity during *yoga-nidrā*, which was particularly pronounced in the occipital areas of the brain during Stage 1.[362] of the practice. At the

---

360 Kjær and Lou (1997).

361 Gosh, A. K. (Mangalteertham, Sannyasi). (1988). Brain Electrical Activity Mapping During Yoga Nidra. In Yoga Research Foundation. (2015). Volume One, *YRF Journals 1989–1990*. Yoga Publication Trust & in Svami, Satyananda. (2006). *Yoga Nidra*. Chapter: Altered State of Consciousness. Bihar: Yoga Publication Trust, pp. 245–253.

362 For a full description of all Stages of the Satyananda Yoga Nidra method, see Part II.

beginning of Stage 3 — Rotation of Awareness Throughout the Body — there was higher bilateral occipital alpha activity.

At the beginning of Stage 6 — Visualisation — an asymmetric distribution of alpha waves was recorded over the occipital region, as well as an asymmetry indicating higher activity over the right hemisphere. Delta wave activity started slowly in the right hemisphere and gradually became more prominent in both hemispheres, indicating a tranquil state by the end of this stage. The emergence of an alpha blockade at Stage 3 suggested an elevated level of alertness, while the distinct slow-rhythmed delta wave pattern at Stage 6 indicated that the mind had entered a deep-sleep-like state. Remarkably, subjects maintained full consciousness throughout the experiment. By the conclusion of Stage 6 (Visualisation), there was a marked synchrony in brain activity, characterised by a very slow and low level of activity, which was visually represented by a blue coloration in the BEAM images across both hemispheres.

Studies utilising neuroimaging methods have shown clear indications that Satyananda Yoga Nidra can promote movement-related neuroplasticity. For instance, research conducted by Lou et al. (1999) demonstrated increased cerebral blood flow — a key parameter for brain activity — in several critical areas: the parietal cortex, which is responsible for sensory processing; the hippocampus, essential for long-term memory formation; and the frontal lobe, which plays a crucial role in attention, executive functions, goal setting, motivation, and strategic thinking. Enhanced activity in these regions is typically observed during the learning and execution of skilled movements.

Additionally, the study by Hobson and Pace-Schott (2002) highlighted another important effect of *yoga-nidrā*: the increase in the neurotransmitter dopamine.[363] This neurotransmitter is pivotal for various brain functions, including movement, motivation, and the regulation of mood. The elevation of dopamine levels during Satyananda Yoga Nidra suggests that this practice not only fosters relaxation but also may enhance cognitive functions and facilitate the learning process by supporting neuroplasticity. Together, these findings underscore the potential of *yoga-nidra* as a beneficial practice for brain health and development, particularly in areas related to movement

363 Dopamine is produced in the basal ganglia, which consists of a neuronal structure that is also activated during sleep.

and cognitive function. Flöel et al. (2005) demonstrated a direct relationship between increased dopamine release and the processes of learning and executing movements. Their findings align with those of Kjaer et al. (2002), which indicated that participants practicing Satyananda Yoga Nidra could achieve states characterised by theta wave EEG readings. During *yoga-nidrā*, these participants exhibited significant increases in dopamine levels. However, since most people are dopamine-deficient, it may be possible that, rather than exclusively effecting the increase in dopamine, the practice of Satyananda Yoga Nidra has a regulatory effect.

The increase in dopamine is particularly noteworthy because it is closely linked to the brain's reward and motivation systems, enhancing the learning process and reinforcing the execution of movements. The ability to reach theta states during *yoga-nidrā* suggests a deep relaxation and heightened receptivity, creating an optimal environment for cognitive processing and skill acquisition. These studies collectively highlight the neurochemical and physiological benefits of Satyananda Yoga Nidra, illustrating its potential to support not only relaxation and stress reduction but also learning and neuroplasticity related to movement and cognitive functions.

In a further study using the H215O-PET method, Kjær, Lou et al. (1999) identified differentiated activity in the posterior sensory and associative cortices during *yoga-nidrā* practice. These areas are known for their involvement in imagination tasks, highlighting the potential for enhanced creative and cognitive processes during the practice. When comparing the resting state of normal consciousness (baseline) to the *yoga-nidrā* state, the researchers observed significant differential activity in several brain regions, including the dorsolateral and orbital frontal cortex, the anterior cingulate gyrus, the left temporal gyrus, and the left inferior parietal lobule. These regions, along with the striatal and thalamic areas, as well as the pons and cerebellar vermis and hemispheres, are associated with an executive attention network.

Interestingly, the main cerebral blood flow remained unchanged in both subjects throughout the examination, suggesting that the brain activity associated with *yoga-nidrā* does not necessarily rely on increased blood flow to signify engagement. Instead, it may reflect a unique state of consciousness that allows for enhanced focus and imaginative capacity without the typical physiological demands of higher cerebral blood flow. This study provides valuable insights into the neural mechanisms underlying the effects of

Satyananda Yoga Nidra on brain function, particularly regarding executive attention and imaginative processing.

The PET image taken before and after the yoga nidra practice in the study by Kjær and Lou (1997) showed significant activations in key areas of the brain, including the forebrain, brainstem, and cerebellum. These regions are crucial for processing signals from deeper emotional and instinctual parts of the brain, as well as for facilitating readiness to act.

During the practice of *yoga-nidrā*, the PET images indicated heightened activity in the visual center located at the back of the head and the tactile center on the top of the head, both of which were in contact with the limbic system. This suggests an enhanced capacity for visualisation and emotional access during the practice, indicating that participants were able to engage more deeply with their emotions and sensory experiences.

Moreover, in some subjects, particularly those who regularly practiced Svāmī Satyānanda's *kriyā-yoga*, there was noticeable activation in the long-term memory center. This implies that their prior yoga training may have enhanced their experience and effectiveness in *yoga-nidrā*. The activation patterns varied across different Stages of the *yoga-nidrā* practice. Specifically, Stage 3 — Rotation of Awareness Throughout the Body — and Stage 6 — Visualisation — saw particularly strong activation in the visual and emotional centres. In contrast, during Stage 5 — where opposite sensations and the experiences of 'happiness' or 'joy' are emphasised — the centre responsible for speech and language comprehension exhibited heightened activity. This suggests that participants were not only visualising but also articulating and processing their emotional experiences in a way that engaged multiple cognitive functions.

Immink (2013) concluded that Stage 3 of Satyananda Yoga Nidra, which involves guiding the awareness through the body, can significantly enhance the learning curve for new physical movements and skills, hastening the acquisition process, which effect then becomes greater with the later and more subtle Stages of practice.

The sequence of particular activation of key brain areas during the different Stages of Satyananda Yoga Nidra practice can be surmised as follows:

Stage 1. Preparation and internalisation (stillness & *pratyāhāra*):

- cessation of movement (limbic system)
- reduction of tactile excitation (peripheral nervous system & somatosensory cortex)
- spatial awareness (posterior parietal cortex)
- grounding (peripheral nervous system & somatosensory cortex)
- reduction, filtering and limiting of auditory excitation (auditory cortex)

Stage 2. *saṃkalpa* (limbic system, prefrontal cortex)

Stage 3. Body Awareness (peripheral nervous system, somatosensory cortex, posterior parietal cortex)

Stage 4. Breath awareness (parasympathetic nervous system, limbic system, posterior parietal cortex)

Stage 5. Pair of opposites (peripheral nervous system, limbic system—especially the thalamus, hypothalamus, hippocampus and amygdala)

- heavy and light, cold and heat, (peripheral nervous system, thalamus, hippocampus)
- hunger and satiety (hypothalamus, hippocampus, amygdala)
- sadness and joy, fear and courage, hatred and love, etc. (amygdala, hippocampus)

Stage 6. Visualisation (occipital lobe, hippocampus, amygdala)

Stage 7. *saṃkalpa* (limbic system, prefrontal cortex)

Stage 8. Externalisation:

- reengagement of auditory excitation (auditory cortex) and spatial awareness (posterior parietal cortex)
- grounding (peripheral nervous system & somatosensory cortex)
- reengagement of tactile excitation (peripheral nervous system & somatosensory cortex)
- introducing movement (somatosensory and motor cortex)

Part Two

Svāmī Satyānanda's *yoga-nidrā*-Method in Detail

CHAPTER 11

The Tantric Principles and *yoga-nidrā*

Tantra is the science of seeing, feeling, knowing the infinite in and through the finite.[364]

Svāmī Satyānanda

GIVEN THAT SVĀMĪ SATYĀNANDA'S *YOGA-NIDRĀ* method is rooted, among other sources, in tantric principles, it is important to first place this technique within the context of the main attitudes adopted in many tantric traditions before examining each Stage in detail. In *A Systematic Course in the Ancient Tantric Techniques of Yoga and Kriya*, Svāmī Satyānanda defines Tantra as the science of expanding personal consciousness and awakening the individual's dormant energy. This is based on a traditional etymology explaining tantra as deriving from the Sanskrit verbs *tanoti* — 'to expand' and *trayate* — 'to release'.[365] Once individual consciousness has undergone certain purification

364 Saraswati, Satyananda, Swami. (2006). *A Systematic Course in The Ancient Tantric Techniques of Yoga and Kriya*. (4th reprint). Munger: Yoga Publications Trust, p. 385.

365 See Part I., Chapter 1. *Indian Schools of Thought, the Tantra subsection*.

processes and expanded, it can transcend its limitations through the awakening of the dormant energy within the body (*kuṇḍalinī-śakti*)—a concept of the subtle yogic physiology derived from the tradition of the *Haṭha-yoga-pradīpikā*.[366] This process is said to liberate individual consciousness from the bonds of existence (*saṃsāra*) and unite it with Transcendent Consciousness (*avyavahārya*).[367]

Tantric traditions often equate mind with consciousness, viewing it as the immaterial aspect of existence. The components which we typically consider to be part of the mind—such as reason, memory, and the power of discrimination—are seen in various tantric teachings as mere expressions of the mind, rather than the mind itself. Experiences arise from the impulses of the organs of perception (*indriyas*)[368] and manifest as thoughts, emotions, and insights. These experiences are material in nature, dependent on matter, and thus inherently limited.[369] When the mind is freed from material identifications, the process of inner insight occurs spontaneously and continuously. A homogeneous, independently functioning mind allows us to recognise infinite reality, which is not constrained by time, space, or objects.

The purpose of tantric approaches is to enable the seeker to experience manifest reality without necessarily renouncing the material world. Instead, the material world serves as a stepping stone to higher, incomprehensible realms. Consequently, Tantra as an approach is, in principle, accessible to everyone. Its essence lies in personal experience through practice. This practice unfolds within the context of daily life by connecting more fully with it and using it as a means to reach higher states of consciousness. As Svāmī Satyānanda describes, Tantra teaches the knowledge and experience of the macrocosm through the instruments of the microcosm.[370] However, traditionally, Tantra has almost always been an initiatory tradition and not something available to the general public.

---

366 See Part I., Chapter 1. *Indian Schools of Thought, the Sāṃkhya and Yoga subsection.*

367 See Part I., Chapter 4. *History and Origins of yoga-nidrā, the Yoga-nidrā as a Synonym for the Fourth State of Lucidity (turīya) subsection.*

368 See Part I., Chapter 1. *Indian Schools of Thought, the Key Elements of Sāṃkhya subsection.*

369 Saraswati, Satyananda, Swami. (2001). *Kundalini Tantra*. Munger: Yoga Publications Trust, p. 1.

370 Saraswati, Satyananda, Swami. (2006). *A Systematic Course in The Ancient Tantric Techniques of Yoga and Kriya*. (4th reprint). Munger: Yoga Publications Trust, p. 385.

The Main Subjects of Tantra

Tantra encompasses a vast array of topics, covering nearly every aspect of human life. The main subjects of Tantra are outlined in, for example, texts such as the *Vārāhī-tantra*[371], but there are innumerable others. These topics include consciousness, the creation and destruction of the physical universe, the worship of deities, the classification of beings, the heavenly bodies — astronomy and astrology, the different levels of existence (*lokas/bhuvanas/tattvas*), the psychic pathways and centres in the body (*nāḍīs* and *cakras*), laws and duties in society (*dharma*), sacred rites, vows and observances (*vrata*), the establishment and consecration of divine forms (*pratiṣṭhā/nyāsa*), magical formulas (*mantras*), magical geometric figures (*maṇḍalas* and *yantras*), symbolic and evocative gestures (*mudrās*), spiritual practices (*sādhanas*), external and internal worship (*pūjā*), fire offerings (*homa*), the consecration of houses, wells, etc., the description of sacred shrines, magical practices, ceremonial rites and initiations (*dīkṣā*), yoga — including *āsana*, *prāṇāyāma*, immersion methods, etc., medicine of all kinds, the use of sexual energy to develop higher consciousness, and much more. According to Svāmī Satyānanda, practical Tantra is generally summarised under three main aspects: *tantra* (which refers to the rules, principles, and system), *mantra* (power — the vehicle of consciousness), and *maṇḍala* or *yantra* (the form of consciousness). These three aspects are said to encompass everything within the material universe. Consequently, every human being can also be viewed as comprising both *mantra* and *yantra* — representing vibration and sacred form.[372] This is a particular way of viewing the person and body as a microcosm of the greater Universe.

The Meaning and Effect of Mantras

'*Mantra*' is a Sanskrit term which encompasses sounds, syllables, words or formulaic sequences of words which produce sound vibrations in specific

371 Ibid., p. 387–388.
372 Ibid., p. 388.

combinations. These vibrations are believed to hold significant power and positively influence consciousness and various aspects of life. In the context of Tantra, a mantra is regarded as a particular sound vibration capable of both extraordinary effects in the material world and of liberating the material and dualistic mind from its bonds. Mantras are not merely linguistic expressions but are deeply intertwined with sound, materiality, and bodily practices. Consequently, mantras have a cumulative effect and are often repeated several times in succession, typically recited daily, at specific intervals, or during particular occasions.

Mantras are said to possess a sonic and resonant effect and, as a rule, a metaphysical or mystical meaning. However, the precise translation of the words comprising various mantras is not necessarily of paramount importance. Many mantras lack conventional meaning (such as *oṃ*, for example); instead, the vibrations generated during their recitation, the way they permeate the body, and/or the intrinsic power they are considered to carry are key elements. These vibrations are believed to heal, harmonise and awaken the body on a subtle level. The sound waves of mantras are thought to resonate with one's own physio-mental system. In this sense, they are used as a vehicle for awakening the deeper aspects within the individual and guiding them on the path to self-realisation, according to the understanding and system of the different Indic traditions.

According to Svāmī Nirañjanānanda, in a common tantric understanding, the body is viewed as energy (*śakti*), appearing as a concrete form within the realm of human perception. This energy is highly reactive to vibrations and is so subtle and sensitive that every thought, idea, and feeling can alter its nature. The vibrations associated with different moods can remodel the body's vital energies, and when a particular mood is strong and dominant, its energy will adjust the body to align with it. Certain mantras are designed to attune the body's vital energies to specific frequencies, enabling them to vibrate in particular ways. As a state of mind gains momentum, the body becomes a conduit for that energy. Thus, one can assume that anxious energy will attract fear, while aggressive energy will draw in aggression, and empathetic energy will foster compassion. One's own quality—whether sattvic (pure, balanced, humble), tāmasic (inert, lethargic, depressed), or rajasic (active, aggressive)—also influences the energy one emits. When reciting a mantra, one should avoid attempting to focus or control the mind. In

Tantra, mantras are rarely employed as a means of concentration; rather, they are believed to have, among others, a purging effect on the mind, initially stimulating its activity as it jumps from thought to thought before settling into the vibration of the mantra and undergoing transformation. The mantra is said to generate significant power within, with the ultimate aim of permeating the entire body and mind with resonant vibrations.[373]

In some tantric traditions, it is recognised that the vibration of particular mantras has its own archetype within the deeper consciousness. As a result, the sound of such mantras can exert a distinct effect on consciousness, differing fundamentally from other sounds that can be produced. The vibrations of mantras generate specific shapes which can even be recorded using modern measuring instruments, resulting in formations such as circles, triangles, squares, and countless combinations of geometric patterns.[374] These shapes are not hypothetical, conjectural, or imaginary; rather, they are archetypes[375].

The geometric representation of a mantra is called a *yantra*. A *yantra* can be used as an object of ritual or immersion and spiritual development, but it needs the associated mantra(s) to be effective, whereas mantra can be practised independently. Therefore, the mantra is the most subtle of all the manifest forms in Tantra, since it does not require any concentration, but it does create a geometric form which transforms the mind when it focuses on it.

In Tantric techniques, mantra and *yantra* are essential parts of spiritual practice.

Expression Instead of Suppression of the Mind

In order to recognise and experience the hidden nature behind the existence of a human being, one should by no means suppress thoughts and feelings of worry, fear, passion, anxiety, etc., but rather deal with them and penetrate to

---

373 Personal notes of the author from a recording of a public lecture in Australia.

374 In the West, researchers have long explored the connection between sound and form, exemplified by Chladni's sound figures from 1787. Today, this subject is being examined by contemporary science, particularly in the field of cymatics.

375 Archetypes are universal images or figures connected with specific emotions, characteristics, and associations, stored within the subconscious. Collective archetypes evoke similar emotions and associations across generations and cultures through socio-psychological learning processes. This term was coined by C. G. Jung in the context of Western psychology.

their origin. The ultimate goal is to uproot them by no longer 'feeding' them with energy. In comparison to Patañjali's teachings, according to which the *kleśas* etc. are to be systematically weakened, in Tantra these emotions and thoughts are themselves regarded as mental energies which should be channelled before attempting to enter into deeper states of immersion. As long as they are not channelled and the mental field is not cleansed, disturbing mental energies will arise during meditation and prove to be an obstacle to progress on the spiritual path.

When during *pratyāhāra* we uncouple the sense perception from its objects, with the aim of preventing the senses from providing the mind with external stimuli, we should then deal with the mind and its stored impressions, along with the thousands of memories and experiences — and Tantra suggests doing this with an attitude of acceptance and understanding. Every thought or impression is mental energy, which is not in itself evaluated as either positive or negative. The evaluation and classification into good or bad, positive, negative, etc. has moral, religious or social roots. We tend to suppress the variegated nature of the mind as soon as we experience negatively connoted situations. We charge such experiences with strong emotions and thereby give them more weight. In this way, we create hostility and internal conflict in our own personality. We become entangled in mental and emotional tensions which rob us of valuable energy for our lives and for further development.

Tantra encourages us to confront the mind, along with all its thought patterns, with full awareness and acceptance. These patterns are inherited from our childhood, our ancestors, and our society, enabling us to function in the world. Attempting to resist, suppress, or reject the mind would be tantamount to gradual spiritual suicide.

Our role is to learn to look 'over the mind's shoulder' with full, but impartial awareness. The mind oscillates between a distant past and an uncertain future, often neglecting the present moment. We can observe this oscillation neutrally from an observer's perspective, without identification, thus granting our mind complete independence and freedom. In doing so, it breaks through its own barriers. However, dwelling in the here and now, with full awareness, must first be cultivated systematically. In Tantra, the path to this experience need not be long or arduous; it is not necessary to exert special effort to attain it. The experience is available in the here and now, present in every moment and situation of life, and must simply be recognised. It is crucially important to understand that this means neither allowing oneself to be wholly possessed by feeling or emotion to the point of losing control, nor striving to become cold and emotionless. When we identify with our feelings or emotions then awareness and consequently control have already been lost. This does not mean that one becomes detached, cold and emotionless either, where awareness and control are also lost. The aim is to engage in life fully while cultivating present, non-judgemental awareness (*draṣṭā-bhava*).

According to a study by Tseng and Poppenk (2020)[376] the human brain experiences approximately 6.5 thought transitions per minute, resulting in more than 6,000 thoughts per day for the average young adult. These predominantly unconscious thoughts create a substantial traffic flow in the brain. During our yoga practice, we should become aware of this traffic congestion without getting emotionally involved or making judgments. Yoga techniques which lead to the *pratyāhāra* state, particularly immersion through mantra, naturally stimulate a surge of thoughts. The aim is to allow these thoughts to flow freely so that the mind can gradually settle into a deeper, more subtle experience. This requires interrupting the sensory impressions which constantly engage us during immersion. The mind becomes isolated, allowing us to observe the endless play it engages in without tiring. As our practice progresses, we gradually achieve a more homogeneous state of mind, characterised by the step-by-step integration of all levels of thought. Therefore, Tantra practitioners do not seek to eliminate certain expressions of the mind while favouring others; instead, they aim to interrupt the insatiable hunger for experience and grow beyond it.

Svāmī Satyānanda studied tantric scriptures which adopt this approach and explored many significant, yet lesser-known practices. After practising and examining them, he developed a method he claimed corresponded to a state described in various tantric and non-tantric texts, which he named *yoga-nidrā*[377]. This method aimed to encapsulate only the essence of the tantric practices, without resorting to the challenging vows and rituals usually associated with them.[378] In this way, by systematising the practice principles

---

376 Tseng, J. & Poppenk, J. (2020). Brain meta-state transitions demarcate thoughts across task contexts exposing the mental noise of trait neuroticism. *Nature communications*. 11(1), 3480. https://doi.org/10.1038/s41467–020-17255–9 (accessed on 07.11.2022).

377 See Part 1, Chapter 4. *History and Origin of yoga-nidrā*.

378 Saraswati, Satyananda, Swami. (1979). The Path of Experience. Satsang (Lecture). *Yoga Magazine*. 1980(3). Munger: Yoga Publication Trust.

from multiple sources, he also distilled the essence of the approach, also leaving out the explicit theistic elements (both dualistic and non-dualistic) of the respective religious, philosophical and yoga traditions he drew upon. Thus, he made the essential Stages of his method accessible to the modern practitioner, without the need for strict observances or restriction to a particular religious or social background.

The Practitioner's Attitude in Satyananda Yoga Nidra: No Need to Wilfully Concentrate

When practising the *yoga-nidrā* method developed by Svāmī Satyānanda, the practitioner should adopt an open and unbiased attitude. As previously mentioned, concentration is often associated with effort and control, particularly in the West. However, *yoga-nidrā* is about entering the practice free of expectations and being open to its effects. It is not about forceful control of the mind and body, which will bring tension instead. During the session, our perception flows fluidly from one point to another, enabling us to delve deeper into our essence.[379] The practitioner's focus should not be on rigidly adhering to the facilitator's instructions but rather on maintaining the uninterrupted flow of perception.

As a result, the incessant chatter of thoughts recedes from everyday consciousness, while the practitioner remains alert and does not fall asleep. In this phase, the initial stages of *pratyāhāra* occur, allowing the practitioner to simultaneously experience the inner observer and their own body. In this state of stillness, the body reduces the signals it sends to the brain, which facilitates both physical and mental relaxation. As physical, mental, and emotional tensions are released, energy (*prāṇa*) can once again flow freely throughout the body and more advanced practices can be undertaken.

---

379 Saraswati, Satyananda, Swami. (2006). *Yoga Nidra*. (12th reprint). Munger: Yoga Publications Trust, p. 27.

CHAPTER 12

Further Important Principles: Yogic Immersion vs 'Meditation'

Yoga-nidrā IS OFTEN MISTAKENLY DESCRIBED in the West as a 'meditation technique'. In modern parlance, however, the term is used indiscriminately to conflate a wide variety of techniques and practices. In order to understand the *yoga-nidrā* state and what it entails, it is essential to examine how the term 'meditation' is used today. Originating from the Latin *meditatio* — meaning 'mental reflection' or 'preparation' — the term 'meditation' is typically used to describe methods which cultivate a mostly cognitive contemplative state. In Western interpretations of yogic immersion (which may be of many types and forms and use different means), 'meditation' often relates to the yogic concepts of the 'interactive mind' (*manas*) and the 'intellect' (*buddhi*), however, the term is not usually used to refer to an experience which engages all aspects of the mind (i.e. the *antaḥkaraṇa*). By contrast, the yogic term '*dhyāna*' (i.e., 'prolonged focused awareness'), for example, describes a state of deep immersion involving the entire mind (or consciousness, depending on the tradition). It denotes a stage/state preceding enlightenment/liberation/spiritual emancipation/awakening rather than a technique or method for achieving these.[380] As previously noted, there exists no single Sanskrit term for 'meditation', which captures all the various states of immersion as an abstraction or an overarching category; instead, distinct terms exist for each particular state/practice.

The Problematic of the Term 'Meditation' in Brief

In the West, the terms 'contemplation' and 'meditation' refer both to a state of focused, absorbed awareness and to a range of practices intended to help us reach such a state. However, 'meditation' is also indiscriminately used as a blanket term for all of the following: a) the different states of immersion, concentration, and contemplation, b) the techniques and methods for entering/achieving them, and c) states which are both achieved by the practitioner themselves and those, which are externally facilitated. In this book, however, an effort has been made to use the respective Sanskrit terms for the different states and methods for achieving them, both for the sake of maximum possible clarity, and to try and dispel the vague mysticism usually associated with the term 'meditation' in the West. This does not mean that the term 'meditation' couldn't or shouldn't be used. The issue is, that yoga (in its higher levels especially) deals with deep and extremely subtle forms of immersion and using a single word to simultaneously refer to all levels thereof, to all techniques and methods for achieving them, across multiple quite different traditions may easily create the false impression in the practitioner that 'anything goes'. That false impression could be that a) the states in question are all the same, and b) that the practitioner is achieving or has achieved such high states of immersion, absorption or enlightenment, which are usually accessible only after, for example, establishing and becoming proficient in the *drāṣṭā* stance, mastering *pratyāhāra*, and having systematically dealt with the different aspects of the mind, for which a qualified and experienced guide

380 It must be noted that *dhyāna* in tantric Buddhist and Śaiva yoga may, in fact, refer to visualisation. This is not the case in this context. Further see the *Tāntrikābhidhānakośa* volume III. entry for *dhyāna*. Goodall, D. & Rastelli, M. (Eds.). (2013). *Tāntrikābhidhānakośa* III, T–Ph: Wörterbuch zur Terminologie hinduistischer Tantren (Reihe: Beiträge zur Kultur- und Geistesgeschichte Asiens, Band 76). Wien: Verlag der Österreichischen Akademie der Wissenschaften, pp. 238–239.

is necessary in the vast majority of cases. It is also not unheard of in Indic traditions that such states may arise spontaneously, but this usually happens to either saints or madmen and occurs only under extraordinary circumstances.

Furthermore, the aims of 'meditation', as commonly understood in the West, and the different states of immersion, as understood in the East and historically, are different. Often, the goal of 'meditation' is suggested to be creating 'peace of mind', 'inner peace', 'to feel connected with your heart', 'to feel connected with myself/oneself', 'to feel connected with everyone', 'to feel connected with the world', 'to be filled with love', 'self-love', 'loving everyone' which build up the expectation of achieving such vague and ill-definable conditions. This is, ironically, diametrically opposed to the process of cultivating the objective observer stance (*draṣṭā*) and actually dealing with the mind in all its aspects. Convincing oneself that one has achieved such 'goals' is what is unfortunately commonly described as 'being spiritual'.

To briefly unpack the above, concepts such as 'loving everyone' or 'to be filled with love' have a distinctly religious Chirstian flavour and one would be hard-pressed to compare them to, for example, Buddhist universal compassion for all beings, which is distinctly different. In Advaita, or in Sāṃkhya, on the other hand, universal love plays no part in achieving liberation. 'Feeling connected with myself/oneself' is equally vague and ill-defined. There is no consensus in the West on the concept of the Self (such as in Vedānta) or the lack thereof (such as in Buddhism). The closest one comes is either Christian belief of the soul, or psychoanalytical concepts such as the ID or the ego.[381] Things such as 'feeling connected with your heart' or 'peace of mind', while marginally more relevant than the former, in an Eastern context would describe either aspects of an immersion practice, preparation for one, or a technique employed in one — not necessarily the aim. 'Feeling connected with the world' comes closest to being similar to the aim of immersion in the East, such as unification with or realisation of the Highest Self, realisation of Emptiness, etc., however, much like the other 'aims' of 'meditation' in the West, what 'connected with the world' is actually supposed to mean is left more or less to the opinion of the practitioner and not subject to objective assessment or criteria. Most Indic systems have such criteria.

381 In Freudian psychoanalysis, the ID is the unconscious source of all innate needs, emotional impulses and desires, including the sexual drive, and the ego is that part of the ID which has been modified by the direct influence of the external world.

Furthermore, Eastern techniques of immersion can be very powerful, even when badly practiced or incomplete and can have equally powerful side effects. These side effects, such as some degree of extrasensory perception, for example, can be a serious problem even if the methods have been applied after proper preparation, under proper qualified guidance, let alone when done in an incomplete, inexperienced and/or unsupervised way. Alternatively, the powerful effect may, in the end, even have a result opposite to the intended one. For example, the expectation to 'feel love' while using Eastern methods of immersion, which by default will force oneself to confront the negativity and the suppressed aspects of the mind, will result in the unwanted effect of feeling that 'my meditation wasn't nice'. Instead of diffusing the negative expressions of the ego, such ill-conceived hybrid practices may well end up cultivating them.

Trying to achieve Western goals with Eastern methods is problematic in many aspects and can even be dangerous, because facing the mind needs systematic preparation and qualified guidance, otherwise it can result in mental and psychological disorders, such as dissociation.[382]

The Benefits of Yogic Immersion: *pratyāhāra*

There are various methods, which can lead to different degrees of immersion, available for practice in yoga. The first immersive state which needs to be systematically mastered is *pratyāhāra*. Techniques of immersion following this method are not necessarily always practiced in complete stillness but sitting, walking, dancing, or through the use of mantras. The Satyananda Yoga Nidra method available for the general practitioner is precisely a *pratyāhāra* practice. In its advanced stages, it has the potential to guide practitioners towards a deeper state of *dhāraṇā*.[383] Consequently, some general concepts and principles relating to the inner attitude necessary for practising immersive techniques need to be discussed first.

382 See Part III., Chapter 17. *Yoga-nidrā and Western Psychology, Yoga-nidrā and Hypnosis*.

383 Maintaining true concentration or the right focus, which leads to a meditative state.

Yogic immersive practices can have many positive effects. The most frequently observed are:

- improved physical health: normalised blood pressure and reduced muscle tension and pain;
- improvements at the psychological level, such as increased mental balance and calmness in general, which in turn support the development of self-regulation and resilience;
- improved mental function — clear and generally more constructive outlook on life, improved memory and increased ability to concentrate;
- supportive effect in finding meaning and increased fulfilment in life, deepening of self-understanding and strengthening of self-acceptance, further development of the ability to live life according to our innate vocation (*dharma*).

Some Important Fundamentals

- **The *āsana***

Sitting in a stable posture is a fundamental aspect of most immersion practices. Preparatory *āsanas* develop the strength and flexibility necessary for maintaining a seated posture over extended periods. The Bihar Yoga *āsana*-series *pavana-muktāsana* 1[384] is particularly effective for this purpose, as its movements enhance flexibility in the joints of the feet, knees, and hips while promoting stability. For beginners, a recommended approach is to start with short sitting sessions, gradually extending the duration over time. Regular practice of the seated position increases both stamina and comfort.

To protect the knee joints, conscious and aware movements into and out of the meditative *asana* are essential. Folded blankets or cushions can

---

384 Saraswati, Satyanana, Swami. (2009). *Asana, Pranayama, Mudra, Bandha*. (reprint). Munger: Yoga Publication Trust, pp. 23–44.

be placed under the buttocks or knees, and meditation stools or chairs may also be used to help maintain an upright back.

- **The *mudrās*[385]**

In meditation practice, the 'hand gesture of knowledge and wisdom' (*jñāna-mudrā*) or 'the inner gesture of consciousness' (*cin-mudrā*) are most commonly used. They help to direct the flow of *prāṇa* in the body and the mind inwards.

- **The sequence (*krama*) of the method**

At the beginning of the practice, we sit in a comfortable and stable *āsana*, developing calmness (*sukha*) and stability (*sthairya*); then we focus the awareness on body stillness (*kāya-sthairyam*), on the breath, collect the mind spontaneously in preparation for a particular immersive technique. This is followed by the technique itself, and finally, we gradually transition back out of the subtle inner dimension of practice by means of a step-by-step externalisation. Each of these phases may last a short or long time, depending on the practitioner's individual needs and proficiency, as well as the specific technique.

- **The awareness: being established in awareness**

During the process of immersion, we 'become aware' and advance towards 'being established in awareness'. That is why, when speaking about deeper stages of immersion, 'awareness' means 'being established in awareness'. Becoming aware involves increasingly realising specific objects of focus, which process may include external elements, such as parts of the body, or it may involve internal aspects, such as mental processes. What currently occupies the mind, and what is it observing?

- **The observer (*draṣṭā*)**

The agent of awareness is the uninvolved observer — the *draṣṭā*. The cultivation of this neutral observer is a direct component of many yoga techniques.

---

385 *Mudrās* are hand and body positions in yoga which direct *prāṇa*.

It is a core aspect of *pratyāhāra* practices, *yoga-nidrā*, *kāya-sthairyam* ('body stillness'), and, in a broader sense, the *draṣṭā* is a feature of all yoga techniques, ideally extending to all life experiences.

The observer's attitude — *draṣṭā-bhāva* — should ideally be maintained throughout the immersion process, from start to finish. To attain and preserve a quiet state of mind (*sukha*), it is essential to develop and refine the ability to observe (*dṛṣṭi*), aspiring to become an uninvolved, impartial witness to all that is experienced during immersion — whether the body, breath, or the stream of thoughts. This results in the process of purifying the mind and aims at observing the object of focus neutrally and attentively, without reacting to, analysing, or attempting to change what is observed. The practice of *pratyāhāra* is also integral to *dhyāna*, ultimately enabling one to remain unaffected by the challenges and complexities of daily life.

With the cultivation of the inner observer, both *pratyāhāra* practice and one's own life can be enhanced by the following abilities:

- increasing disidentification[386] with the distractions caused by sense perceptions and the mind as a prerequisite for achieving the state of *pratyāhāra*;
- 'undisturbed sitting', regardless of the experiences which occur during practice (or in everyday life), without falling back into emotional attachments or identifications;
- purification (*śodhana*) of the mind by releasing thoughts, emotions and experiences which would otherwise remain trapped or suppressed within us;
- developing a better understanding of the Self, the mind and emotions by observing the underlying patterns of the mind in our lives.

- *pratyāhāra*

The term *pratyāhāra* refers to the state which arises when the mind focuses away from external sense objects. In the usual waking state, the mind is directed outward, following sensory perceptions — what one sees, hears,

386 On the fundamental differences between disidentification and dissociation and its significance, see Part III., Chapter 17: *Yoga-nidrā and Western Psychology*, the subsection on *Dissociation vs. Disidentification*.

smells, tastes, and physically experiences. The initial phase of immersion practice involves observing and gradually neutralising the mind's engagement with sensory activities, ultimately withdrawing awareness from thoughts about the world, which preoccupy us as objects, concepts, and their associated feelings, fantasies, and so forth. Through this process, sensory perceptions can be trained to follow the mind. Dreaming and daydreaming are familiar examples of *pratyāhāra*-like states, where there is, however, little to no control over the process.

- **The focused state of being (Concentration)**

'Meditation' is often linked to concentration. However, concentration is generally associated with mental effort, willpower (*icchā*), and the suppression of unwanted impressions — resulting in a state of mental tension which can actually hinder immersion. However, the concentration aimed for in yogic immersion is instead a calm, mentally focused state of being, which arises gradually and naturally as a result of systematic practice rather than something which is practiced.

- **The process of mental purification**

Purification (*śodhana*) of the mind is an essential outcome of *pratyāhāra*. Just as *āsanas* and other *haṭha-yoga* purification practices cleanse the body, specific immersion practices purify the mind on multiple levels. This mental purification involves observing the mind's activities and releasing emotional and thought patterns which have a restrictive effect. The process can be intense, often presenting a broad spectrum of unexpectedly emerging images and emotions. For this reason, a gradual introduction to immersion practice and to the act of observing is of great importance.

- **Regularity of the practice**

Regularity of practice (*abhyāsa*) is essential, as the cumulative effects become evident only with consistent practice; little can be achieved through occasional practice alone. One should aim to establish a habit of practicing regularly, which contributes to a healthy, fulfilled, and balanced life.

• Trust and motivation

For the practice to bear fruit, it is essential to practise regularly, with complete trust (*śraddhā*) in the process and with dedication (*pratiṣṭhā*). Maintaining regularity in daily life can be challenging, so it is important to find ways to keep motivation refreshed. Inspiration may come from reading spiritual texts, listening to lectures by masters (*satsaṅga*), and, above all, from spending time with like-minded individuals (*saṅga*)—those who pursue similar goals and share similar perspectives.

> PLEASE NOTE: As mentioned above, immersion practices can be quite intense and should be gradually introduced into your yoga practice programme. It is highly advisable to seek the guidance of a qualified teacher. Certain techniques are contraindicated for people who are overly introverted or prone to depression, or who suffer from other symptoms of mental imbalance. For these individuals, guidance from a qualified teacher would be necessary and useful—even before they begin any immersive practice.

CHAPTER 13

Svāmī Satyānanda's *yoga-nidrā* Method

Approach Towards Practising *yoga-nidrā*

Svāmī Satyānanda's *yoga-nidrā* method induces a state in which all levels of being are more open to our awareness. To enable this, the *yoga-nidrā* method follows a fixed, systematic sequence which should remain unchanged from the initial to the advanced stages of the practice. The practitioner is systematically guided from the external level of perception into deeper levels of inner awareness and back to externalisation again. Each distinct, logically structured step remains clearly recognisable to the practitioner.

The benefits of *yoga-nidrā* extend beyond relaxation, restored vitality, and psycho-emotional purification, all of which arise naturally with correct practice. *Yoga-nidrā* also offers a means to address longstanding thought and behavioural patterns, unresolved negative memories, emotions, and desires. Through *yoga-nidrā*, we can experience deeper aspects of the Self and discover our vocation in life. As habitual thought and feeling patterns (*kleṣas*) and forms of old conditioning (*saṃskāras* and *pratyayas*) dissolve, the intuitive and creative aspects of our Self are gradually revealed.

To progress effectively through the stages of *yoga-nidrā*, self-study (*svādhyāya*) is essential. It is beneficial to take time to become aware of personal insights and to identify tools which help confront harmful or troubling old patterns and feelings. The more consciously we engage in this process, the more we allow our unconscious thoughts and feelings to surface into conscious awareness. This enables us to discern precisely which feelings, desires, and beliefs are beneficial and which have a destructive impact and, therefore, should and can be released.

> Without professional guidance and support from a teacher during the practice, you may find yourself stuck in an endless loop of what you already know about yourself. Constantly reflecting on your issues in the same manner tends to yield the same results.

Our task is to explore new ways of thinking and acting which constructively and effectively support us on the path to greater awareness. Ideally, these approaches should encompass both the conscious and subconscious aspects of our minds, illuminating our thoughts and actions while motivating us to persist on this path. This change rarely occurs simply through reading a book. Intellectual knowledge, without practical application, as well as practice without study, are both insufficient in yoga; we learn and continually develop through our direct experience, and deepen our understanding of that experience by study.

Attitude and Preparation

Yoga-nidrā is practised in the corpse posture (*śavāsana*[387]) in which the body is best supported by the floor. In this pose, the deep muscles can also completely relax. It is important to actually lie on the floor, not in bed or on a mattress or other soft surface, as residual tension remains in the muscles and body which cannot be completely released on a softer surface. In *śavāsana*, all joints and

---

387 For a detailed description of *śavāsana*, see Part III, Chapter 19. *Absence of Tension Through śavāsana and yoga-nidrā.*

body parts are brought into the position which is most comfortable. Physical contact and sensory stimulation of the brain are reduced to a minimum.

Ideally, one should do a few preparatory *āsanas* before lying down in *śavāsana* to release stiffness and general tension in the body, such as the series of *pavana-muktāsana*[388]. He also recommends *sarvāṅgāsana, halāsana, matsyāsana, paścimottānāsana, bhujaṅgāsana, śalabhāsana, naukāsanai*[389] or a few repetitions of *sūrya-namas-kāra.*[390] *Trāṭaka* (gazing at a point, usually at the red tip of the ignited wick of a candle) increases the effectiveness of *yoga-nidrā* when done beforehand. Alternatively, *śāmbhavī-mudrā* (focusing on the eyebrow centre) or *nāsikāgra-dṛṣṭi* (focusing on the tip of the nose) can be practised[391].

Swami Satyananda's recommendations for practising *yoga-nidrā*[392]

Yoga-nidrā should not be practiced immediately after meals.

- The important point in *yoga-nidrā*, as well as other meditation practices, is that you must not allow yourself to fall asleep. In *yoga-nidrā* sleep tries to overpower you. [...] If sleep comes, concentrate on the body or on the sleep itself as if it is trying to possess you and you are watching it.
- If images arise before your mind, go on watching them.
- In *yoga-nidrā*, when you feel that you are unconscious, it actually means that you are conscious of being unconscious, but if you sleep, if you lose your consciousness, then it is *nidrā*, sleep, and not *yoga-nidrā*. Therefore, in *yoga-nidrā* the mind is not allowed to concentrate

388 These, Svāmī Satyānanda developed on the basis of an already existing series of 'subtle exercises' (*sūkṣma vyāyāma*) by Svāmī Dhīrendra Brahmacārī and, some say, exercises from traditional Indian dance and the martial arts. However, there is no known reference for this claim. See Saraswati, Satyanana, Swami. (2009). *Asana, Pranayama, Mudra, Bandha*. (reprint). Munger: Yoga Publication Trust, for more details.

389 See *Asana, Pranayama, Mudra, Bandha* for detailed descriptions and instructions regarding the practice and contraindications of these *āsanas*.

390 Saraswati, Satyananda, Swami. (2006). *Yoga Nidra*. (12th reprint). Munger: Yoga Publications Trust, p. 76.

391 Saraswati, Satyanana, Swami. (2013). *Yoga Nidra – Water the Roots* 4. Munger: Yoga Publications Trust, p. 7.

392 From ibd., p. 7–8.

or unite at one particular point, but it is made to move from point to point.

- It is always better to practice *yoga-nidrā* either with someone (a teacher) or with the help of a recording. If one practices *yoga-nidrā* by oneself without a guiding facilitator or recording, there is a problem. You will retain your memory, your intellectual awareness throughout the practice and that should not be the case. The instructions should be the same, but it is better if they are recorded. Day after day, the same technique should be repeated. The emphasis, the sentences, the arrangement, everything should be the same point by point; nothing should differ.
- The individual consciousness becomes so sensitive and receptive during the practice of *yoga-nidrā* that if you try to influence yourself you can (as in Stage 2—*saṃkalpa*). This indicates the importance of the deeper layers of the consciousness. There are much deeper, higher and more potential states of individual awareness than we are aware of at this moment. Every state of consciousness has its own limitations of experience. The particular state of consciousness in which we exist now is more limited than the subconscious state which one usually experiences in *yoga-nidrā*. In this psychic sleep there is a greater possibility to induce a new system of thinking, a new process of adjustment and also an absolutely new process of tranquillity.[393]

Further Thoughts on Why the Practice of *yoga-nidrā* Should Be Led by an External Facilitator

Perhaps the question would naturally arise, why, like with any technique, one shouldn't start to practice *yoga-nidrā* by guiding oneself after having gained some experience with the practice being led by a facilitator? After all, many traditional yoga texts and approaches focus on the need for individual practice and effort, so why can't Svāmī Satyānanda's *yoga-nidrā* method be practiced on one's own?

393 See Part II. Chapter 14. *Foundation of the Eight Stages*, Stage 2 – *saṃkalpa* – *the Essence of yoga-nidrā*.

> *Yoga-nidrā* being led by an external facilitator eliminates the need to keep track of the complex sequence of shifts of awareness and visualisations which would undoubtedly cause tension and steal focus away from its proper objects and thus lessen or completely eliminate its beneficial effects.

Although there is no historical source specifically teaching *yoga-nidrā* as a technique facilitated by an external guide, the principle itself is well-established in various tantric traditions. In many schools of Śaiva and Śākta Tantra, for example, disciples are often guided through initiation and ritual by a qualified master, resulting in profound leaps in spiritual development and attainment. This approach bypasses the rational, waking state of mind, allowing direct access to deeper levels of consciousness. Similarly, in the narrative of the *Mārkaṇḍeya-purāṇa*, Yoganidrā, although an aspect of Viṣṇu's, consciousness is still a force which exerts an external influence on him, rather than it being actively initiated by him.[394] Inversely, if such practices are attempted on one's own, there are great dangers which are difficult to avoid, including permanent madness.

The difference between subliminal suggestion, propaganda or hypnosis and *yoga-nidrā* is that the latter is done consciously, with awareness, the practitioner is in complete control and the facilitator does not attempt to influence them in any way.[395] Reviewing again the complex yoga path outlined by Patañjali, it becomes clear that, although possible, the solitary pursuit of extinguishing the *citta-vṛttis* through personal effort is a complex and serious undertaking, likely achievable only by the most dedicated yogins. In contrast, Svāmī Satyānanda's *yoga-nidrā* method places the responsibility of tracking the stages of practice and their specifics in the hands of an experienced, qualified facilitator. This allows the practitioner to focus solely on maintaining awareness of the object they are guided to observe at any given moment. By employing this approach effectively, he has significantly eased access to progress along the yoga path, which had been heavily restricted by the need to arduously practice for many long years in order to get to the stage where one can directly address the *citta-vṛttis* by *dharaṇa*, *dhyana* and *samadhi*, as is, for example, in Patañjali's system.

---

394 See Part I. Chapter 4. *History and Origins of yoga-nidrā, the subsection on The Goddess Yoganidrā and the Sleep of Viṣṇu.*

395 See Part III. Chapter 17. *Yoga-nidrā and Western Psychology; Yoga-nidrā and Hypnosis.*

The Eight Stages of Svāmī Satyānanda's *yoga-nidrā* Method — an Overview

Svāmī Satyānanda's *yoga-nidrā* method[396] integrates principles from tantric techniques, guiding awareness without requiring deep prolonged one-pointedness with regard to any single point or Stage of the practice. Awareness moves from the gross to the subtle sheaths of being — from the sheath of the physical body (*annamaya-kośa*) to the sheath of vital energy (*prāṇamaya-kośa*) and the mental-emotional sheath (*manomaya-kośa*) to the wisdom sheath (*vijñānamaya-kośa*) and the bliss sheath (*ānandamaya-kośa*)[397]. This progression can be approximately mapped as follows:

Stage 1 (Preparation) for *yoga-nidrā*: our awareness moves in the area of *annamaya-kośa*.
Stage 2 (*saṃkalpa*): *manomaya-kośa* is addressed.
Stage 3 (Rotation of Awareness Through the Body): the subtle connections between *anamaya-kośa*, *prāṇamaya-kośa* and *manomaya-kośa* are utilised.
Stage 4 (Breath Awareness): the awareness is connected with *prāṇamaya-kośa* and prepared for the next Stage.
Stage 5 (Pairs of Opposites): *manomaya-kośa* is addressed.
Stage 6 (Visualisation): the transition from *manomaya-kośa* to *vijñānmāyā-kośa* becomes possible.
Stage 7 (*saṃkalpa*): reaffirms our resolve at the *manomaya-kośa* level, and the final
Stage 8 (Externalisation): leads our awareness back to *annamaya-kośa*.

Each of the eight Stages, aside from Stage 2 (*saṃkalpa*), is in itself a tantric 'meditation'. The Satyananda Yoga Nidra technique which is appropriate for most people focuses on the process of *pratyāhāra* — the purification of impressions stored in the subconscious. Advanced *yoga-nidrā* stages and techniques such as *dhāraṇā-yoga-nidrā* can be learned from an experienced master.

---

396 See Part I. Chapter 5. *Pratyāhāra as Foundation for yoga-nidrā.*

397 See Part I. Chapter 8. *Pañcakośa – the five shells of being.*

Stage 1—Preparation

After the body is settled in *śavāsana*, the observer stance, known as *draṣṭā-bhāva*, is adopted. The sense perceptions and the mind are gradually drawn into *pratyāhāra*, and this state is further deepened throughout the practice. In this way, awareness is prepared for the experience of *yoga-nidrā*. In the first stage, principles of the tantric method of *kāya-sthairyam*, or body stillness, is applied, where awareness is systematically guided through the body to cultivate a deeper physical stillness and a certain disidentification with the physical body. Further, the awareness is deepened through elements of the tantric technique *antar-mauna*, the 'inner silence'. Without the facilitator explicitly instructing practitioners to relax, relaxation naturally unfolds as awareness is directed through the body—from the breath to the senses, to sounds, to touch, and so forth. After some time, the mind gradually loses interest in external stimuli, comes to rest, and is systematically guided into the initial stage of *pratyāhāra*, the withdrawal of the mind from external sensory objects.

Stage 2—Resolve (*saṃkalpa*)

Saṃkalpa is an essential element of the practice and a powerful tool for constructively remodelling one's personality and attitude to life. It is a concise, positive statement of intent or vow which builds strength and direction within the mind's framework. Choosing the *saṃkalpa* carefully is crucial, and it should not be changed until it has fully manifested in one's life. Practising *yoga-nidrā* harmonises and integrates the brain's right and left hemispheres, bridging conscious thought and unconscious awareness. The *saṃkalpa* influences habitual patterns, giving the subconscious a directive to shift and reshape inner structures. In a state of deep stillness and relaxation, the *saṃkalpa* finds its way into the subconscious, charged with full trust and strong willpower, alongside the conviction that it is already taking root in one's life. One should avoid dwelling on how the intention will be realised and refrain from holding specific expectations. We first create our reality on a spiritual-mental level, so that the *saṃkalpa*, generated internally during *yoga-nidrā*, can manifest in life seemingly of its own accord.

Stage 3 — Rotation of Awareness Throughout the Body

This stage of *yoga-nidrā* can be traced back to the practice known as '*nyāsa*' — applied in both Vedic ritual and later tantric practice — in which awareness is directed through various parts of the body, each linked to a corresponding mantra. Svāmī Satyānanda adapted this technique, making it accessible by replacing the mantra with the name of each body part. It is essential to follow the same sequence when moving through the body to prevent any disruption of the subconscious mind. No concentration is required; awareness is simply directed through the body parts in rapid succession while the body remains completely still. The body parts mentioned should be felt and visualised, and the names of the body parts should be repeated internally. This unifies body and mind, facilitating the release of prāṇic (vital-energetic) blockages. At more advanced levels of practice, it evolves to include mentally repeating the specific mantras for each body part.

The sequence developed by Svāmī Satyānanda begins with the right thumb and moves to the fifth toe of the right foot; it then follows a circuit from the left thumb to the fifth toe of the left foot, continuing along the back of the body — from the heels to the back of the head, or sometimes starting from the buttocks to the back of the head, and then moving from the head and facial features down the front of the body. At this stage, consciousness is connected to the body sheath (*annamaya-kośa*), the vital energy sheath (*prāṇamaya-kośa*), and the mental-emotional sheath (*manomaya-kośa*). This establishes *pratyāhāra* of the physical body.

Stage 4 — Breath Awareness

In this stage, awareness is directed at subtler levels, focusing on the natural movement of the breath within specific areas: at the navel, centre of the chest, the throat pit, the 'frontal passage'[398] (the front of the body from the navel to the throat), and the nostrils. The breath is observed in its natural flow, without any attempt to alter or control it. Counting backwards mentally (starting from 11, 27, 54, or 108 breaths) helps to deepen relaxation, though the goal is not to reach one, but rather to sustain an uninterrupted

398 See Part II. Chapter 15. *Awareness of the Subtle Breath in yoga-nidrā*.

awareness of the breath. This breath awareness enhances both relaxation and immersion, linking awareness to the vital energy sheath (*prāṇamaya-kośa*). In this way, *pratyāhāra* is initiated from the subtle body and sustained into the next Stages.

Stage 5 — Pairs of Opposites

At this stage, immersion and disidentification are further deepened at the level of feelings and emotions. Physical or emotional sensations are deliberately recalled, fully experienced and then neutralised in pairs of opposite physical sensations such as heaviness — lightness, cold — warmth and, in advanced stages, in emotions such as pain — pleasure, sadness — joy, etc.

Our lives are often governed by attraction (*rāga*) and aversion (*dveṣa*). We are drawn to what we perceive as pleasant and seek to avoid what we find unpleasant, oscillating between attachment and aversion as a dual aspect of all life experiences. One of the primary aims on the spiritual path is to transcend this duality in order to achieve inner maturity. Cultivating the ability to recall impressions and memories, along with the simultaneous experience of contrasting sensations is a valuable skill on this path. Adopting the stance of the *draṣṭā* — the uninvolved observer — stimulates and integrates the neural pathways of the brain's two hemispheres above what is possible in ordinary states.[399] This process creates a better balance and integration between brain centres, fostering harmony between our inner and outer environments. In turn, it enhances our ability to consciously integrate emotional and physiological responses, manifesting in daily life as refined sensory perception, emotional stability, and greater inner balance.

The mind, however, quickly becomes saturated by any evoked feeling and spontaneously shifts to a neutral or opposing sensation. Therefore, each sensation should be experienced only briefly. In this Stage, awareness is connected to the mental sheath (*manomaya-kośa*), which supports the *pratyāhāra* of the mind.

---

399 See Part IV. and Part V. for an overview of scientific studies concerning the different psycho-physiologcal effects of *yoga-nidrā*.

Stage 6—Visualisation

The Stage of visualisation enhances inner awareness. The facilitator names and rapidly repeats images of archetypes—free of connotations, meaning they are neither positive nor negative—such as images of nature, everyday objects, or symbols representing the elements. This practice aims to bring the underlying contents of the subconscious and unconscious mind to the surface of consciousness. These archetypes can provoke the purification of disturbing or painful mental material. Our mental material typically remains closed to perception, leading to subconscious tension which may contribute to illness and inner stress. This process helps release stored experiences, both negative and positive, and promotes mental relaxation. However, it is not a practice of concentration, nor does it engage the rational, analytical mind. The stance of *draṣṭā*—the uninvolved observer—is maintained throughout, and is what is essential.

> The visualisation stage of *yoga-nidrā* is often misunderstood. It is not a fantasy journey, a guided imagery journey[400], visualisation meditation, inner voyage of healing, etc., nor should it contain suggestive images. The symbols used in *yoga-nidrā* are universal archetypes neutral in nature, and the facilitator must carefully select them to avoid causing confusion for the practitioner. These archetypes are named in rapid succession to help keep the practitioner in a receptive and aware state. Initially, visualising these images may prove challenging, but this ability will develop with time and practice.

This phase of the practice can also strengthen memory and foster creativity. According to Svāmī Satyānanda, this stage guides the mind towards focused awareness (*dhāraṇā*) and, in more advanced stages, to prolonged immersive focused awareness (*dhyāna*). In these advanced stages, there is a conscious experience of the visualised object emerging from the unconscious, with no further distracting images arising.[401] Consciousness is linked to the mental-emotional sheath (*manomaya-kośa*) and the wisdom sheath

400 A technical term used in fields such as hypnotherapy and positive psychology.

401 Saraswati, Satyananda, Swami. (2006). *Yoga Nidra*. (12th reprint). Munger: Yoga Publications Trust, p. 57–58.

(*vijñānamaya-kośa*), facilitating deeper immersion in *pratyāhāra*. The ultimate goal is to reach the bliss sheath (*anandamaya-kośa*) and the fourth state of consciousness, known as *turīya*.

Stage 7—Resolve (*saṃkalpa*)

At the end of the practice, the subconscious is highly receptive to the 'planting' of the resolve, and the *saṃkalpa* is repeated in the same manner as at the beginning, with complete faith and conviction that it will be fulfilled. This reinforces the resolve within the subconscious.

Stage 8—Externalisation

The awareness is now gradually led back outwards in reverse order, by returning to the external sounds, the environmental stimuli and the physical body, and connecting with them.

In the next chapter, we will examine each Stage of Svāmī Satyānanda's *yoga-nidrā* method in detail and explore their origin.

CHAPTER 14

Foundations of the Eight Stages

Stage 1 — Preparation

After settling into *śavāsana*, the observer stance (*draṣṭā-bhāva*) is adopted, and the senses gradually withdrawn into *pratyāhāra*. The practice begins with the tantric technique of *kāya-sthairyam* (body stillness), guiding awareness through the body in order to cultivate stillness and detachment. Elements of *antar-mauna* ('inner silence') further deepen the awareness, allowing relaxation to naturally unfold. As attention moves from the breath to the senses, the mind is disengaged from external stimuli, entering the initial stage of *pratyāhāra*.

Stage 2 — *saṃkalpa* — The Essence of *yoga-nidrā*

> *Anything in life can fail you, but not the saṃkalpa made during yoga-nidrā. […] The resolve you make at the beginning of the practice is like sowing a seed, and the resolve at the end is like irrigating it.*[402]
>
> Svāmī Satyānanda

The Sanskrit term *saṃkalpa* encompasses will, determination, intention, goal, wish, idea, desire, resolution, intention, decision[403], dedication; embodying a focused willpower which directs thought with clarity. In Satyananda Yoga Nidra, *saṃkalpa* is its core, serving as an effective means of planting personal intentions into the subconscious. Through this process, individuals can positively and constructively reshape their personality and outlook on life.

The *saṃkalpa* Concept in Yoga

Manas naturally moves within the bounds of dualistic variegated ideation (*saṃkalpa-vikalpa*).[404] In *jñāna-yoga* the play of thoughts, *saṃkalpa-vikalpa*, is considered a function of the mind: pondering, brooding, doubting, planning, playing through all possibilities. The aim here is to observe this play of *saṃkalpa-vikalpa* in one's own mind continuously, to detach oneself from it and to enter into the pure consciousness which lies beyond all thinking, willing and feeling. This process is integrated into both spiritual practice and daily activities.

In some yoga texts, saṃkalpa stands for deliberate thought or determination. For example, in *Bṛhadāraṇyaka-upaniṣad* (2.4.11), the seer Yājñavalkya explains that the mind is the point of convergence of all thoughts (*saṃkalpa*).[405] The much later text *Yogavāsiṣṭha* also describes *saṃkalpa* as 'ideation', or

402 Saraswati, Satyananda, Swami. (2006). *Yoga Nidra*. (12th reprint). Munger: Yoga Publications Trust, p. 24–25.

403 Huchzermeyer, Wilfried. (2015). *Das Yoga-Lexikon*. Karlsruhe: Verlag W. Huchzermeyer, p. 246.

404 As mentioned before, this expression can also be understood as the pair of 'determination and indetermination'; See Part I., Chapter 4. *Yoga-nidrā as a Synonym for the Highest State of Immersion – samādhi*.

405 Olivelle, Patrick. (1998). *The Early Upaniṣads: Annotated Text and Translation*. New York/Oxford: Oxford University Press, p. 69.

'imagination', but notes that what it produces is very similar, at least in appearance, to a manifestation of Supreme Reality in a yogic experience:

> *ākāśasphuradākāras saṃkalpapuruṣo yathā* |
> *pṛthvyādirahito bhāti svayambhūr bhāsate tathā* || 3.2.52 ||

> Like a visualised[406] personage (*saṃkalpa-puruṣa*), He (Brahmā as Creator), the Self-existing One appears thus: He has the visionary form of shimmering space [itself], [so He] shines forth [as having a form, yet] free from Earth and the other [gross Elements].

> *na dṛśyam asti no draṣṭā paramātmani kevale* |
> *svayaṃ cittvāt tathāpy eṣa svayambhūr iti bhāsate* || 3.2.53 ||

> There is no Object of Observation, there is no Observer in the Union in the Supreme Self—the Self-existing One appears by Himself out of the state of being Mind/Consciousness Itself.

Saṃkalpa understood as 'ideation' in this context is not considered ultimate, but it is similar to the Ultimate in appearance. Even though *saṃkalpa* is part of a more conditioned, differentiated level of reality, it has a direct connection to Ultimate Reality in the form of consciousness. From an Advaita point of view, such manifestations would be considered the mere externality of the *brahman* and more of an impediment to proper realisation, but from a tantric point of view, these manifestations of the multiplicity of Reality are considered useful tools (both: *māyā*). A difference must therefore be made between the meaning of *saṃkalpa* as 'imagination' or 'ideation' in the dualistic sense and *saṃkalpa* as 'determination' within the context of a yogic spiritual endeavour. Once both indetermination (*vikalpa*) has been extinguished and determination (*saṃkalpa*) has become no longer necessary—that is when the root of variegated ideation (*saṃkalpa-vikalpa-mūla*) is truly severed. Once that occurs, the actualisation of states such as *yoga-nidrā* becomes truly accessible, rather than just being briefly glimpsed through some practice or other. Therefore, the principle of *saṃkalpa* as 'determination', 'resolve' or 'inner

406 Also 'willed into existence'.

vow' can, in fact, be used to help one progress along the spiritual path, until such a level is reached, where *saṃkalpa* is no longer the adequate tool for that purpose, i.e. states of absorption where duality dissolves completely. This is especially true in the case of regular practitioners.

In Chapter 6 of the *Yogavasiṣṭha* it is explained that the mind (*manas*) and the vital energy (*prāṇa*) are interwoven. If one is restrained, the other is also subdued. *Manas* projects its very own imaginative willpower (*saṃkalpa*) onto the 'mental canvas', which is driven by the power of the root desire (*vāsanā*). Spiritual seekers strive to control the fluctuating vital energy and to calm the mind. The most direct way to achieve this is to transcend the powerful force of the root desire (*vāsanā*).[407] The ultimate goal on the path to *samādhi* (or *yoga-nidrā* state) is to then free the mind from all *saṃkalpa*, that is, to gradually extinguish all thoughts and desires directed towards a goal. This is also a very high state of consciousness, which is only achievable by the most diligent and rigorous of practitioners. Another meaning of *saṃkalpa* refers to the decision to perform a ritual or ascetic act for a specific spiritual purpose.

In modern times, parallels are often drawn between the concept of *saṃkalpa* and the practice of autosuggestion[408]. The repeated self-affirmations during autosuggestion aim at self-induced influence on the psyche[409], in order to transform a certain thought into a conviction or a fact. The techniques of autogenic training, various methods of mental training and the concept of positive thinking have developed from this. However, there are marked differences between *saṃkalpa* and autosuggestion which will be discussed below.[410]

---

407 Feuerstein, Georg. (2008). *The Yoga Tradition – Its History, Literature, Philosophy and Practice* (3rd edition). Arizona: Hohm Press. p. 491.

408 Autosuggestion (Greek-Latin): self-influence. The doctrine of autosuggestion was developed by the French pharmacist Émile Coué in the 19th century.

409 Psyche (Greek) – 'soul'; in Western psychology, the totality of all mental properties and personality traits of a person (sensation, feeling, thinking, etc.).

410 See Part III. Chapter 17. *Yoga-nidrā and Western Psychology*; *Yoga-nidrā and Hypnosis*, the subsection on *Suggestion in Hypnosis vs. in yoga-nidrā*.

The Meaning and Effect of *Saṃkalpa* in *Yoga-nidrā*

The principle of *saṃkalpa* as applied in Swāmī Satyānanda's *yoga-nidrā* method goes beyond mere wishful thinking; it is a vow with transformative power, a commitment to support our path towards the realisation of Ultimate Reality. In this practice, *saṃkalpa* engages and mobilises all forces (*śaktis*) of the mind.[411] Awareness of the parts of the physical body during *yoga-nidrā* brings *prāṇa-śakti* along with it to produce a certain subtle effect. Similarly, a *saṃkalpa* focuses the awareness on a particular point in the sub- and unconscious, where it has the same effect, but on an even subtler level. It works to unify and stabilise the mind, shifting it away from gross thought patterns by integrating subconscious, obstructive, and destructive elements. This process directs the mind with firm focus, strengthening willpower and aligning it toward a single purpose.

> *Saṃkalpa increases the sensitivity and the potentiality of the mind. It increases the willpower and, initially through a form of positive suggestion, it takes you to the psychic dimension where the mind is sensitised, the faculties of the mind have a lot of force and suggestions have a lot of force. In the initial stages, saṃkalpa is used to focus the mental energies, later it builds up psychic energy. To begin with, externally it may look like a form of auto-suggestion but it prepares the ground for inner harmony. It sharpens the faculties of the mind. [...] So, it is sensitising the mind to deal with the energies within, which is the purpose of saṃkalpa. Also, it focuses the mental energies to a point where they become powerful like a laser beam.*[412]
>
> Svāmī Nirañjanānanda

Once we have recognised and formulated our *saṃkalpa*, we should regularly recall it, activating and nurturing it in our subconscious. Through the practice of *saṃkalpa*, it is activated and charged with energy and potency—*saṃkalpa-śakti*. The *saṃkalpa-śakti* includes the three higher energy aspects necessary to manifest the *saṃkalpa*, namely *icchā* (the force of the will to act), *jñāna* (the force of the knowledge of how to act) and *kriyā* (the force

---

411 See Part I. Chapter 9. *Māṇḍukya-upaniṣad and yoga-nidrā.*

412 Saraswati, Niranjanananda, Swami. (1997). *Yoga Sadhana Panorama*, Volume 2. Munger: Yoga Publication Trust, p. 92–93.

of acting).[413] They are the prerequisites for accessing the subtle realms of the mind and for interrupting the dispersing mechanism of *saṃkalpa-vikalpa*.

Svāmī Satyānanda explains that *saṃkalpas* grow increasingly powerful with consistent yoga practice, as the mind is gradually purified through *yoga-nidrā* and other techniques. For an advanced *yogin*, a stage is eventually reached where all *saṃkalpas* naturally come to fruition. This phenomenon is symbolically depicted in yogic texts as the *kalpavṛkṣa* or *kalpataru* — the 'wish-fulfilling tree'. This transformative state is achieved when one attains the level of awareness associated with what in later centuries came to be known as the *anāhata cakra*, the subtle centre of unconditional love and boundless joy located in the heart space.

Svāmī Satyānanda says in one of the few preserved original audio recordings of him guiding a *yoga-nidrā* practice:

> *These resolves* [saṃkalpas] *change the course of your destiny, your life and your personality. Therefore, do not be in a hurry to make a* saṃkalpa *now and here. Do not make ordinary* saṃkalpa *[...]. What do you want to be? What do you want to achieve? Very few people know this. Therefore, at this point of* yoga-nidrā, *before the practice begins,* saṃkalpa *or a resolve has to be made [...]. Anything in life can fail but not* saṃkalpa. *A resolve* [saṃkalpa] *made before* yoga-nidrā *and the same resolve* [saṃkalpa] *made at the end of* yoga-nidrā *will never fail [...].* Saṃkalpa *is like a boon, which you receive from a higher power and therefore do not ask for ordinary things. Do not ask for the trivial objects of the world.*[414]

The Interrelation between *Saṃkalpa* and the *Antaḥkaraṇa*

From the viewpoint of Yoga Psychology,[415] the imprinting of a beneficial thought or mental programme in the subconscious serves to counteract and neutralise disruptive or obstructive mental patterns. The negative imprints operate like a powerful undercurrent, subtly yet persistently drawing mental

---

413 Rama, Swami. (1988). *Path of Fire and Light*, Volume II. Honesdale: Himalayan Institute Press, p. 78–79 and pp. 117–122.

414 Recorded during a seminar in Antwerp, undated.

415 See Part I. Chapter 6. *Antaḥkaraṇa – Structure of the Mind According to Yoga Psychology*.

energy and focus into their influence and away from other areas. Often, it is almost impossible to resist this pull, and these imprints tend to drain mental resources, leading away from positive outcomes. By establishing a constructive *saṃkalpa* or determination, however, these counterproductive currents can be gradually diminished, allowing mental energies to realign towards more desirable goals.

The practice of *saṃkalpa* simultaneously removes negative mental programmes and consciously imprints positive determinations into the subconscious and/or unconscious mind. As one properly sets and reinforces the *saṃkalpa*, the mental space which was once occupied by limiting patterns is cleared, allowing the new, constructive patterns to take root and guide the mind's direction. This dual process of removal and imprinting fosters a constructive shift in thought, behaviour, and perception, gradually replacing obstructive mental patterns with a purposeful alignment.[416]

In cognitive behavioural therapy (CBT), this constructive shift, construed there as a transformative ability, is termed 'brain plasticity', which refers to the brain's capacity to override outdated neural pathways and consciously establish and reinforce new, beneficial ones. In a similar vein, the practice of *saṃkalpa* becomes most effective when the subconscious mind is more receptive — specifically, in the transitional state between waking and sleeping. During typical waking consciousness, the mind (*manas*) is busy with various thoughts and tasks, creating a barrier which limits access to the subconscious mind and its flow of energy. Conversely, in sleep states, awareness fades, making it difficult to reinforce or imprint the *saṃkalpa*. The ideal state, therefore, lies in this intermediate phase, where the conscious mind is calm but open, allowing deeper access to and impression upon the subconscious for lasting change.

Through *yoga-nidrā*, *manas* (the thinking mind) is quieted by disengaging perception from the external sensory input, releasing physical tension, and calming active thoughts, along with the interplay of *saṃkalpa* (determination, vow) and *vikalpa* (doubt or mental distraction). This calming occurs via habituation[417], achieved by a steady and sequential shifting of awareness throughout the practice. As the awareness returns to bodily

416 Panda, Nursing, Charan. (2011). *Yoga-Nidra*. (2nd edition). New Delhi: D.K. Printworld (P) Ltd., p. 91.

417 In psychology, habituation refers to the gradual decrease in an individual's responsiveness to a stimulus which is repeatedly presented and perceived as insignificant. As the stimulus proves to

sensations repeatedly, perception begins to classify these sensations as insignificant, ultimately 'forgetting' them. This filtering out of external stimuli facilitates a shift of attention inward. In the hypnagogic state — between wakefulness and sleep — the subconscious aspects of *manas* become especially open to *saṃkalpa*, allowing it to take deeper root.

According to Nursing Charan Panda, once the *saṃkalpa* is stored in the subconscious, it leaves an impression in the *smṛti* (memory), which remains inaccessible to the ordinary, conscious recall. A deep layer of *manas* (the mind) then activates *ahaṃkāra* (the sense of 'I' or ego) to carry out this 'auto-command' through the conscious mind, along with all bodily systems and organs. This execution happens on an unconscious level, requiring no active perception by either the bodily systems or the conscious mind itself.

Ahaṃkāra, or the sense of 'I'-ness, has the ability to generate strong inclinations toward attachment and action (*pravṛtti*) due to its freedom in choosing responses. These tendencies fuel the *kleśas* (afflictions or obstacles), which then lead to *karmans* (actions and their consequences). In *yoga-nidrā*, the practitioner's determination is embedded by repeating the *saṃkalpa* (resolve), thus counteracting the pull of *pravṛtti*. This repetition weakens the habitual inclinations of attachment and helps align the mind with the new, positive direction set by the *saṃkalpa*, gradually overcoming the automatic drives toward ingrained patterns.[418]

While in classical autosuggestion, the affirmation is also ideally repeated in near-intermediate states, such as having just woken up, falling asleep, or having relaxed, in *yoga-nidrā* there is the purposeful use of a precise moment which is reliably known to be where the mind is prepared to be receptive. In contrast to CBT, which uses calm reflection, sometimes with visualisation and behavioural rehearsal, the *saṃkalpa* is used in a state of calm, when the conceptual mind is passive. However, both share the feature that the message must be formulated in a positive way.

---

be meaningless, the mind begins to disregard it, gradually fading it out from conscious awareness. Over time, the reaction to such a stimulus may eventually cease altogether.

418 Panda, Nursing, Charan. (2011). *Yoga-Nidra*. (2nd edition). New Delhi: D.K. Printworld (P) Ltd., pp. 95–96.

Phrasing the *Saṃkalpa* and Practical Advice for its Application

> *A resolve or saṃkalpa is made during the practice of yoga-nidrā. It should be something of immense importance to you. Resolves are short sentences of moral significance to be embedded in the subconscious [...] Such resolves can change your whole life. They will certainly come true if you repeat your resolve with enough conviction. By this method you can change old habits and cure certain mental illnesses. Saṃkalpas can have a spiritual objective like 'I shall become more aware.' Your saṃkalpa or resolve should be repeated several times during the practice.*[419]
>
> Swāmī Satyānanda

The *saṃkalpa* repeated during Satyananda Yoga Nidra should be a concise, positively phrased resolve expressed in the present tense, preferably in one's mother tongue. It should be carefully selected, as it encapsulates the practitioner's intention or goal. The *saṃkalpa* should not be altered frequently, but rather maintained until it manifests in daily life. It is important to choose a *saṃkalpa* which reflects the entirety of one's personality and aligns with a clear direction in life—one which brings fulfilment, harmony, and constructive change. Ultimately, the *saṃkalpa* is a vow, which serves to guide the practitioner along the spiritual path, helping them to realise their vocation.

In a state of deep relaxation and stillness, the *saṃkalpa* is more effectively imprinted in the subconscious especially, when the practitioner charges it with strong willpower and conviction, trusting that the fulfillment of the intention has already been set in motion. The key is not to question the *how*—the method or means by which the intention will come to fruition. Instead, the focus is on mentally and spiritually setting the trajectory and live with what could be described as 'the questions'[420] of life. As the *saṃkalpa*

---

419 Saraswati, Shankardevananda, Swami. (n.d.). *Sankalpa and Yoga Therapy*. Yoga Magazine. 1999(9). http://www.yogamag.net/archives/1990s/1999/9909/9909skyt.html (accessed on 22.05.2023).

420 Inspired by Rilke, Rainer, Maria. (2011). *Letters to a Young Poet*. Penguin Edition Nr. 103. London: Penguin Classics, p. 26–27 'Letter IV: currently in Worpswede near Bremen, on 16th July 1903 [...], *and I should like to ask you, as best I can, dear Sir, to be patient towards all that is unresolved in your heart and to try to love the questions themselves like locked rooms, like books written in foreign tongue. Do not now strive to uncover answers: they cannot be given to you because you have not been able to live them. And what matters is to live everything.*

is nourished internally during *yoga-nidrā*, it can manifest in a variety of ways, often beyond the conscious mind's expectation, allowing for flexibility and openness to the unfolding process.

> It is important that *saṃkalpa* is not confused with the modern concepts of 'positive thinking', 'autosuggestion' (as mentioned previously), or 'the law of attraction'. While these approaches are based on the idea that 'like attracts like', i.e. that imagining something will somehow magically manifest it into existence, the method of *saṃkalpa* works by influencing one's view and attitude towards a goal, objective or life itself, which then finds its expression in one's thought patterns and behaviour. While the former tries to influence the external world with the power of imagination, the latter works directly with the structure of mind to consciously shift one's outlook to or direction in life. This is also why great care must be taken when choosing and continuously using a *saṃkalpa*. Furthermore, a *saṃkalpa* does not work magically on its own—it must be supported by discipline and personal responsibility.

In everyday life, the *saṃkalpa* serves as an essential support for the mind, guiding our actions and decisions. An important practice is to review the day at its end, contemplating how the personal *saṃkalpa* was expressed throughout the day. This contemplation helps bring awareness to the process of the resolve being embodied. It is natural to occasionally stray from the path of *saṃkalpa* fulfilment, and when this happens, it is important to offer ourselves compassion and support through self-study.

When we recognise that we have deviated from our intended course, we can pause and ask ourselves: What could I have thought, said, or done to stay aligned with my *saṃkalpa*? Visualising a new response or action allows us to experience it emotionally and physically. This practice helps us consciously choose to react differently in the future, reaffirming our resolve and remaining true to our intentions. Even when not actively working, the *saṃkalpa* causes heightened awareness with regard to its subject and thus works in a more subtle, indirect way.

Live the questions for now. Perhaps then you will gradually, without noticing it, live your way into the answer, one distant day in the future.'

Once the seed of the *saṃkalpa* is deeply planted in the subconscious, the mental faculties begin to align in support of its fulfilment. This directional power of the *saṃkalpa* helps dissolve the mental conditioning which holds us back from awakening to our true nature. It provides clarity and strength, guiding us toward personal growth.

> It is important to keep the *saṃkalpa* to oneself and not share it with others, as doing so could dissipate the energy which has been cultivated. The doubts and scepticism of others may unconsciously trigger the *saṃkalpa-vikalpa mechanism*—the internal conflict between intention and doubt—which can undermine the process. The power of *saṃkalpa* thrives when we are attuned to our true needs and desires. To fully benefit from this practice, we must avoid letting insecurity or scepticism interfere with the process, allowing the intention to unfold naturally and powerfully. However, this also means one shouldn't fall into blind single-mindedness—as with everything in Yoga, awareness and balance are key.

One's own attitude is of particular importance for the success of the *saṃkalpa*:

- *your own desire*—a clear, strong feeling of purpose. (Do I truly want to achieve this goal with all my heart?);
- *your own trust and will*—the more you are convinced of your goal and the possibility of achieving it, the more likely you are to succeed. (Do I really believe in this goal?);
- *acceptance*—the willingness to accept what you are striving for and to allow it into your daily life;
- *cultivate honesty with yourself* with the help of the *draṣṭā* stance—being objective and non-judgemental toward yourself, your true feelings and aspirations, which helps you with realising what obstructs you in the process;
- *give yourself permission*—sometimes we prevent ourselves from reaching our goals by not allowing ourselves to reach it, because it might be frightening, among other reasons.

When deciding on the *saṃkalpa*, the Bihar Yoga System usually suggests the SWAN technique[421] (Strengths, Weaknesses, Ambitions, Needs), as a tool to analyse and assess oneself in order to better formulate one's goals. Svāmī Nirañjanānanda developed this method to provide a systematic way for gaining clarity about which areas of one's personality and life should be developed.

STAGES OF THE *SAṂKALPA*

A *saṃkalpa* can exist on different levels and evolve through various stages. At its core, each person carries a primary *saṃkalpa*, which is aligned towards the role or vocation in life towards which they aspire, either consciously or unconsciously. However, most people are unaware of this central *saṃkalpa* and are seeking purpose and direction. The practice of cultivating *saṃkalpa* in *yoga-nidrā* is, ultimately, about discovering this primary goal, which can be spiritual, psychological, or worldly in nature. This is done by making sure to, at each stage, consciously select a *saṃkalpa* which resonates deeply with our whole being. It should feel authentic and truly meaningful. To find our primary *saṃkalpa*, we need time for introspection and contemplation, allowing ourselves to tune into what we genuinely wish to achieve in life and why—what will bring us deep satisfaction, contentment, and fulfilment.

> Finding one's primary *saṃkalpa* may take time and patience—sometimes even years. It is important not to rush the process. In some cases, the first step could even be to set the *saṃkalpa* of discovering the right *saṃkalpa* for oneself. This introspective journey ultimately helps us align with our true purpose, guiding us towards greater clarity and fulfilment in life.

In certain situations in life, it can be helpful to apply a short-term or 'mini' *saṃkalpa*, especially in cases where the individual is facing a specific challenge, such as an illness, or when the original *saṃkalpa* seems too broad or distant. These smaller, more focused intentions can serve as a temporary anchor to address immediate concerns or provide clarity in times of uncertainty.

---

421 For further reading: Saraswati, Niranjanananda, Swami. (2013). *Yoga Nidra – Water the Roots* 4. Munger: Yoga Publications Trust and Satyadharma, Swami. (2013). SWAN Meditation – Theory and Practice. Munger: Yoga Publication Trust.

For example, if one is dealing with a physical or emotional setback, a mini *saṃkalpa* could be something like 'I am healing and restoring my health' or 'I am resilient and capable of overcoming this challenge.' These short-term resolves help direct the mind and energy towards the immediate need, offering a grounded sense of control and purpose.

However, once the situation has been addressed or resolved, the practitioner should return to their original *saṃkalpa*, the broader, long-term intention aligned with their deeper purpose. This ensures that the *saṃkalpa* practice remains rooted in one's true, overarching goal, keeping the individual focused on their *dharma* and life's true direction, while also giving space to address short-term needs when necessary.

In summary, the *saṃkalpa* should:

- resonate with you;
- be as short and clear as possible;
- be worded positively;
- be formulated in the present;
- be expressed in your own words and in your mother tongue;
- be emotionally appealing;
- be treated as if it is already fulfilling itself.

Examples of possible formulations (and the obstructive thought patterns which may limit them):

- I trust in myself and know that I can do what I set out to do. (vs. 'Whatever I start, I fail.');
- I trust in my body's healing powers. (vs. 'I'm sick, I feel bad.');
- I am strong and trust in myself. (vs. 'I feel powerless and weak.');
- I trust I will find true meaning in life. (vs. 'Nothing makes sense.');
- Everything I experience contributes to my inner growth. (vs. 'Why does this have to happen to me?');
- I accept all my feelings as a part of myself. (vs. 'I don't want this...');
- I have the strength and the confidence to determine my own life. (vs. 'Everything is too much for me, I can't do it.');
- I am at peace with what I have and trust that I can obtain everything I need. (vs. 'If only I had this and that, then...');

- I recognise and appreciate the good things in my life. (vs. 'I feel bad, I'm unhappy.');
- I am capable of rising up to the challenge. (vs. 'I feel out of my depth.');
- I express my [positive qualities].;
- I am developing [...], etc.

> If you find it difficult to formulate a *saṃkalpa*, you can just make a *saṃkalpa* for finding your *saṃkalpa*.

Svāmī Śaṅkaradevānanda, a disciple of Svāmī Satyānanda's and a medical doctor, recommends[422] the use of *saṃkalpa* as a therapeutic tool, especially in situations of illness or suffering. Under these circumstances, it can be difficult for individuals to maintain a clear sense of purpose or recall the reasons behind their actions, particularly when dealing with lengthy or challenging therapies. The healing process can often feel drawn-out or uncertain, which can lead to frustration or a lack of motivation.

To support the healing process, Svāmī Śaṅkaradevānanda suggests using focused *saṃkalpa* phrases designed to reinforce the connection between the individual's healing process and their deeper, spiritual intention. These therapeutic *saṃkalpa*s are simple yet powerful, aimed at encouraging the body and mind to align with the process of healing.

Examples of therapeutic *saṃkalpa*s might include:

- I will become stronger;
- I will be healthier;
- I make myself strong and overcome all obstacles;
- My immune system is getting stronger every day.

and similar phrases that can help you feel your own strength.

Svāmī Śaṅkaradevānanda advises against rigid rules, such as the blanket instruction to 'never use the future tense' when formulating a *saṃkalpa*. He points out that, while a present tense formulation like 'my immune system

---

422 Saraswati, Shankardevananda, Swami. (n.d.). Sankalpa and Yoga Therapy. *Yoga Magazine*. 1999(9). Munger: Yoga Publication Trust. http://www.yogamag.net/archives/1990s/1999/9909/9909skyt.html (accessed on 22.05.2023).

is fighting cancer' can sometimes generate underlying doubts or uncertainties, in some cases, using the future tense may be more fitting. The future tense could be appropriate, especially if it serves to convey determination and resolve. However, when doing so, it is crucial to ensure that the *saṃkalpa* emphasises willpower, not just the future event.

For example, a *saṃkalpa* like 'I will become healthier' involves more than just an abstract future outcome. It also carries the inherent idea that the individual must begin taking action now, setting into motion the necessary steps toward achieving that health. This formulation is considered an 'unlimited' *saṃkalpa* because it suggests continuous improvement in health, with no end point, making the goal open-ended and ever-evolving.[423] However, one should consider carefully whether this form would be just as apt in one's mother tongue, if it is not English — subtle differences in meaning can be found in all languages, which can make a literal translation difficult.

Svāmī Śaṅkaradevānanda highlights that a truly effective *saṃkalpa* should be rooted in something fundamental and deeply important to the individual. When this central goal is achieved, it often results in the simultaneous fulfilment of other goals. This ultimate *saṃkalpa* can be seen as the key to healing, for it reflects an overarching desire for well-being and wholeness which encompasses all aspects of life.

Moreover, Svāmī Śaṅkaradevānanda addresses a common challenge for long-term yoga practitioners: the tendency for certain aspects of practice to become unclear or forgotten over time. He suggests that when such lapses occur, it's often because the individual has lost sight of their *saṃkalpa*.

> As Svāmī Satyānanda notes, while many things in life may falter or fail, the *saṃkalpa* pursued with deep determination, persistence, and sincerity remains steadfast. It is the reminder of what we truly want to accomplish, acting as a guide on our path to healing and fulfilment. Ultimately, everyone carries their own personal *saṃkalpa*, even if they are not consciously aware of it, and this intention can help direct and shape their life journey.[424]

423 Ibid.
424 Ibid.

Stage 3 — Rotation of Awareness Throughout the Body

The rotation of awareness through the body, which involves guiding the awareness from one body part to the next, is a consistent sequence in Stage 3 of the *yoga-nidrā* practice. The order of the mentioned body parts and the repetition sequence remain constant. The practitioner mentally repeats the name of each body part while becoming consciously aware of it and visualising it. In this manner, each part of the body in *yoga-nidrā* is stimulated through the rotation of awareness, similar to the tantric technique of *nyāsa*.

Nyāsa — A Tantric Technique and Root of *yoga-nidrā*

Nyāsa means 'the ritual placement of mantras on the body or on the deity's vehicle (*vahana*) in order to anchor the power of the mantra there'[425]. *Nyāsa* has its roots in both Vedic ritual and later Tantric practices. It is a historical practice which has been used and developed further by Tantra. The ritual placement of deities onto objects, figures, or bodies using mantras was traditionally the duty of a Vedic priest, and later, this responsibility extended to the tantric practitioners (*sādhakas*) themselves. In both instances, this process is performed in a specific order, systematically 'consecrating' body parts in a predetermined sequence. The *yoga-nidrā* method represents Svāmī Satyānanda's interpretation of this ancient practice.

Practising *nyāsa* involves establishing one's own body as the sacred abode of the divine. The term itself means 'to place', 'to insert' or 'make an impression with the mind (on a single point)'. *Nyāsa* is performed as an essential part of certain Vedic and Tantric rituals. During these practices, the priest or tantric master touches different parts of their or the disciple's body while seated, reciting specific mantras and thus 'placing' them within the body — or, in a yogic context, feeling or experiencing them. This process is supposed to activate the *prāṇa*.

The process of *nyāsa* is intended to facilitate the infusion of subtle power — an aspect of the divine — into the material body, resulting in

425 Goodall, D. & Rastelli, M. (Eds.). (2013). Tāntrikābhidhānakośa III, T–Ph: Dictionnaire des termes techniques de la littérature hindoue tantrique. *A Dictionary of Technical Terms from Hindu Tantric Literature. Wörterbuch zur Terminologie hinduistischer Tantren.* (BKGA 76.) Vienna: VÖAW, p. 342.

transforming that body or vessel into a container for the divine. A mantra is recited while focusing on a specific part of the body, and this energy is 'placed' by touching that area with a specific hand gesture (*hasta-mudrā*). This practice 'charges' the body part with energy and consecrates it with mantric power (*mantra-adhiṣṭhāna*).

The practice of *nyāsa* is conducted in a meticulously systematic manner to effectively distribute psycho-spiritual energies throughout the body. This process requires expanding one's awareness beyond the physical form to engage with the deeper layers of the personality. From a yogic standpoint, cultivating the quality of *sattva* in the mind (*buddhi*) is essential for this expansion. *Sattva* embodies clarity, purity, and harmony, enabling practitioners to connect more profoundly with their inner selves and facilitate the transformative effects of *nyāsa*.

There are various forms of *nyāsa* practice. As a foundation for Stage 3 of his *yoga-nidrā* method—the Rotation of Awareness Through the Body—Svāmī Satyānanda refers, for example, to techniques from the *Mahānirvāṇa-tantra* (ca. 1700 CE), namely the *aṅguṣṭhādi-hṛdyādi-saḍaṅga-nyāsa* (5.121–126) and *pītha-nyāsa* (5.127–135). According to the first technique—*nyāsa* of the six fingers, beginning with the thumb and so forth (*aṅguṣṭhādi-saḍaṅga-nyāsa*), mantras are placed on the hands as follows:[426]

- both thumbs: *hrāṃ aṅguṣṭhābhyāṃ namaḥ*
- both index fingers: *hrīṃ tarjanībhyāṃ svāha*
- both middle fingers: *hruṃ madhyamābhyāṃ vaṣaṭ*
- both ring fingers: *hraiṃ anāmikābhyāṃ hūṃ*
- both little fingers: *hrauṃ kaniṣṭhikābhyāṃ vauṣaṭ*
- both palms and back of the hands: *hraḥ karatalakarapṛṣṭhābhyāṃ phaṭ*

And *nyāsa* of the six parts of the body, beginning with the heart and so forth (*nyāsa* of the six fingers, beginning with the thumb and so forth (*hṛdyādi-saḍaṅga-nyāsa*) on the upper body, as follows:

426 Avalon, Arthur (Woodroffe, John G.). (1953). *Tantra of the Great Liberation* [*Mahanirvana Tantra*] – *Translation and Commentary*. Madras: Ganesh & Co. Ltd., pp. 116–120.

- heart: *hrāṃ hṛdayāyā namaḥ*
- head: *hrīṃ śirase svāha*
- crown: *hruṃ śikhāya vaṣaṭ*
- upper body ('armour', or *kavaca*): *hraiṃ kavacāya hūṃ*
- three eyes: *hrauṃ netratrayāya vauṣaṭ*
- two palms: *hraḥ astrāya phaṭ*

In the second technique—*pītha-nyāsa* (5.127–135), mantras, symbols and visualisations are placed in particular parts of the body in a very specific order.

First, the Lotus of the heart (*hridayāmbujo*) is established by visualising in succession:

- *adhāre śakti* (the supporting force): *adhāre-śaktaye namaḥ*
- the tortoise (*kūrma*; the support): *kūrmāya namaḥ*
- the serpent Śeṣa (the supporter): *śeṣāya namaḥ*
- the Earth (pṛthivi; the supported): *pṛthivyai namaḥ*
- the Ocean of Ambrosia (*sudhāmbudhi*; the situation): *sudhāmbudhaye namaḥ*
- the Isle of Gems (*maṇi-dvīpa*; the location): *maṇi-dvīpāya namaḥ*
- the Pārijāta tree (*pārijāta-taru*; the central axis): *pārijāta-tarave namaḥ*
- the Sunctum of the Wish-fulfilling Jewel (*cintāmaṇi-griha*; the abode): *cintāmaṇi-grihāya namaḥ*
- the Jewelled Altar (*maṇi-mānikya-vedikā*; the place): *maṇi-mānikyavedikāyai namaḥ*
- the Lotus Seat (*padmāsana*; the seat of the Goddess in union with the Self): *padmāsanāya namaḥ*

Then, one proceeds to eight other parts of the body, before returning to the lotus of the heart:

- right shoulder (*dharma*; the universal law): *dakṣa-skhandhe dharmāya namaḥ*
- left shoulder (*jñāna*; knowledge): *vāma-skhandhe jñānāya namaḥ*
- right hip (*aiśvarya*; sovereignty): *dakṣa-kaṭau aiśvaryāya namaḥ*
- left hip (*vairagya*; non-attachment): *vāma-kaṭau vairagyāya namaḥ*
- mouth (*adharma*; absence of dharma): *mukhe adharmāya namaḥ*

- left side (*ajñāna*; absence of knowledge): *vāma-pārśve ajñānāya namaḥ*
- navel (*anaiśvarya*; absence of sovereignty): *nābhau anaiśvaryāya namaḥ*
- right side (*avairagya*; absence of non-attachment): *dakṣa-pārśve avairagyāya namaḥ*

After which the practitioner proceeds to internal *nyāsa* of the pericarp, filaments and the petals of the heart lotus (*cakra*)—the *pīthas*, before doing particular *prāṇāyāma*, ritual worship (*pūjā*), and *dhyāna*.

The sequence of the *nyāsa* described in the *Mahānirvāṇa-tantra* may be interpreted as corresponding to the creation of a three-dimensional *yantra*, in which the body is conceptualised as the *yantra* itself. The first two steps—*nyāsa* of the fingers and hands, and *nyāsa* of the heart and putting on the armour is the preliminary observance or cleansing and protecting the space, where the *yantra* will be created. Then, first, the step of 'piercing the centre' (*bindu-bhedana*), i.e. establishing the core or source of power, is done through the *nyāsa* of the abode of the deity (*pītha*). After, this is followed by 'drawing of the outline/base' (*bhūpūra/bhūmi-parigraha*) by *nyāsa* of four foundational qualities and their opposite counterparts in eight points in the body, surrounding the *bindu* (the lotus of the heart).

This ritual allows the practitioner to cultivate awareness of each part of the body, effectively bestowing consciousness upon them, by placing various mantras systematically on specific body parts by touching them in a predetermined order. Thus, *nyāsa* can facilitate the release of tension and lethargy, promoting re-integration of consciousness and energy (subtle and gross). As the practitioner engages in this process, they not only deepen their connection to their physical form but also activate the flow of *prāṇa* (vital energy).

> Svāmī Satyānanda recognised the potential of these traditional techniques and implemented them in such a way that they could be used by anyone, even those who are not familiar with mantras. This effective practice was no longer kept hidden as a tool for secret rituals, but was, in this way, made widely accessible. In his *yoga-nidra* method, the ritual components are dispensed with, but the effect remains.

Svāmī Satyānanda deliberately removed the explicitly religious and ritual elements of *nyāsa* in his *yoga-nidrā* technique.[427] The basis of his *yoga-nidrā* method is the cultivation of a focused awareness, which was also the prerequisite for performing *nyāsa*. *Yoga-nidrā* thus shares the roots of its essentially yogic method of managing body and mind with other traditions, such as the tantric ones.

The principle of *nyāsa* permeates the entire *yoga-nidrā* method. In Stage 3, when awareness is rotated around the different body parts, the name of the respective body part is mentally repeated instead of the mantra. Through this process, the practitioner's own body becomes a kind of 'object', allowing the mind to detach (*pratyāhāra*) from identification with the body and enabling the practitioner to gain distance from their body. Despite the absence of mantras, the effect and intensity of *nyāsa* are retained.[428]

In Stage 5 of Svāmī Satyānanda's method, pairs of opposite sensations are evoked. In this Stage, the experience of opposites — such as enduring heat and cold, akin to the external ascetic practices of *tapas* in Patañjali's system — is internalised. *Yoga-nidrā* consistently translates into an inner practice which involves feeling opposites without relying on an external source. This experience is generated from within, representing another aspect of *pratyāhāra*[429] which has been integrated into the *yoga-nidrā* practice. In Patañjali's system, during the state of '*pratyāhāra*, where the senses are withdrawn from external objects of perception and imitate the form of the mind' (*YS* 2.54). In this process, sensory perception reflects the activities of the mind rather than transmitting information received from external stimuli. Consequently, it can be inferred that the flow of vital energy (*prāṇa*) is also influenced by directing attention to specific parts of the body during the practice of *yoga-nidrā*, owing to the interconnectedness of awareness, sensory

427 When external ritual was internalised in the form of yogic practices, symbolic and iconic elements representing aspects and sequence of the external ritual were often preserved in the form of images and specific visualisations. Without dispensing with the core principles and aims of these, Svāmī Satyānanda removed the religious and culture-specific symbolic environment, leaving the very essence of the practice, so that it is not bound by any religious or cultural baggage and thus accessible to anyone willing to try. See also Part I., Chapter 5. *The Stages of pratyāhāra*.

428 See also Part I. Chapter 5. *The Stages of pratyāhāra*.

429 See Part I., Chapter 7. *Pratyāhāra – The Purification Process of the Impressions of the Subconscious*; *Pratyāhāra Stages*; Mircea Eliade coined the term 'ritual interiorisation' in this context.

perceptions and perception through the physical organs. A similar approach can be observed in the practice described in the *Yoga-yājñavalkya* (7.2–7).[430]

In later yogic systems, *prāṇa* is regarded as subtler than the physical body but grosser than the mind. In this context, it is reasonable to conclude that focusing attention on a specific point naturally draws *prāṇa* to that location. Through this process, the body's vital energies can be directed to flow in a particular manner, and the systematic control of this flow may yield various effects, including the facilitation of unimpeded *prāṇa* flow throughout the body. Since *yoga-nidrā* exists neither in a lethargic (tāmasic) unconscious state (*nidrā*), nor in an active waking state (*jagrat*), it can be inferred that a balanced (sattvic) quality prevails in the mind (*buddhi*) during the practice of *yoga-nidrā*.[431]

> In psychotherapy, hypnotherapy, and mental management techniques, the term 'body scan' is widely used for a sequence assumed to be similar to Stage 3 — Rotation of Awareness Throughout the Body — of Swāmī Satyānanda's *yoga-nidrā* method, albeit with different applications. The practice has become increasingly popular in the West, both as a stand-alone meditation technique and when incorporated into body-oriented therapies. The body scan is generally regarded to originate in the Buddhist tradition of *vipassanā* and is attributed to the Theravāda Buddhist teacher U Ba Khin (1899–1971), who dedicated himself to the 'body-oriented awareness' centred on developing awareness of one's own mortality and transience and rooted in early Buddhism. However, although the body scan and Stage 3 of *Satyananda Yoga Nidra* may appear very similar on the surface, they are distinct techniques, often incorrectly assumed to be identical.

THE *NYĀSA* TECHNIQUE AND THE *MOTOR HOMUNCULUS*

This Stage of the practice is particularly important and highlights a clear connection between recent findings in modern neuroscience and the *yoga-nidrā* method developed by Svāmī Satyānanda. By directing awareness to different

430 See part I. Chapter 5. *Pratyāhāra as Foundation for yoga-nidrā*, the subsection on *The Stages of pratyāhāra*.
431 See Part I. Chapter 3. *The Eightfold yoga-path of Patañjali* (The dissolution (*nirodha*) of the *vṛttis*, *pratyaya* and *saṃskāras*).

parts of the body, the corresponding neuronal centres in the somatosensory cortex are activated. This aligns with the theoretical increase in *prāṇa* flow when similar methods are employed in yoga or Tantra. The nerve centres for the addressed body parts can be localised in a specific arrangement on the cortex, which is illustrated by Penfield's motor and *sensory homunculi*[432].

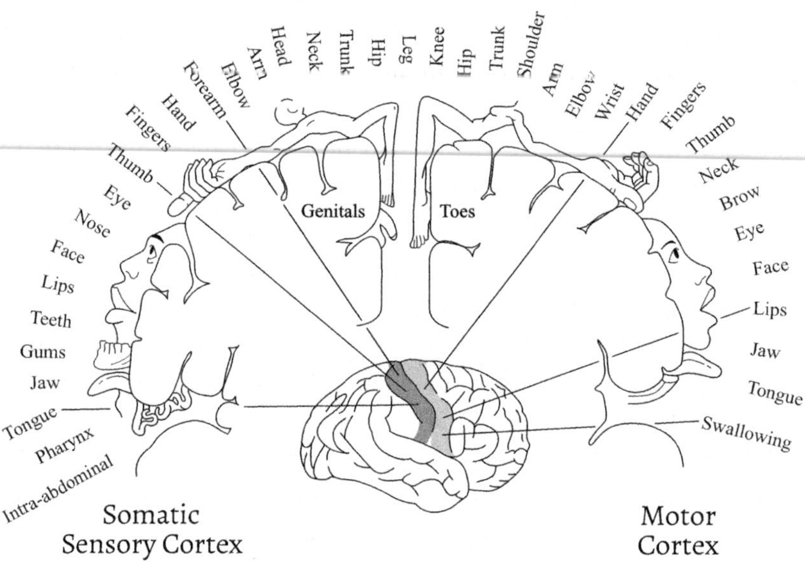

FIGURE 13: Motor homunculus[433] symbolic visualisation.

The *motor homunculus* represents the neuromotor processing of various parts of the body, while the *sensory homunculus* illustrates the sensitivity of these parts. The *motor homunculus* can be considered a neural mirror-image of the physical body. The more densely innervated, or sensitive, the areas of a body part are, the larger their representation on the surface of the somatosensory cortex. This leads to a model of a small human with disproportionate body parts, which are enlarged in the model to symbolise their prominence on the cortex and to visualise their importance in communication with the outside world. The sequence of rotation of the awareness through the body aligns with this, emphasising the hands, feet, and face. Swāmī Satyānanda

432 The concept of the *motor homunculus* comes from the research of Dr. Wilder Penfield, was first published in 1951 and is still used today in medicine and neuroscience almost unchanged.

433 *Motor homunculus* symbolic visualisation. Image by © Immanuel Stürzebecher

thus integrated Western scientific knowledge about the nervous system and incorporated Penfield's *homunculus* into the sequence of various body parts in the *nyāsa* principle utilised in his *yoga-nidrā* method.

When practicing *yoga-nidrā*, we focus on these specific areas by 'touching' the body parts with our awareness. The awareness rotates through the body and thus stimulates the corresponding neural centres in the brain. It is particularly important to maintain the same order while rotating the awareness since all body parts are addressed in exactly the same sequence as they are mapped on the *motor* homunculus.[434] The body parts activated during *yoga-nidrā* lie in a continuous line on the cortex. Similar to the tantric technique of *aṅguṣṭhādi-ṣaḍaṅga-nyāsa*, the conscious awareness of the body parts in *yoga-nidrā* always begins with the right thumb.

In contrast to a neurosurgical procedure which stimulates specific points in the brain with electric impulses, *yoga-nidrā* stimulates the entire surface of the brain through heightened body awareness. By consciously and systematically becoming aware of different parts of the body, all neural pathways to the brain are 'purified'. From a yogic perspective, this practice enhances the *prāṇa* current along the *nāḍis*, allowing it to flow more freely. According to Swāmī Satyānanda, the resulting energetic homogeneity in the brain facilitates an immediate disconnection of awareness from the input of the sensorimotor channels of perception, leading to a subjectively perceived sense of relaxation, relief, or a feeling of 'letting go'.[435] This creates a synergy where the relaxation experienced in the body also allows the mind to release tension.

The term 'relaxation' is usually used to signify bodily relaxation as a primary effect and mental or subtle relaxation as secondary. However, in Satyananda Yoga Nidra, the primary relaxation is that of the central nervous system, where the body (i.e. the periphery) follows along. This approach ensures that both body and mind release tension, whereas if one were to only concentrate on bodily relaxation, without proper *pratyāhāra*, the mind would remain in an active or agitated state and deep relaxation would not be possible (similar

434 The idea of the *śavayātrā* exercise, also known as the '61-point exercise', which Svāmī Rāma Bhāratī taught at the Himalayan Institute as a subtle form of relaxation which leads to deep states of consciousness, is very similar. It is based on the 61 *marmasthānas* – energy points in the body, which are known from Āyurveda. The sequence of the body parts addressed differs slightly from the method of Svāmī Satyānanda.

435 Saraswati, Satyananda, Swami. (2006). *Yoga Nidra*. (12th reprint). Munger: Yoga Publications Trust, pp. 35–38.

to rajasic sleep as described by Vācaspati[436]). It must once again be noted that this is an effect of the practice, but not its goal.

Stage 4 — Awareness of the (Subtle) Breath in *yoga-nidrā*

> *Awareness of the breath not only promotes relaxation and concentration, but also awakens higher energies and directs them to every cell of the body. It assists pratyāhāra from the subtle body in the practices that follow.*[437]
>
> Svāmī Satyānanda

Stage 4 of Svāmī Satyānanda's *yoga-nidrā* is breath awareness. It marks the completion of the physical relaxation process and serves to deepen the practitioner's awareness on a more subtle level. By directing the mind's attention to the natural flow of the breath, the practitioner begins refining their sensitivity to the more subtle dimensions of the breath, particularly the *prāṇa*, or vital force.

This heightened awareness has a purifying, revitalising, and healing effect on the body's tissues and cells, promoting overall well-being. The process helps facilitate mental stillness and calm, further deepening the body's relaxation. As the practitioner continues to focus on the natural breath without attempting to control or alter it, they begin to experience the *prāṇamaya-kośa*, or the subtle energy sheath which, according to yogic theories of subtle physiology, sustains and nourishes the physical body.[438]

Mechanics of Breath Awareness in *yoga-nidrā*

During Stage 4, breath awareness is cultivated by consciously observing the natural rhythm and flow of the breath, without any effort or interference. The breath flows in and out effortlessly, allowing the practitioner to become more attuned to subtle *prāṇa*. However, it is important to keep in mind that

436 See Part I. Chapter 4. *Yoga-nidrā as a Synonym for the Highest State of Immersion – samādhi*.

437 Saraswati, Satyananda, Swami. (2006). *Yoga Nidra*. (12th reprint). Munger: Yoga Publications Trust, p. 71.

438 See Part I, Chapter 8. *Pañcakośa – The Five Sheaths of Being*.

what we are talking about here is awareness *with* the breath and not *of* the breath, and the term 'breath awareness' is used to refer to that on occasion for the sake of convenience.

> At this Stage, it is crucial to simply observe the breath as it is, without attempting to manipulate it. Any attempt to control or change the breath would shift the focus back to the physical aspect of breathing, interrupting the deeper level of immersion that this Stage of *yoga-nidrā* aims to cultivate. Instead, the practice encourages observing the breath as a natural, ongoing process, allowing the awareness to deepen into the more subtle energies of the body.

To maintain awareness and prevent falling asleep during this process, the practitioner is encouraged to focus continuously on an inner object, in this case, the breath. Svāmī Satyānanda suggests a technique of counting backwards from a specific number as a tool to anchor the mind and keep it alert. The purpose of the counting is not to reach a particular number, but to sustain uninterrupted focus and prevent the mind from drifting into sleep or distraction, thus extending the hypnagogic state. If the awareness of the breath falters or the practitioner loses focus, they should simply restart the counting process.

Numbers considered sacred[439] such as 11, 12, 27, 54, 108, or 1008 are commonly used as starting points for the counting. These numbers hold significance in many spiritual traditions, adding a layer of significance to the practice. The act of counting in this manner not only helps keep the mind focused and alert but also trains the practitioner's ability to maintain concentration and awareness over longer periods, even at a subtle level. This practice enhances mental discipline and contributes to the deepening of the overall *yoga-nidrā* experience.

As the practice of *yoga-nidrā* progresses, the practitioner's awareness deepens, enabling them to sense more subtle energy currents in the body which are typically beyond ordinary perception. Initially, the focus is on the physical sensation of breathing—the rise and fall of the breath within

439 In Indian numerical mysticism, certain sacred numbers symbolise the divine and the basic principles of creation.

the body. However, as the practitioner becomes more attuned to the flow of breath, their awareness gradually expands to include the subtle currents of *prāṇa* (vital energy) which circulate throughout the body.

At this Stage, breath awareness transitions into *prāṇa* awareness. The practitioner begins to perceive the *prāṇa* as it moves along the *nāḍīs* (energy channels) and the *cakras* (energy centres) of the body, fostering a deeper connection to the subtler energy sheath of existence, or *prāṇamaya-kośa*.

This Stage of awareness lays the groundwork for more advanced yogic practices, such as *dhāraṇā* (concentration), *prāṇa-yoga-nidrā* (an advanced *yoga-nidrā* practice involving deep *prāṇa* awareness)[440], *kriyā-yoga* (the yoga of balancing the psycho-physiological movements of the mind)[441], and *prāṇa-vidyā* (knowledge or mastery of *prāṇa*). By refining the awareness of *prāṇa* in *yoga-nidrā*, the practitioner prepares themselves for these higher practices, where mastery of subtle energy currents can lead to profound states of immersion, healing, and spiritual awakening.

The focus of awareness with the breath during *pratyāhāra-yoga-nidrā*[442] can be directed in one of the following ways:

- awareness of the spontaneous movement of the navel with the breath;
- beginning with awareness of the spontaneous movement the navel, then successively shifting the awareness to the centre of the chest and then to the throat pit together with the natural breath;
- directing the awareness along the anterior psychic passage[443] between the navel and throat with the natural breath;
- awareness of the movement of the breath in the nostrils;
- *anuloma-viloma*—mental alternate nostril breathing.

---

440 See Part I. Chapter 8. *Pañcakośa – The Five Sheaths of Being*.

441 The term *kriyā-yoga* is used by Svāmī Satyānanda to refer to the system of practices he developed to that purpose. As with many other Sanskrit terms, depending on the tradition and context '*kriyā-yoga*' can refer to many different practices and systems (such as the *kriyā-yoga* of the tradition of Paramahaṃsa Yogānanda Giri), which do not necessarily have much overlap or commonality.

442 See Part I. Chapter 8. *Pañcakośa – The Five Sheaths of Being*; Part II. Chapter 12. *The Benefits of Yogic Immersion: pratyāhāra*.

443 In subtle yoga physiology, aside from the central vital energy channel (*suṣumnā*) and the left (*iḍā*) and right (*piṅgalā*) channels, other subsidiary prāṇic pathways exist as well. One such pathway runs along the front of the body in the centre, mirroring the *suṣumnā* which runs centrally inside the body, following the inside of the spine. Working with this anterior psychic passage is the first stage at which one must learn to practice before proceeding towards working with the other channels and the *cakras*.

Directing the awareness along the anterior psychic passage in conjunction with the natural breath is a breath awareness practice from the *kriyā-yoga* technique *ajapā-japa* within the Bihar Yoga system. *Ajapā-japa* means 'recitation of the non-recited', here understood to refer to continuous repetition, and includes the flow of the awareness with the natural breath between the navel and throat, as well as the awareness of the *prāṇa* and the vibrational power of the 'breath mantra' — *so 'ham*. In Śaiva and Śākta yogic practice the *ajapā* or *haṃsa* mantra — understood as *ahaṃ saḥ* ('I am He.') — takes the inverted form *so 'ham* (inhalation-exhalation), meaning 'He am I', the repetition being performed with a view to identifying oneself with Śiva.[444] This is described in texts such as the *Vijñāna-bhairava-tantra* verse 156, which reads:

> *ṣaṭśatāni divā rātrau sahasrānyekaviṃśatiḥ* |
> *jāpo devyāḥ samuddiṣṭaḥ sulabho durlabho jaḍaiḥ* || 156 ||

> [Exhaling (*haṃ*), inhaling (*saḥ*)] 21 600 times over a day and a night[445] — it is [this] mantra-repetition of the [Supreme] Goddess, which is taught in full [in this Tantra]. It is easily attainable [by the knowledgeable] and difficult to reach for the ignorant. (156)[446]

The *haṃsa*-mantra refers to the utilisation of the unconscious, reflexive repetition which occurs with every breath. Every human being repeats this mantra unconsciously 21,600 times a day and night, corresponding to the number of breaths one typically takes in a 24-hour period.

In the context of the *Vijñāna-bhairava-tantra*, the *haṃsa*-mantra is said to be a manifestation of the divine sound, representing the goddess Parā ('The Supreme'), and is thus considered a transcendental and secret form of knowledge (*parā-vidyā*). This mantra is not merely a sound but a spiritual practice. It holds the key to unlocking the highest experiences of spiritual realisation, as it connects the practitioner to the universal rhythm of the breath, which in turn links them to the divine.

---

444 Brunner, Héléne; Oberhammer, Gerhard; Padoux, André (eds.). (2000). *Tantrikabhidhanakosa I: Dictionaire des termes techniques de la litterature hindoue tantrique – A Dictionary of Technical Terms from Hindu Tantric Literature – Wörterbuch zur Terminologie hinduistischer Tantren*. (BKGA 35.) Vienna: VÖAW, p. 97.

445 I.e. a 24-hour period.

446 Translation from the Sanskrit: Georgi Krastev.

Svāmī Satyasaṅgānanda, comments that, despite its simplicity, the traditional understanding is that the full significance and power of the *haṃsa*-mantra can only be revealed through *guru* initiation. The *guru*, as a spiritual teacher or guide, imparts this sacred knowledge, enabling the seeker (*sādhaka*) to consciously tap into the mantra's effective potential. The process of initiation brings the practitioner into a deeper, experiential understanding of the breath-mantra, offering the possibility of profound spiritual awakening and connection with the divine essence of life itself.[447] However, in *yoga-nidrā* this principle is simplified in order for it to not necessitate initiation and thus makes it more widely accessible.

For example, the *anuloma-viloma* technique, also known as mental alternate nostril breathing, is a highly effective practice which can be done in *yoga-nidrā* for balancing the mind and purifying the subtle energy channels (*nāḍis*). It follows the same principle as the 'purification of the energy channels' (*nāḍi-śodhana*) technique, where the practitioner directs the flow of breath from one nostril to another in succession through closing and opening them with the help of a hand *mudrā*. However, in *anuloma-viloma* this is done purely mentally, without physical control of the nostrils, which means that although the practitioner imagines the breath moving through the nostrils, they do not physically alter or control their natural breathing rhythm. This method of breathing serves as a bridge to deeper practices, including visualisation (Stage 6 of Satyananda Yoga Nidra), by refining the awareness and helping to integrate mind and body.

The process begins with guiding the awareness during inhalation through the left nostril, using the power of imagination, until the practitioner's awareness is sensitised to feel the flow of *prāṇa*. After inhaling, the practitioner mentally shifts the awareness of breath to the right nostril during the exhalation. The cycle then alternates: after exhalation through the right, awareness is guided with inhalation through the right nostril, followed by awareness of exhalation through the left nostril, and so on. This alternating flow of breath awareness through the nostrils is not only a physiological process but also facilitates the purification (*śuddhi*) of the subtle energy channels or *nāḍis*, which are believed to carry *prāṇa* (vital energy) throughout the body.

---

447 Sarawati, Satyasangananda, Swami. (2004). *Sri Vijnana Bhairava Tantra – The Ascent*. Munger: Yoga Publication Trust, p. 424.

Effects on the Subconscious

The practice of *anuloma-viloma* aims at cleansing the energy channels but also helps in purifying the subconscious of deep-seated impressions (*vāsanas*), *samskāras*, and emotions. As the mind becomes calm and the breath balanced, various thoughts, images, and emotions may arise. These fleeting mental impressions are a natural occurrence during deep relaxation, and they provide insight into the subconscious mind. However, it is important not to become attached or identified with these thoughts.

To maintain a focused and non-reactive state of awareness, practitioners use two key tools:

1. Counting backwards: This helps anchor the awareness in the present moment, preventing the mind from wandering or getting lost in the arising thoughts or emotions.
2. The *draṣṭā* attitude: The concept of *draṣṭā* refers to the observer aspect of consciousness—which manifests as the mind which simply observes without attachment or judgment. By cultivating this attitude, the practitioner does not engage with the passing thoughts or emotions but instead remains detached and aware of them without identifying with them.

This combination of breath control, mental focus, and non-identification with fleeting impressions prepares the practitioner for deeper states of immersion and visualisation, enabling them to access and refine their inner consciousness in *yoga-nidrā*.

Stage 5 — Pairs of Opposites in *yoga-nidrā*

> *Imagining certain feelings within the body can trigger off various memory centers and bring up deep-rooted memories, experiences and events from our subconscious and unconscious mind.*[448]
>
> Svāmī Nirañjanānanda

Stage 5 (opposite sensations) of *yoga-nidrā* addresses this level of dualistic perception. Intense, opposite physical sensations or opposite emotions are now consciously accessed, fully experienced internally, rather than induced by external stimuli,[449] and thus weakened during this stage. This is in contrast to the usual state of mind where the consciousness is involuntarily carried by the current of changing conditions and emotions and is characterised by identification with them.

During this Stage, the facilitator guides the practitioners' awareness towards pre-selected specific pairs of opposite sensations. In the initial and moderately advanced forms of *yoga-nidrā* practice, the pairs of opposite sensations should relate to the physical realm of perception, such as heaviness and lightness, cold and heat, hunger and thirst, etc. It is in the more advanced forms, that pairs of sensations from the mental realm, such as pain and pleasure, grief and joy, or hatred and love, are introduced systematically. However, these advanced forms should be practised only under the guidance of an experienced teacher and with caution, as the emotions which can arise and are confronted by the practitioner can sometimes be very intense.

Opposite Sensations in Yoga and Tantra

Our subjective experience of the external world is shaped by joy and suffering, which we perceive as a pair of opposites. In everyday life, desires and aversions are triggered by sensory impressions and the identifications which arise with them. When we encounter something pleasant, we desire to repeat the experience; when we come across something unpleasant, we feel aversion.

---

448 Saraswati, Niranjanananda, Swami. (2012). *On the Wings of the Swan*. Part 1. (2nd edition). Munger: Yoga Publication Trust, p. 48.

449 See Part I. Chapter 5. *The Stages of pratyāhāra*.

This constant involuntary movement between *rāga* (attraction) and *dveṣa* (aversion), or liking and disliking, creates suffering and personal drama in us. On the subjective level of reality, these opposites always coexist—where there is pleasure, pain is also present. Regardless of our attitude towards these feelings, opposing emotions simultaneously affect the unconscious.

> In the context of Satyananda Yoga Nidra two approaches to spiritual advancement can be observed: as discussed previously, in Patanjali's system the impeding modifications of the mind (*citta-vṛttis*) are neutralised (*niruddha*) by means of discipline and the *draṣṭā*-stance. Patañjali's system works by the practitioner seeking to neutralise the roots of bondage and suffering by quieting the manifest activities of the mind and cultivating concentration. The tantric approach, on the other hand, works through harnessing the innate capacity of mind and expanding awareness instead. Stage 5 of Satyananda Yoga Nidra utilises rather the second approach.

Svāmī Satyasaṅgānanda explains that, in order to gain knowledge about something, one must observe it neutrally and with awareness. The experience of duality should ultimately be transcended, but to transcend it, one must first become aware of what is being transcended, rather than it being ignored or suppressed. For an objective experience, disidentification is necessary—separating the awareness into subject (the observer) and object (the observed). That is why the approach from Patañjali's system is used at the beginning. The use of the dual perspective is actually essential in the early stages of spiritual practice (*sādhana*), before inner knowledge (*vidyā*) can be attained.[450] In the tantric approach there is no conceptual assessment—phenomena are not ultimately qualified as 'good' or 'bad', 'positive' or 'negative' in the emotional sense, but are seen as more or less useful tools, resources and energies to be harnessed by the practitioner in order to achieve their goals. They are regarded as the myriad manifestations of the Divine—many, but non-separate (*abheda*).

Ultimately, everything in life can be taken as a practice which can lead to the realisation of the unity of existence—that all is one reality.

---

450 Sarawati, Satyasangananda, Swami. (2004). *Sri Vijnana Bhairava Tantra – The Ascent*. Munger: Yoga Publication Trust, p. 138–139.

For example, the 14th century *haṭha-yoga* text *Yogabīja* (verses 89–90) explains how yoga ultimately unites all dualities:

yo 'pānaprāṇayor yogaḥ svarajoretasos tathā ||
sūryācandramasor yogo jīvātmaparamātmanoḥ || 89 ||

evaṃ tu dvandajālasya saṃyogo yoga ucyate || 90ab ||[451]

The union of *apāna* and *prāṇa*, one's own *rajas* and semen,
the sun and moon, the individual soul (*ātman*) and the supreme soul (*brahman*), (89)

and in the same way the union of all dualities, is called *yoga*. (90)[452]

The earlier Śaiva *Vijñāna-bhairava-tantra* also discusses transcending dualistic perception in verses 19–20:

na vahner dāhikā śaktiḥ vyatiriktā vibhāvyate |
kevalaṃ jñānasattāyāṃ prārambho 'yam praveśane || 19 ||

śaktyavasthāpraviṣṭasya nirvibhāgena bhāvanā |
tadāsau śivarūpī syāt śaivī mukham ihocyate || 20 ||

Just as the force (*śaktiḥ*) of ignition cannot be imagined (i.e. meditated upon, cultivated, conceived of) separately from fire (*agni*),
only when such an undertaking has been entered (engaged) into with the knowledge [of this truth], (19)

when one has arrived at that [level of] visionary cultivation characterised by non-discrimination which is within the realm of [Supreme] Śakti,

451 Muñoz, Adrián. (2016). Yogabīja: A critical transcription of a text on haṭhayoga. In: *Nova Tellvs*, 33/2, p. 142.
452 Mallinson, J. and Singelton, M. (2017). Roots of Yoga. London: Penguin Classics, p. 23.

[only] then is [this state] itself She-who-has-the-form-of-Śiva, [and is hence] referred to as 'the face of Śiva'. (20)[453]

In Tantra, the goal is not to widen the gap between opposites such as love and hate, life and death, etc., but to unite them at the centre, allowing unity to be experienced in that way. This principle is applied across all aspects of existence in Tantra, whether it is the flow of breath in the form of inhalation and exhalation, or the two opposing vital energies of *prāṇa* (upward) and *apāna* (downward), which move in opposite directions within the body, or the concepts of time and space, or energy and consciousness.[454] In verse 126, the *Vijñāna-bhairava-tantra* explains how the focus of awareness on the space between two opposites serves to effectively eliminate the idea of difference and duality:

na dveṣam bhāvayet kvāpi na rāgam bhāvayet kvacit |
rāgadveṣavinirmuktau madhye brahma prasarpati || 126 ||

One should conjure no aversion anywhere, nor any affection at all –
It is in that middle [which is arrived at] when attraction and aversion have been let go of, that Brahman sets in. (126)[455]

Although the overall approach differs, transcending opposites through experiencing them in order to achieve balance is also present in Patañjali's system at least in the realm of physical sensation. There, aside from the 'heat of practice' (*sūtra* 2.1), tapas or 'ordeal' can also refer to the voluntarily enduring of opposing sensations such as heat and cold, the desire for food or drink, standing and sitting, etc. Furthermore, achieving a 'stable and comfortable posture' (*āsana*; *sūtra* 2.46) is tantamount to having mastered the realm of opposing physical sensations (*sūtra* 2.48), wherefore practicing *tapas* in this form is no longer a necessity.

Detaching oneself from attraction and aversion does not imply an indifferent or passive approach to life. On the contrary, it enables a more conscious,

453 Translation from the Sanskrit: Georgi Krastev
454 Sarawati, Satyasangananda, Swami. (2004). *Sri Vijnana Bhairava Tantra – The Ascent*. Munger: Yoga Publication Trust, p. 373–374.
455 Translation from the Sanskrit: Georgi Krastev.

attentive, free, and active participation, through engagement with the true and not the subjective nature of reality. Through this pure presence, we can empower the mind to become the master of itself. Or, as Svāmī Satyānanda puts it:

> *Yoga-nidra* thus develops control of the emotional reactions and autonomic responses. This [...] is reflected in daily life as increased perceptual awareness, emotional control and an increasingly conscious destiny.[456]

The Effect of the Awareness of Opposite Sensations on the Brain

Stage 5 of the practice connects us to an evolutionarily old area of the brain—the 'emotional' brain or limbic system, which, among other things, interacts with the hypothalamus—the control centre for the entire autonomic nervous system. The limbic system, which is composed of several structures, is a 'switchboard' for instincts and is a part of the brain which is essential for our survival. Here, we will address a particular part of the limbic system, our emotional 'accelerator'—the almond-shaped amygdala with its multiple nuclei, situated in the medial temporal region of the brain. Signals are sent between the amygdala and the hypothalamus via the stria terminalis pathway. This primarily influences the body's autonomic functions—such as breathing and blood circulation—and adapts them to the respective situation. 'The amygdala also projects in a reciprocal fashion to brain stem nuclei involved in the autonomic changes that accompany fear and stress related responses. [...] The connections between the amygdala and the hypothalamus and visceral brain stem nuclei explain the complex physiological responses that occur with mood changes in general, specifically fear and the 'fight-or-flight' response.'[457]

The hypothalamus plays two essential roles in this. On the one hand, it fulfils psychosomatic and somatopsychic functions, and on the other, it is the most important brain region for maintaining homeostasis and for making

---

456 Saraswati, Satyananda, Swami. (2006). *Yoga Nidra*. (12th reprint). Munger: Yoga Publications Trust, p. 42.

457 Friedman, Joseph H. Kelvin; Chou, L. (2007). Mood, Emotion, and Thought. In: Christopher G. Goetz. *Textbook of Clinical Neurology*, Chapter 3. (3rd edition). Amsterdarm: Saunders Elsevier, p. 35.

the necessary adjustments to the organism when it is under stress. Thus, the hypothalamus, as the centre of the autonomic nervous system, reacts to strong emotional stimuli from the amygdala to trigger the production of adrenaline in the adrenal glands, thus preparing the body for danger. Even the slightest disturbances of this extremely important forebrain area can have a direct effect on our ability to survive.

As discussed before, since in *pratyāharā* the senses are uncoupled from their sense objects, i.e. there is little to no reaction to external stimuli, the other natural source of information — memory and its associated emotional information, become more prominent in the activity of the mind, but also much more accessible to the awareness, since the distraction usually provided by those external stimuli is eliminated. The connection between emotion and memory, as well as the interrelation between and the physical responses to the two are largely regulated by the limbic system, and the amygdala and the hypothalamus in particular. This is a region of the brain responsible for the emotional evaluation of experiences and usually precedes the higher-function decision-making processes in the cerebrum.

The amygdala plays a major role in:

- the fear response, anxiety and aggression;
- learning through rewards and punishment;
- unconscious memory and habituated actions (riding a bike, tying your shoe laces, etc.);
- recognition of and reaction to social cues (facial expression, tone of voice, etc.);
- emotions related to parenting and bonding, the emotional valency of memories;
- addiction.

The hypothalamus plays a major role in:

- regulating body temperature and blood pressure;
- feelings of hunger and thirst, as well as the sense of fullness when eating;
- mood;

- sex drive;
- the production of dopamine, prolactin, oxytocin;
- regulating the circadian rhythm;

The hypothalamus and the amygdala, together with the entire limbic system, play a major role in controlling many vital functions such as

- Triggering feelings such as anger and aggression and their physical expression;
- Maintaining homeostasis (temperature, blood pressure, osmolarity);
- Regulating body temperature;
- Autonomic regulation of food and water intake;
- Maintaining wakefulness and sleep patterns or the circadian rhythm;
- Controlling the functions of sex drive and reproduction.

Environmental and intrapsychic stimuli, as mediated by the hypothalamus, initiate mental and emotional responses that in turn trigger physiological responses throughout the body. Through this connection with the limbic system, our physiological and hormonal reactions are directly influenced by our emotions. Thus, our limbic system regulates our affective and instinctive behaviour towards the environment as well as our memory. The incoming sensory information is stored and coordinated in the limbic system, where it finds its emotional response. Although human behaviour is controlled by the entire nervous system, the limbic system controls most of its involuntary aspects.

As we address various opposing sensations, such as heaviness—lightness, heat—cold, pain—pleasure, etc. in our *yoga-nidrā* practice, we stimulate the hypothalamus and the limbic system at the same time. By identifying with these different sensations and emotions, we develop instinctive or habitual reactions to how we feel. By practicing systematic directed awareness of them, we gradually uncouple the stimuli from the emotional reactions and thus disidentify with them, much in the same way as when the senses are uncoupled from their sense objects in the initial stages of *pratyāhāra* and thus they start to imitate the mind.

Over time, this level of practice can help us maintain and even strengthen our homeostatic balance by giving us some control over our unconscious, normally uncontrollable functions. With repeated practice, a new neural circuit between different areas is established in the brain which normally never work simultaneously. The activated circuit enables us to perceive two previously contrary experiences of consciousness in immediate succession, with the aim of balancing our basic instincts. By deliberately activating them, we learn to control their functions, which generally occur unconsciously. This process is very profound, because gradually we will be able to mitigate our own autonomous and emotional reactions by means of their respective contrasting sensations.

This practice also strengthens willpower on an emotional level. At this stage, memories of deep feelings can also be released. Through the detachment and liberation of these memories, an even deeper emotional sense of relaxation can occur. The greater the tension between the two opposites, the greater the energy which emanates from them and can be released. We can think of this process as a pendulum movement in which the pendulum, instead of always moving to the left and right, settles in the middle area and the extremes are gradually surpassed.

Stage 6 — Visualisation in *yoga-nidrā*

> *The technique of visualisation in yoga-nidrā is an important practice for unlocking the stored up contents of the unconscious mind which normally only manifest during dreams.*[458]
>
> Svāmī Satyānanda

The use of visualisation practices is characteristic of Tantric yoga. Deep immersion — *dhyāna* — historically in Tantra this often included the active visualisation of a deity (*bhāvanā*) and the awareness of its qualities and attributes. The descriptions of these visualisations can be highly complex and sophisticated, often interweaving symbolism and mantras with theology and metaphysics. Stage 6 of *yoga-nidrā* — visualisation — is also based on such tantric practices.

---

458 Saraswati, Satyananda, Swami. (2006). *Yoga Nidra*. (12th reprint). Munger: Yoga Publications Trust, p. 43.

This last, inwardly-directed Stage of *yoga-nidrā* leads to deep mental relaxation, thus completing the *pratyāhāra* process. Awareness is directed towards *cidākāśa*, the 'space/opening of consciousness'. In this space, the practitioner is able to perceive (often referred to as 'seeing') the contents of the mind which are gradually released from the subconscious in the form of inner images. At this stage of the practice, the practitioner awakens and perceives images, symbols and patterns, with the help of prompts provided by the facilitator. Since the images used often have a universal meaning and yet can evoke strong individual associations, they spontaneously lift the hidden contents of the deep subconscious into conscious awareness. It is essential to understand that this is neither a fantasy journey nor hypnosis[459] — nor should content from these techniques be used.

Although the term 'visualisation' suggests the active imagination of the image of something visible, the *pratyāhāra-yoga-nidrā* technique actually involves more than just imagining images. Nor is this a purely visual experience. It also encompasses sounds, smells, bodily sensations, feelings and emotions. In fact, these inner, spontaneously arising 'images' emerge from our mind rather than being created under the influence of input from our physical senses or, in more profound states reached by the experienced practitioner — even without conceptualisation. The technique facilitates the natural, spontaneous emergence of such experiences, and not active imagination or visualisation in the usual sense. Rather than supplying input to the mind, the facilitator merely creates the right environment for the mind to display its own content.

As described above, the various levels of consciousness can be reached in the *pratyāhāra* state during *yoga-nidrā* because the boundaries between the conscious, subconscious and unconscious become loose and translucent. Visualisation (cultivation) in this state promotes the development of awareness of the Self and relaxes the mind by clearing it of disturbing or painful impressions. This allows the subconscious to be purified (*śodhana*). Although a deep relaxation naturally occurs when practising *yoga-nidrā*, the primary goal of the *pratyāhāra-yoga-nidrā* technique is to release such disturbing impressions and to free the subconscious of them. This increases

459 See Part 3. Chapter 20. *Yoga-nidrā and Western Prychology; Yoga-nidrā and Hypnosis – A Comparison of the Fundamental Similarities and Differences.*

mental energy, capacity and focus for further meditative states. This practice strengthens the ability of our mind on many different levels. In addition to its purifying effect on the subconscious, it also promotes the development of our imaginative capacity. The visualisation Stage is usually concluded with an image which evokes a deep sense of peace and tranquillity.

The visualisation Stage can lead the mind to *dhāraṇā*, and in advanced stages of *yoga-nidrā*, it can immerse it in *dhyāna*, where there is a conscious experience of the visualised object in the unconscious, there is no longer any distinction between the conscious and the unconscious, and no more distracting images arise.

During the practice of *yoga-nidrā*, one experiences the connection with the different layers of consciousness in a more aware manner, depending on the depth of the level of experience. In waking consciousness, relaxation, a comforting experience, or sleep can all occur. When the subconscious is engaged in the further stages of the practice, one experiences an apparent suspension of gravity, as the perception temporarily detaches itself from the body image. This can also cause further, different subtle sensations.

At this Stage, the transition of perception and awareness from *manomaya-* to *vijnānamaya-kośa* occurs. Occasionally, it is possible to penetrate to the core of the unconscious, where the latent contents (*saṃskāras*) of the mind, which we usually do not consciously experience, can be perceived.

Effect and choice of images and symbols

In *yoga-nidrā*, various images and symbols are used to bridge the gap between the waking state and the deeper layers of the mind at the boundary between the subtle body — the subconscious — and the causal body — the unconscious. They are like catalysts which provoke a reaction in the unconscious. One can consider them as a kind of archiving programme on the computer which decodes and releases the impressions stored in the subconscious, which we cannot 'unzip' and view without them. Confronting these impressions can be very challenging for the practitioner if they take the form of painful memories, unfulfilled desires, conflicts, fears, complexes and neuroses. The process of visualisation enables us to become a neutral observer of these reactions and to purify the mind of these limiting impressions. These pratyayas and *saṃskāras* are the silent and invisible root causes of most of our suffering.

The images suggested by the facilitator serve to activate the deeper layers of the mind through spontaneous associations. These images do not have to be related to each other, connected by a thematic thread or progressing like a story. They should be delivered in rapid succession, repeated two or three times, and kept very brief. The practitioner should perceive the succession of symbols and images without judgement, as if watching a film.

In this process, it is not necessary to recognise or analyse the released impressions. These impressions can often arise as an unclear image, sound, thought or feeling. While the *saṃskāras* within conscious memory are arranged in a specific, coherent and personal-logical order, while in the subconscious and unconscious they do not follow any clearly comprehensible order. When these images are viewed objectively rather than subjectively, the ego temporarily becomes inactive — it no longer identifies with the inhibitions, likes or dislikes which reinforce its individual nature.

> *The symbols used form two categories. Firstly, there are the conditioned symbols, which are associated with our day-to-day social, cultural, religious and moral experiences. These would vary for persons of different localities, countries and [peoples] and the images used from a certain cultural situation may be completely meaningless to the practitioner whose mind has been conditioned by other types of symbols. Then there are the universal symbols (as described by Jung) such as mantra, yantra and mandala, which form part of the consciousness of every man, woman and child, irrespective of social, religious and cultural traditions. These symbols form the 'collective unconscious' mind of mankind, and symbols used in this area invoke very deep responses.*[460]
>
> Svāmī Satyānanda

All images should be carefully chosen by the facilitator, taking into account the participants or group of participants to be guided. Apparently harmless images can have a strong effect.

Svāmī Satyānanda indicates two categories of images to be used:

---

460 Ibid., p. 45–46.

- conditioned images — social, cultural, religious and moral symbols which have different meanings depending on origin, culture, location, etc.;
- universal symbols — archetypes as described by C. G. Jung, which are part of the 'collective unconscious' and the consciousness of all cultures, e.g. mantra, *yantra*, *maṇḍala*.

As long as the mind is not focused and directed, visualisation can be difficult; the scattered mind cannot hold the attention long enough for an image to emerge. To develop the ability to visualise, Svāmī Satyānanda recommends:

- visualising familiar objects, daily routines and events which have left a strong impression;
- visualising the objects as large as possible in the mental space;
- first giving the images a dynamic expression and then moving on to static images.

The visualisation in *yoga-nidrā* can be of two different types: *pratyāhāra* and *dhāraṇā*. The beginner to intermediate level visualisation is practised with a *pratyāhāra* focus. At advanced stages of the technique, the focus can be deepened to *dhāraṇā*-visualisation. However, this more advanced practice should only be practised after proper preparation and under the guidance of an experienced teacher.

Cidākāśa — The space of consciousness

Cidākāśa or *cittākāśa* is composed of two words — *cit*(*ta*) (mind/consciousness) and *ākāśa* (space, the element of ether). It represents the inner firmament, the consciousness which forms the inner space and in which all experiences during *dhāraṇā* and *dhyāna* take place. This means that a consciousness which is all-encompassing expands in all directions, so that one can experience oneself as an all-pervasive consciousness.

When we withdraw our awareness from the realm of gross, external perception, we initially experience darkness (*tamas*) — until gradually the impressions and archetypes which have accumulated and deposited in the causal body or in the unconscious emerge. While our eyes are closed in deeper immersion, we can become aware of the infinite space within ourselves and our existence, although we cannot see our physical body with closed eyelids. In the infinite space of the *cidākāśa*, we can experience the inner aspects of the individual Self (*puruṣa*).

The 'physical' space of *cit(ta)* is located behind the eyes or at the level of the cranial cavity, directly behind the frontal bone. It can only be experienced when both the thinking mind and the intellect cease their normal functions in interaction with the senses. Therefore, while focusing on *cidākāśa*, the inner awareness should be brought into the space behind the closed eyes. Everything we experience in it should be witnessed without getting involved with the impressions and images or the thought flow.

At first, it can be very difficult to recognise or 'see' anything other than darkness in the inner space. With practice, we gradually begin to perceive images which correspond to the impressions hidden deep within us, accumulated in the subconscious and unconscious. Therefore, during *pratyāhāra* visualisation, the practitioner may see whatever the suggested symbols are, according to their 'inner material'. It is essential to let the impressions arise spontaneously, without trying to visualise them. In order to remain present in this space, we should practice daily for several months. It therefore takes a correspondingly long time for the stored images of the subconscious to be cleared in *pratyāhāra-yoga-nidrā*, so that the mind can later clearly distinguish the symbols mentioned in *dhāraṇā-yoga-nidrā*. Although we may not experience anything in *cidākāśa* at the beginning, this does not mean that there is nothing in the inner space. We will always arrive at some experience, but it depends a lot on how regularly and with what conviction we practice.[461]

In *Vijñāna-bhairava-tantra* verse 85, the practice of focussing the mind in the space of *cidākāśa* is described as follows:

---

461 Saraswati, Satyananda, Swami. (2002). *Dynamics of Yoga – The Foundations of Bihar Yoga*. Munger: Yoga Publication Trust. (2nd reprint), pp. 122–129.

līnaṃ mūrdhni viyat sarvam bhairavatvena bhāvayet |
tat sarvam bhairavākāratejastattvaṃ samāviśet || 85 ||

Being absorbed in the cranial vault, [the practitioner] should cultivate/ visualise all Space as being of the nature of Bhairava,[462]
[that is,] all that — as completely permeated by the brilliant reality of Bhairava's form. (85)[463]

Stage 7 — *saṃkalpa* and Stage 8 — Externalisation

At the end of the practice, when the subconscious is highly receptive, the *saṃkalpa* is repeated with full faith and conviction to firmly embed the resolve, after which awareness is gradually externalised in reverse order by reconnecting with external sounds, environmental stimuli, and the physical body.

462 Bhairava is the name given to the Absolute, the transcendent God in particular streams of Śaivism. He is usually wild, wrathful and terrifying.

463 Translation from the Sanskrit: Georgi Krastev.

Part Three

Fields of Application of Satyananda Yoga Nidra in Today's Society

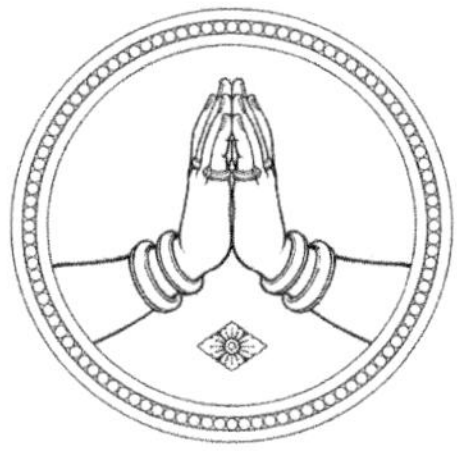

CHAPTER 15

Effects of Stress and the Importance of Relaxation

THE DEMANDS OF CONTEMPORARY SOCIAL existence on the individual are constantly increasing. The accelerating speed of communication, the development of related technologies and the alienation from Nature and other human beings are also increasing exponentially, and our senses are constantly being overstimulated. The human mind can often hardly process the amount of impressions, the flood of information, the resulting thoughts and feelings. Instead, it stores them mostly unconsciously. These experiences then turn into constant subliminal tensions which we can usually neither resolve nor process, and which we ultimately take with us into our sleep every day. As a result, our body and mind can no longer recover, we still wake up exhausted, and the fatigue remains with us throughout the day. The energies of body and mind are permanently scattered, creating a vicious circle.

The Body's Functions Under Stress

When under stress, the organism activates the sympathetic nervous system, which in turn triggers the primitive 'fight-or-flight' response. Without sufficient relaxation, the body remains in a permanent state of agitation, which gradually leads to eventual exhaustion. On a biochemical level, this means that our body continuously releases stress hormones, including adrenaline and cortisol, as well as other related compounds, rather than doing so only intermittently when required. When adrenaline levels rise, mental and muscular tension increases. Negative and destructive emotions, thoughts or experiences, which also provoke the production of stress hormones, can eventually lead to psychophysiological and somatic disorders.

Signals are sent to the muscles via the sympathetic nervous system, causing them to respond with tension and overactivity, thereby disrupting natural muscle tone. In this way, the body is ready to put thoughts and affects[464] into action. However, in our daily lives, we usually suppress our frustration and negativity; tensions remain unresolved and the body remains in a constant 'fight' mode. This results in enormous energy consumption, which usually leads to, at the very least, chronic fatigue.

The large energy consumption brought about by constant muscle tension leads to an increase in blood circulation, erratic breathing and heart rate. To maintain the muscles of the extremities in a state of heightened readiness, the body mobilises energy from the internal organs and the associated musculature. This interrupts normal organ function. Likewise, the entire endocrine system must inevitably run at full speed to cope with such an increased demand for bodily functions. Since this condition is not sustainable, we often resort to secondary means to help us cope with the stress and tension—coffee, alcohol, food, extreme sports, drugs, etc.

The gut is one of the most important parts of the immune system and, with its independent enteric nervous system[465], is considered to be our 'second brain'. It extends over more than 100 million nerve cells. The number of

464 A technical term in psychology, an affect is the underlying experience of feeling, emotion, attachment, or mood.

465 The enteric nervous system (ENS) is one of the three divisions of the autonomic nervous system (ANS), the others being the sympathetic nervous system (SNS) and parasympathetic nervous system (PSNS). It is an independent regulatory system that is, however, influenced by signals from the SNS and the PSNS.

nerve cells in the gut is far greater than those in the entire peripheral nervous system combined, and is four to five times the number of nerve cells in the spinal cord alone. Ninety percent of these cells in the gut are involved in transmitting information to and from the brain via the vagus[466] nerve. The gut nervous system plays a significant role in modulating our emotions through its connection with the brain. Approximately 90–95% of the body's 'happy hormone' serotonin is synthesised in the enterochromaffin cells of the intestinal mucosa, where it plays key roles in regulating gut motility and communicating with the central nervous system via the gut–brain axis.[467] Medical professionals are already trying to treat depression and mood swings by improving bowel function. The gut requires a great deal of energy to perform its functions. If the sympathetic nervous system remains activated far beyond 'emergency situations', the gut is deprived of this energy, which can lead to illnesses such as digestive problems and local serotonin deficiency. As a result, other psychosomatic illnesses can develop and the entire immune system is permanently weakened.

Our body has a perfect regulatory system for relaxation and regeneration — our sleep. However, the accumulation of our subconscious everyday tensions prevents us from having deep, restful and relaxing sleep. It has been scientifically proven that sufficient sleep is vital to allow our entire system sufficient rest and regeneration. The WHO (World Health Organisation) recommends that adults get eight hours of uninterrupted sleep, every night.[468] However, there are hardly any people who get to enjoy a sleep pattern like that. Most of us are woken by the sound of our alarm clock, and so we jump into our day and perform mentally and/or physically throughout the day until at some point we fall into bed tired. We take the day's unresolved mental tensions with us to bed, sleep restlessly, sleep remains superficial, and many people do not sleep through the night.

Constant stress inhibits the production of serotonin, which in turn is necessary for the production of the 'sleep hormone' melatonin. The result is poor sleep-quality, insufficient sleep and an interrupted circadian rhythm (the

---

466 The vagus nerve is a cranial nerve which creates a pathway interfacing with the parasympathetic control of the heart, lungs, and digestive tract.

467 The most important sites for serotonin production are the enterochromaffin cells of the intestinal mucosa.

468 Walker, Matthew. (2017). *Why we sleep – unlocking the power of sleep and dream*. New York: Scribner, p. 3.

sleep-wake cycle). This has serious consequences for our brain, ranging from poor concentration and memory to increased risk of developing Alzheimer's disease. Even if we get too little sleep for just one week, our body's blood sugar level, for example, can become so unbalanced that a blood test could show that we are prediabetic. Unfortunately, sleep cannot be compensated for and a lack of sleep can cause the body's ageing processes to progress rapidly. So, according to scientific studies, there really is such a thing as beauty sleep.[469]

Excessive weight gain or weight loss can be further symptoms of tension and lack of sleep. Some people tend to eat more when their body lacks energy or when they are tense, and they gain weight uncontrollably. Others, on the other hand, lose their appetite when they are tense and unintentionally lose weight.[470]

In his book *A Systematic Course in The Ancient Tantric Techniques of Yoga and Kriya*, Svāmī Satyānanda differentiates between general physical and mental as well as emotional tension. In his view, the causes of this tension are internal or external in nature, but fundamentally they are an expression of 'wrong' thinking about other people and our environment. The factors which prevent us from living in peace with our environment are fear, hatred, dislike, jealousy, etc. These negative feelings have been accumulating in us since the moment of our birth, unconsciously influencing our everyday lives and subsequently leading to disharmony and disturbed homeostasis in the body and a disturbed mind. Identifying with problematic situations causes enormous mental tension. When we reflect and brood, we experience those problems over and over again, becoming more and more absorbed in them and constantly recreating the same unfavourable biochemical and muscular state. We use a lot of energy to assert ourselves against our environment and constantly live in a state of tension with our surroundings. As a result, our systems function non-stop in a kind of emergency mode, which leads to the dispersion of our energies, the distraction of our attention and our resources in all possible directions. Becoming aware of these unconscious programmes which control our lives and reprogramming them is a central task on the path towards balance and well-being in everyday life.

---

469 Ibid., p. 13.
470 Ibid., p. 14.

Recent research in neurophysiology expands this classical understanding of the stress response by describing not only the sympathetic 'fight-or-flight' reactions but also the so-called 'freeze' or 'shutdown' mode, which is mediated by the dorsal branch of the vagus nerve. When sympathetic overactivation becomes chronic and the organism perceives no possibility of successful fight or escape, the body may shift into this parasympathetically dominated immobility response. This freeze state, characterized by tonic or atonic muscular collapse, is accompanied by dissociative mechanisms in the brain that serve short-term survival but lead, in the long run, to a persistent fragmentation of experience and to an inability to act.[471]

In this condition, physiological energy is not released outward through movement but locked inward, resulting in chronic dissociation, emotional numbing, and functional disconnection from the environment and from one's own inner states. The person remains 'frozen' between sympathetic hyperarousal and vagal 'shutdown'. Over time, this pattern undermines the organism's capacity for self-regulation, subjective relatedness, and relaxation. In psychological terms, it manifests as constant distraction, exhaustion, and a loss of embodied presence.[472]

Within this neurobiological context, the practice of Satyananda Yoga Nidra can be understood as a systematic process of re-engaging the vagal system in a regulated way. Through conscious withdrawal of the sense perception from the sense objects (*pratyāhāra*) and the cultivation of the witness attitude (*draṣṭā-bhāva*), the practitioner gradually re-establishes safe interoceptive awareness. This allows the nervous system to oscillate naturally between sympathetic activation and parasympathetic restoration without falling into collapse. Over time, the capacity for self-soothing, emotional integration, and relational openness is restored.

---

471 See: Porges, S., W. (2011). *The Polyvagal Theory: Neurophysiological Foundations of Emotions, Attachment, Communication, and Self-Regulation*. New York: Norton and Dana, D. (2018). *The Polyvagal Theory in Therapy: Engaging the Rhythm of Regulation*. New York: Norton.

472 Schauer, M., & Elbert, T. (2010). Dissociation following traumatic stress. *Zeitschrift für Psychologie*. 218(2), 109–127. https://doi.org/10.1027/0044-3409/a000018 (seen on 07.10.2025).

The Concept of 'Relaxation' in Yoga

Relaxation as such is not conceptually present in pre-modern Yoga; the associated practices come from Western psychology. In Yoga, a state of the absence of tension in the mind (*citta-viśrānti*)[473] is rather regarded as a neutral prerequisite for certain yogic practices. During the late nineteenth and early twentieth centuries, various techniques were developed within the Western therapeutic milieu to promote relaxation in patients facing the increasing stresses of industrial society. By the second half of the twentieth century, a secularised form of Yoga had emerged, emphasising its positive effects on both physical and mental health. In classical Yoga, however, relaxation is regarded less as an ultimate goal than as a side effect or intermediate stage—one element within the broader process of yogic practice.

Svāmī Satyānanda further recognised that genuine recuperation and rejuvenation require the regular release of accumulated tensions in both body and mind. Although deep relaxation may appear simple, it is in fact profoundly challenging for many individuals. We must relearn how to let go, to relax, and to allow the body-mind complex to rest. When ordinary sleep is insufficient to restore balance due to chronic restlessness and tension, specific yogic techniques—particularly *śavāsana* and *yoga-nidrā*—can provide effective means of renewal.

Promoting relaxation, or more accurately—a tension-free state, is a basic approach or a preliminary stage of all Yoga techniques to be practiced in a modern environment, not only because we live more healthily through relaxation, but because we can only penetrate to the deeper levels of existence and train and sharpen our perception in a tension-free state. Such a state is also a prerequisite for immersion, and thus for our spiritual development.

It is not possible to enter into immersion when we are tense. Tension dissipates our energy, whereas a tension-free state allows us to focus our physical and mental resources and helps us achieve emotional balance. The aim to live in the here and now, to be more aware and conscious, is the basis of yoga.

473 *Haṭha-yoga-pradīpikā* 1.34. (See below).

Practicing *āsanas* with awareness, for example aligned with the breathing rhythm, connects body and mind and has the same calming effect as the practice of *prāṇāyāma*, extended time in *śavāsana*, turning inwards and centring oneself while sitting, and focusing on the breath for a few moments in everyday life. Through the practice of *yoga-nidrā*, subconscious tensions can be released and the process of self-healing in the body can be activated without having to make any conscious effort. Satyananda Yoga Nidra offers people of today a method which can be easily integrated into their busy lives.

CHAPTER 16

Absence of Tension Through *Śavāsana* and *Yoga-Nidrā*

Relaxation techniques start by taking your consciousness away from emotionally charged thoughts and directing it to activities that are emotionally neutral, such as the awareness of your breath or different parts of your body. It is almost impossible for anyone to remain or to become tense and angry when their attention is directed towards their big toe. In this way, relaxation techniques stop the ceaseless and futile cycle of brooding on problems. Simultaneously the muscles are consciously relaxed.[474]

Svāmī Satyānanda

In the Bihar Yoga system, *śavāsana* and *yoga-nidrā* release the body's state of tension by gradually turning the mind away from external sensory stimuli naturally, through becoming aware of the sensory channels and perceptions,

474 Satyananda, Swami. (2006). *A Systematic Course in The Ancient Tantric Techniques of Yoga and Kriya*. (4th reprint). Munger: Yoga Publications Trust, p. 32.

and by remaining aware of the various sensory impressions and sensory stimuli.[475] The connection between stimulus and brain is interrupted for the duration of the practice by systematically guiding the practitioner into disidentification[476], which allows the sympathetic nervous system to gradually relax and stops the sending of activation impulses to the muscles.

śavāsana — the Corpse Pose

uttānaṃ śavavad bhūmau śayanaṃ tac chavāsanam |
śavāsanaṃ śrāntiharaṃ cittaviśrāntikārakam || *Haṭha-yoga-pradīpikā* 1.34 ||

When the back, like that of a corpse, has the ground as its bed—that is the 'corpse pose'.
The 'corpse pose' eliminates [bodily] fatigue and abates the weariness of the mind.

Śavāsana is one of the most important *āsanas* in Bihar Yoga and is used as a short awareness phase in *āsana* practice. *Śavāsana* is effective in some preliminary *prāṇāyāma* practices or simply in between or as a longer awareness practice.

Posture: In a supine position. The body lies symmetrically in a straight line with the heels placed hip-width apart, with the toes loosely falling to the side. The pelvis is tilted slightly upwards so that the lower back can relax better. The arms rest outstretched beside the body without touching it; the palms face upwards, rotated slightly outwards. The fingers are loosely curled. The shoulders are down and the shoulder blades are flat on the floor. The chin is

---

475 *śavāsana* and *yoga-nidrā* – Stage 1.

476 Disidentification is achieved by the practitioner being systematically guided into the observer stance (*draṣṭā*) during the practise and becoming absorbed in it. It is an attitude of neutral, yet active awareness in which all impressions and mental processes are perceived without judgement, without the need to act.

tucked in towards the chest so that the neck can lengthen and let go. The head is balanced and aligned with the spine. The lips and eyes are gently closed.

Although *śavāsana* appears very simple, the details of the pose should be considered, such as making sure that the body is lying symmetrically. If there is any tension in the body, it should be felt and consciously released so that the body can completely adopt a tension-free position and the breathing can flow freely. This preparation is part of the *āsana* and is of great importance.

Aids: For neck problems or tinnitus, a folded blanket or thin cushion can be placed under the head to raise it slightly. For back problems, a bolster or rolled-up blanket can be placed under the hollow of the knees to provide support for the lower back.

Śavāsana should be practised on the floor and not in bed or on a soft surface so that both superficial and deep muscles can completely let go. Its effect is increased when it is practised after dynamic *āsana*s or after *āsana*s such as *naukāsana* (the boat pose), in which many muscles of the body are activated. The physical and mental stillness in *śavāsana* can then occur more deeply.

Benefits: Although *śavāsana* is a static pose, it has a profound effect on several aspects of our wellbeing. All bodily systems slow down, and there is simultaneous relaxation of all psycho-physiological systems. In *śavāsana*, the mental level as well as the physical level are freed from tension. Impressions stored in the subconscious, which lead to unconscious tension, are also released. The origin of many diseases is stress or tension; with regular practice of *śavāsana*, the body, especially the nervous and immune systems, recover. In a tension-free state, the self-healing properties are stimulated and body and mind are allowed to regenerate.

As soon as the gross physical body enters a tension-free state, subtle planes of existence, such as the *prāṇamaya-kośa*, are also stimulated. Furthermore, by practising *śavāsana*, the mind is trained to remain alert and aware in a state of rest. A prolonged *śavāsana* practice is therefore an excellent preparation for deepening the awareness and may further lead into immersion.

General Effects of *yoga-nidrā*

Satyananda Yoga Nidra is usually practised in *śavāsana*, as sensory stimuli can be most easily reduced in this pose. In *śavāsana*, the organism can come into a tension-free state very effectively because the entire body—in comparison to classical meditation postures or other *āsanas*—rests on the floor without the use of muscle strength.

Yoga-nidrā can also be practised by those with some mental health issues[477], even while sitting, with eyes open if necessary. Pregnant women should enter *matsyakriḍāsana* (flapping fish pose)[478] or, if they are more advanced in their pregnancy, lie on their side, supported by cushions, or in another comfortable position.

In *yoga-nidrā*, the mind naturally disidentifies from the body during the rotation of awareness throughout the different body parts (Stage 3) as well as during breath awareness (Stage 4), and the muscles relax. The parasympathetic nervous system is thus reactivated, muscle cells, nerve cells and blood vessels, etc. can regenerate, and the various areas of the brain are protected from the constant influx of sensory information from the body and the environment and come to a rest.

Svāmī Satyānanda also explains the effect of coming to rest on the brain[479]—many ailments are caused by restrictions imposed on the body by the more highly developed areas of the brain. When consciousness disengages from the body, evolutionarily older brain regions or subordinate neural centers, such as the spinal cord, can perform their functions unimpeded by the higher developed brain centers. The subordinate centres then begin to restore balance in muscle tone. Balance in the endocrine system is also restored.

When the mind has also come to a state of stillness as a result of this process, we are in a more balanced mood and the adrenaline level in the blood remains low. The lessened release of adrenaline in turn reduces emotional

---

477 In the case of serious psychological problems, the treating psychotherapist should be consulted. *Yoga-nidrā* is generally not recommended for people who are very introverted or clinically depressed.

478 See Saraswati, Satyananada. (2009). *Asana, Pranayama, Mudra, Bandha*. Munger: Yoga Publication Trust., p. 91–92.

479 Saraswati, Satyananda, Swami. (2006). *A Systematic Course in The Ancient Tantric Techniques of Yoga and Kriya*. (4th reprint). Munger: Yoga Publications Trust, p. 32–33.

and mental irritability, as well as the willingness to engage in conflict. This results in a reduction in stress and anxiety, thus halting the release of adrenaline. The whole body can recover and regenerate, and the vicious circle of constant tension is broken.

A key principle for the success of the practice is how alert and aware we remain during the process. The more aware we are during the practice, the more profound the effect. According to Svāmī Satyānanda, the regenerating effect of an hour of *yoga-nidrā* practice on the mind can be equated to about four hours of deep sleep.[480] The mind needs a certain amount of time to move from relaxation to deep relaxation. The minimum practice time to achieve this state is about 20 minutes for the average adult. That is why a *yoga-nidrā* session lasts at least 20 minutes.

This chapter exclusively concerns itself with the effects of *yoga-nidra* on stress reduction and deep release of tension from body and mind. However, it should not be forgotten that one of the most important goals of *yoga-nidrā* is to achieve and master the state of *pratyāhāra*.

- **Prevention and Lasting effects**

The described effect of these practices only lasts for a certain period of time in our daily lives, usually only until we are exposed to a problematic situation again. Then the vicious circle of chronic stress and tension begins all over again.

To prevent the recurrence of tension, we should try to neutralise and transform our mental reaction programmes stored since birth. The integral yoga approach and in particular the *pratyāhāra* and *svādhyāya* techniques can be helpful in achieving this. For this reason, in the integral yoga approach, the *svādhyāya* techniques are implemented as a supporting element of *sādhana*.

The most important principle for stress and tension prevention with the help of *yoga-nidrā* is regular, daily practice, as the effects accumulate over a period of time. Just like with chronic sleep deprivation, sleeping for three days straight would not 'compensate' for the effect of two consecutive weeks or more of lack of sleep.

480 Saraswati, Satyananda, Swami. (2006). *Yoga Nidra*. (12th reprint). Munger: Yoga Publications Trust., p. 14.

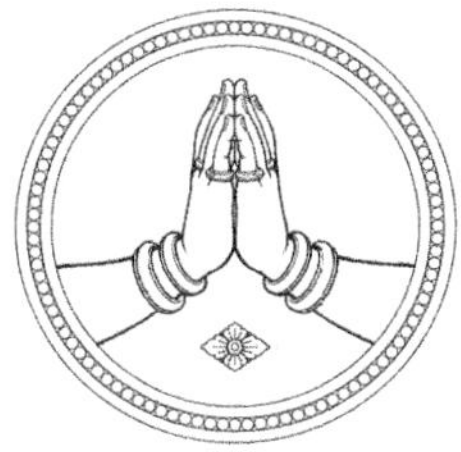

CHAPTER 17

Yoga-nidrā and Western Psychology[481]

In recent decades in the West, there has been increased research interest in the effects of Eastern immersion techniques on the body and mind, including *yoga-nidrā*. The results of such research are particularly significant when discussing the application of *yoga-nidrā* in the fields of psychology and psychotherapy.

In the context of traditional schools of Yoga, human beings should be understood holistically, including inherent consciousness, and not, as is often the case with scientific studies done in the West, reduced to mechanistic-causal functional units—automata. Scientific research of the brain and its biology tends to only take into account what is measurable at any particular time. The scientific instruments at our disposal can measure physical phenomena, but not psychological or mental ones. Although mentally active forces, but also many physical processes, cannot yet be empirically, conclusively and falsifiably measured, such an approach nevertheless increases the risk of seeing people only as the sum of their functional units as seen

481 This chapter is written with the support of Mag. Stephan Schmidmayer – a clinical and health psychologist, psychotherapist and certified Satyananda Yoga Nidra facilitator.

through the lens of such measurements. However, the mechanistic view unnoticeably present in the background of many studies usually presupposes that psychological and mental phenomena are reduceable to the physiological phenomena observed taking place in the brain. Psychophysiological measurements only capture indirect, third-person correlates of subjective experience, and therefore consciousness can never be fully translated into neurophysiological data.

Pointing this out is by no means meant to suggest a rejection of the scientific method or empirical enquiry. On the contrary—many of the techniques and approaches which we find in the Indian traditions are the result of trial and error over thousands of years. Of course, they are not completely 'scientific' in the modern sense of the word and tend to favour theological reasoning rather than what would be understood as a rigorously scientific approach today. That being said, much of science tends to rely on axioms, i.e. discovered principles which, however, often cannot be empirically proven (such as mathematical axioms), or no longer questions its own paradigms. An exchange between science and spiritual traditions would be desirable, taking care to ensure that such a discourse takes place under meaningful conditions and that power or domination struggles are avoided on both sides of the dialogue. Indeed, both scientific approaches and spiritual traditions are subject to the risk of reductionism, oversimplification and a certain blindness to a preconceived ontology.

The reductionist approach has also been applied to research on *yoga-nidrā*. As already discussed[482], brain waves and brain reactions have been clinically measured using an electroencephalogram (EEG) and body reactions have been measured using electrodermal activity (EDA) to explore the effect of the technique. However, if this research approach is used in the West as the only scientific method capable of proving the effectiveness or lack thereof of certain 'meditation' techniques or *yoga-nidrā*, then this would be a one-sided, mechanistic approach to the fundamentally holistic yoga context.

However, the discussion about which methods and approaches are appropriate is also a point of contention within Western psychotherapy. This is because, unlike cognitive behavioural therapy which is dominant in

---

482 See Part I. Chapter 10. *Brain Activity and States of Consciousness During yoga-nidrā.*

university psychology but also not without controversy[483], psychodynamic[484] and humanistic[485] schools of psychotherapy reject a purely reductionistic and quantitative-scientific methodology, preferring instead hermeneutics and phenomenological methods. Furthermore, systemic therapy approaches are often based on constructivism. Some psychoanalysts, especially from the Anglo-Saxon world (e.g. Mark Solms[486]), have tried to use neuroscientific findings for psychoanalysis (without reducing it to them). They have, on the other hand, been most criticised by those who follow the French psychoanalyst Jacques Lacan or the Frankfurt School of Critical Theory, who see the attempt to incorporate neuroscience as ineffective and as an attempt to adapt psychoanalysis to trends in the medical establishment.[487] However, many initially psychoanalytically-oriented psychotherapists, such as the German Alfred Lorenzer[488], now take a balanced middle position which recognises both hermeneutic and neuroscientific research approaches.

Nevertheless, Western science is by no means uniformly reductionist. Contemporary research — for example in neurophenomenology, embodied cognition theory, and the enactivist movement — actively integrates physical, neural, and subjective dimensions of experience (Varela[489], 1996; Thompson[490], 2007; Gallagher[491], 2017). Such developments demonstrate that science is increasingly opening itself to the holistic orientation that methods such as *yoga-nidrā* and its predecessors have long pursued.

---

483 For a concise but well-researched summary of the current controversy on this topic, see Burkeman, Oliver. *Therapy wars: the revenge of Freud*. https://www.theguardian.com/science/2016/jan/07/therapy-wars-revenge-of-freud-cognitive-behavioural-therapy (accessed on 10.01.2022).

484 These include psychoanalytic and deep-psychology therapy methods, such as the classic ones established by Sigmund Freud, Alfred Adler and Carl Gustav Jung, but also newer methods such as Mentalisation-Based Therapy or Transferential Focused Therapy.

485 For example, Carl Rogers' client-centred therapy, Jacob Moreno's psychodrama and Fritz and Laura Perls' gestalt therapy. cf. Kriz, Jürgen. (2014). *Grundkonzepte der Psychotherapie* (7th edition). Weinheim: Beltz

486 Solms, Mark; Kaplan-Solms, Karen. (2005). *Neuro-Psychoanalyse – Eine Einführung mit Fallstudien*. (2nd edition). Stuttgart: Klett-Cotta.

487 See: Lindemeier, Alexander. (2015). Neuropsychoanalyse. Modeerscheinung oder Rückkehr zu den Freud'schen Urkonzepten?. [online publication]. In Springer. Interview partners: Stephan, Doering & August, Ruhs. *Neuropsychiatrie*. (29). 39–42. https://doi.org/10.1007/s40211-015-0137-y (accessed on 11.01.2022).

488 Lorenzer, Alfred. (2022). *Die Sprache, der Sinn, das Unbewusste*. Stuttgart: Klett-Cotta.

489 Varela, F. J. (1996). Neurophenomenology: A methodological remedy for the hard problem. *Journal of Consciousness Studies*. 3(4), pp. 330–349.

490 Gallagher, S. (2017). *Enactivist Interventions: Rethinking the Mind*. Oxford University Press.

491 Thompson, E. (2007). *Mind in Life: Biology, Phenomenology, and the Sciences of Mind*. Harvard University Press.

Recent contributions by John Vervaeke, Bernardo Kastrup, and Michael Levin each advance a more nuanced understanding of consciousness, meaning, and self-organisation.

John Vervaeke[492], through his theory of relevance realisation, conceptualises consciousness as a dynamic interplay between brain, body, and environment—an approach that makes an effort to transcend classical subject-object dualism and resonates with key aspects of yogic notions of awareness and embodiment.

Bernardo Kastrup[493], in his formulation of analytic idealism, posits that consciousness constitutes the fundamental basis of reality—a position which aligns with certain streams of Indic philosophy while maintaining philosophical rigour within a contemporary analytic framework.

Michael Levin[494], through his research on bioelectrical self-organisation, demonstrates that cells and tissues exhibit forms of intelligent communication and purposiveness, thereby supporting a processual, non-mechanistic conception of life.

An additional noteworthy contribution comes from Andrés Gómez-Emilsson[495] and the Qualia Research Institute (QRI), who are developing mathematical and information-dynamic models to describe the structure of subjective experience (qualia). Their aim is to capture the qualitative dimension of consciousness scientifically, without reducing it to neural processes. This approach may be understood as a form of formal phenomenology—an attempt to build a bridge between experience and measurement.

---

492 Vervaeke, J. (2019). *Awakening from the Meaning Crisis* [Lecture Series]. University of Toronto.

493 Kastrup, B. (2018). *The Idea of the World: A Multi-Disciplinary Argument for the Mental Nature of Reality*. Iff Books.

494 Levin, M. (2021). Bioelectric signaling: Reprogrammable circuits underlying embryogenesis, regeneration, and cancer. *Frontiers in Cell and Developmental Biology*. 9, 661879.

495 Gómez-Emilsson, A. (2020). *A Future for Qualia Formalism: Toward a Science of Consciousness*. Qualia Research Institute.

Interpretatio Occidentis vs. Interpretatio Orientis?

Integral psychological approaches attempting to bridge the gap between modern Western psychology and ancient Eastern teachings are currently being used more and more frequently.[496] Some of these approaches draw on the idea that reality is a continuous projection of pure consciousness onto the physical plane. In that context, understanding of consciousness is derived from the experience of altered states of consciousness. An alteration in consciousness is taken to involve a qualitative change in its perceptual, cognitive and conative aspects, as well as in the processes which mediate between stimulus and reaction.[497]

In addition to the holistic approaches which attempt to understand and explore the various aspects of consciousness, the two different timelines of human development and perception — historical and mythical — should also be considered. While history, which deals with sequences of physical and experienced events, moves along the linear historical timeline, the perception of reality, according to Mircea Eliade[498], can be assigned to a mythical *illud tempus* timeline, the 'that time', on which the human consciousness and the emotional development of the individual are organised.

Our subjective reality is unconsciously influenced, among other things, by the culturally-contingent mythical consciousness of 'sacred time' (*illud tempus*) and 'sacred space'. According to Eliade, this is the so-called 'myth of eternal return', which expresses the eternal human need to connect with the 'higher' or 'primordial', to imitate and ultimately to reunite with it. Thus, in all cultures and traditions everyday actions are usually given sacred meaning and thereby what we nowadays consider the 'profane' everyday life is elevated to a 'sacred' act — nothing is without sacred significance. With this state of mind, the subjective reality of the individual is oriented towards an archetypal and exists in a timeless present, in which chaos becomes cosmos and history becomes reality. The individual feels part of the whole. Over the past

496 There are approaches in Western psychotherapy that integrate Buddhist concepts and then use different terms for them.

497 Kumar, Kamakhya. (2013). *A Handbook of Yoga-Nidrā*. New Delhi: D. K. Printworld Ltd., p. 35–36.

498 See Eliade, Mircea. (2018). *The Myth of the Eternal Return: Cosmos and History*. Princeton: Princeton University Press.

few centuries, the West has increasingly severed itself from this *illud tempus*-time axis and has taken the opposite direction — sacred actions have been made mundane (e.g. popular advertising and the near worship of material goods, or media consumption and self-representation in social media). The individual is given the role of 'creator' and is thus pushed into egocentrism and loneliness. This development creates a void in modern man, as man is consumed by this consumerism. If we think in mythical terms, man himself is sacrificed. In the East, however, this development is progressing somewhat more slowly and mythical time still has a significant place and value in society. That is why, in recent centuries, the 'civilised' West has repeatedly looked eastwards to remember the *illud tempus* lost in materialism, in an attempt to fill this endless void.[499] However, this is not an argument for some intrinsic supremacy of East over West, or *vice versa*. It is not an argument that 'civilised man' needs to be educated by the 'noble savage' in the spirit of thinkers such as Jean-Jacques Rousseau or Friedrich Hegel, nor for the legitimacy of 'different ways of knowing' as explained by theorists such as Bell Hooks. Neither is it an argument for the supremacy or deplorableness of Western civilisation, such as it is. This is also not an argument in favour of what can be observed in the East itself nowadays, namely the tendency towards a particular kind of cultural supremacy and grandomania and the twisting of science in favour of such views. Instead, it is an argument for the rigorous, objective scientific study of phenomena, which includes taking into account natural perceptual and phenomenological variability.

The modern use of Yoga is often extracted from its philosophical and cultural background — why has this happened, how, and for what purpose?

One of the places where the idea of universalistic interreligious dialogue can be traced to is the religious liberalism of some of the Mughal rulers of India. The cohabitation of the varied traditions of Sufism and Indic religious and philosophical traditions produced a blend which contributed towards the eventual crystalisation of perennial philosophy (*philosophia perennis*) — the

---

499 Ibid.

theosophic idea that all religious traditions share a common core. This 'Secret Doctrine' as Helena Blavatsky called it is a good example of 'bricolage' as conceptualised by Claude Lévi-Strauss in The Savage Mind (1962) to describe a mode of 'mythical' thought in which an individual uses whatever is available to them — a finite and heterogeneous set of materials and ideas — to create something new. Teachings such as perennial philosophy, however, elevate philosophical-religious bricolage to the level of gnosticism, ultimately becoming a major precursor of New Age movements and thinking, which still defines them today. Yogic traditions especially, along with other Indic schools and their texts and philosophy, were one of the sources drawn upon by this movement for their greater doctrinal variety and theories of subtle physiology and personal spiritual transcendence. Unbeknownst to many contemporary yoga practitioners, many of the institutions and materials they have acquired their knowledge from in a Western context are downstream of these phenomena of global religious and socio-cultural history and (often unconsciously) carry its 'baggage'. Ironically, it is the attitude of 'anything goes' and self-styled authority which is to a greater or lesser degree the product of this heritage which has drawn criticism for its 'cultural appropriation', while in reality it often does not at all reflect the culture and tradition it is accused of appropriating. This is, of course, combined with the real problematic of the heritage of the history of colonialism and the notion of the supremacy of greater Western civilisation over other cultures, which is, unfortunately, often merely reduced to twentieth century notions of racism and associated with national-socialist ideology, while actually ignoring deep and multi-faceted historical factors and complex intercultural and inter-civilisational dynamics which have taken place over millennia. This is another expression of the tendency towards oversimplification. A further expression of this modern and profoundly complex problematic is the fact that being native does not equal being intricately knowledgeable about one's culture, in this case, yoga. At the same time movements such as perennial philosophy and its descendents have attempted to claim they are universalist — for anyone and for anywhere, while in reality this often gets expressed into profiteering, manipulation, social engineering or confusion, be it intentional or collateral. Therefore, we must disambiguate the usual colonial framing of 'native knowledge' and 'colonial power' as innate and as innately forming an oppressed-opressor narrative from the real world dynamic of the complex cultural legacy of colonial history and modern dynamics of authoritativeness with regard to traditional cultural, religious and philosophical lineages, practices and views.

No tradition of Yoga has ever said that it is supposed to only be practiced by Indians. We need to, as a prerequisite, try to study and understand the philosophical views of yoga and their history in order to be able to apply it in any meaningful way. Being Indian doesn't necessarily mean one is knowledgeable of and experienced in yoga, but being a non-Indian and demanding one is a *yogin* without having done the necessary work beforehand is equally inadequate.

'Yoga' is not a protected term and yet there are organisations in the West claiming that they have the authority to certify yoga schools and teachers for a particular number of hours in training more in order to further the narrative of their own claim to authority and authenticity, than try and draw on the traditions of yoga more profoundly. Naturally, this is not to say that studying at an Indian institution guarantees quality by default — this is by no means the case. Therefore, every practitioner has the responsibility, if they are truly set on studying properly, to do their research and seek out the appropriate institution or teacher for that purpose — Eastern or Western.

Yoga-nidrā and Psychotherapy

In psychotherapy, a comparison is often made between Western hypnosis and Eastern methods of immersion, especially *yoga-nidrā*. Interestingly, it is often specifically the representatives of cognitive behavioural therapy which emerged from an orientation towards the mere elimination of symptoms, who 'discovered' so-called 'mindfulness' techniques from the Buddhist tradition,[500] but also from Yoga[501] for themselves, while they are discussed less

500 For example, in the context of so-called 'Dialectic Behavioural Therapy', which was designed in particular for patients with borderline personality disorder. cf. Linehan, Marsha. (1996). *Dialektisch-Behaviorale Therapie der Borderline-Persönlichkeitsstörung*. München: CIP-Medien.

501 See Mitzinger, Dietmar. (2009). *Yoga in Prävention und Therapie. Ein Manual für Yogalehrer, Therapeuten und Trainer*. Köln: Deutscher Ärzte-Verlag.

among those who subscribe to a psycho-dynamic approach.[502] In humanistic psychotherapy, the Gestalt-therapeutic concept of 'mindfulness', for example, is based on Zen Buddhist concepts. Hypnosis as a method can be integrated more or less well into all four basic orientations of psychotherapy (cognitive-behavioural, psychodynamic, humanistic, systemic[503]), but more easily into the first two. In the humanistic and psychodynamic schools, however, its use is more controversial.[504]

Secular forms of Swāmī Satyānanda's *yoga-nidrā* method have now been used in Western psychotherapy for decades.[505] In those contexts, the research approach of *interpretatio occidentis* is applied with an 'outsider's' view, excluding the *interpretatio orientis*. Thus, *yoga-nidrā* has been completely removed from its original philosophical and psychological context and set as a stand-alone method for bringing about physical and mental relaxation in a quasi-mechanical way. Individual Stages of the technique are even practiced in isolation. In particular, Stage 3 — Rotation of Awareness Throughout the Body[506], Stage 5 — Pairs of Opposites and Stage 6 — Visualisation have been specially modified and thus transformed from their classically neutral form into an individualised, subject-oriented one. The generally-held argument here is that this secularisation would release *yoga-nidrā* from its culturally-coloured context and thus make it more available to Westerners. However, this reasoning is not coherent, as Swāmī Satyānanda's original technique never contained ritual or religious elements to begin with so that it would be accessible for people of all cultures, despite the fact that the traditional

---

502 The German trauma therapist Luise Reddemann, for example, is an exception; cf. Reddemann, Luise. (2016). *Mitgefühl, Trauma und Achtsamkeit in psychodynamischen Therapien*. Göttingen: Vandenhoeck & Ruprecht, or Erich Fromm's examination of Zen Buddhism, cf. Fromm, Erich. (2020). *Zen-Buddhismus und Psychoanalyse. Berlin*. Suhrkamp Verlag. However, similarities between the attitude of the analyst's 'free-floating attention' and classical awareness concepts have also been discussed; cf. Anderssen-Reuster, Ulrike. (2007). *Achtsamkeit in Psychotherapie und Psychosomatik*. Stuttgart: Schattauer Verlag.

503 See Kriz, Jürgen. (2014). *Grundkonzepte der Psychotherapie* (7th edition). Weinheim: Beltz.

504 This is reflected, for example, in the fact that there is state-recognised, depth-psychology-oriented training in 'hypnosis psychotherapy' in Austria, while in Germany the psychotherapy guidelines for health insurance companies do not allow the use of hypnosis in psychodynamic procedures. Cf. *Richtlinie des Gemeinsamen Bundesausschusses über die Durchführung der Psychotherapie* (Psychotherapie-Richtlinie), p. 19. https://www.g-ba.de/downloads/62-492-2400/PT-RL_2020-11-20_iK-2021-02-18.pdf (accessed on 13.01.2022).

505 In the 1970s, Dr Richard Miller was the first to clinically apply a secularised form of Satyananda Yoga Nidra in his psychotherapeutic practice.

506 See Text Box on body scan in Part II. Chapter 14. *Foundations of The Eight Stages; Stage 3 – Rotation of Awareness (Throught The Body)*.

basis in terms of the theoretical framework and approach was retained as its essential foundation.

The fundamental difference between the original methods and their modified applications in Western psychotherapy lies in their focus and goal. The latter aims at the therapeutic effect of a method in its adapted version and no longer at the spiritual development of the person, who is only seen as a patient in this context. However, since the system, form and goal of the technique are so heavily modified and not applied holistically (i.e. embedded in a *sādhana*), the question arises as to whether the term *yoga-nidrā* can still be used for such practices at all. The perspective of *interpretatio occidentis* is an external view of something foreign and unknown, which is adapted for the Western world view by means of familiar formulations and interpretations. In this case, the 'side effects' of the original method become the goal — treating symptoms. Since the fundamental goal of *yoga-nidrā* is spiritual evolution and the focus is on inner growth, with continuous practice, such symptoms are said to gradually dissolve by themselves. By contrast, Western psychology is a foreign concept in many respects in India, although it has been present there academically and clinically for more than a hundred years.[507]

It should be mentioned here, however, that even in classical, 'non-directional' psychoanalysis, the aim is not merely to cure individual symptoms, but to help the patient find their inner truth — in many hundreds, sometimes even thousands of therapeutic sessions. In contrast to this, there are modified psychoanalytical methods which help people to overcome conditions that cause them suffering in a much shorter period of time. This modification of the method is often criticised by advocates of 'non-directive' psychoanalysis as an adaptation to the wishes of health insurance companies for methods which are as 'efficient' as possible, but less sustainable.[508] Humanistic psychotherapists, on the other hand, argue that the other methods represent a deficient model of the human being. They place more trust in the powers of 'self-healing' and the tendencies towards personal growth present

507 See Languani, Pittu. (2004). *Asian Perspectives in Counseling and Psychotherapy*. New York: Brunner-Rutlege Verlag.

508 See Cremerius, Johannes. (1990) Die hochfrequente Langzeitanalyse und die psychoanalytische Praxis. Utopie und Realität. *Psyche – Zeitschrift für Psychoanalyse*. 44A(1), 1–29. https://pep-web.org/browse/PSYCHE/volumes/44A?openNotificationModal=false (accessed on 13.10.2022).

in every individual, attempting to activate these through 'experience-centred' methods instead of focusing on the problems and disorders of the client.

Undoubtedly, these different approaches each have their own justification and respond to different needs which are addressed by psychotherapy. People look for help for their psychological problems and do not always have the will or the time and mental resources for a deeper transformation. However, they may achieve the conditions for this transformation if certain basal problems can be overcome.

> Psychotherapist and practising Buddhist Jack Engler observed[509] that even people who are spiritually advanced can still have serious psychological problems and deficiencies. This view was also held by the Indian psychoanalyst Sudhir Kakar, who studied traditional Indian psychosomatic healing systems and spirituality and compared European and Indian approaches to healing the body and mind.[510]

Satyananda Yoga Nidra and Hypnosis — A Comparison of the Fundamental Similarities and Differences

When viewed through a modern Western lens, *yoga-nidrā* is frequently compared to hypnosis. It is not uncommon for yoga teachers to deliver *yoga-nidrā* instructions using hypnotic intonation and language — sometimes unconsciously, at other times under the assumption that this approach is not only acceptable but beneficial and appropriate. This tendency is often linked to contemporary notions of 'wellness'.

This section aims to clarify both the similarities and the fundamental differences between hypnosis and *yoga-nidrā*. Although both methods are practiced with closed eyes and use deep relaxation and altered states of

509 Engler, Jack. (2003). Being Somebody and Being Nobody: A Reexamination of the Understanding of Self in Psychoanalysis and Buddhism. In Jeremy D. Safran (Ed.). *Psychoanalysis and Buddhism. An Unfolding Dialogue*. Boston: Wisdom Publications, pp. 35–79.

510 Kakar, Sudhir. (1991). *Shamans, Mystics and Doctors: A Psychological Inquiry into India and its Healing Traditions*. Chicago: University of Chicago Press.

consciousness, they differ profoundly in purpose, method, and underlying philosophy. Hypnosis primarily serves therapeutic or behavioural aims by influencing unconscious processes, whereas *yoga-nidrā* is an immersive method intended to awaken conscious awareness within all layers of the being. What appears similar on the surface is, in fact, rooted in two distinct paradigms — one psychological and instrumental, the other immersive and focused on cultivation.

As with any method or practice, its effectiveness and integrity depend on the clarity of intention and understanding of both the practitioner and the facilitator. If the practitioner is not aware of what they are doing, or why they are doing it, the technique inevitably loses its phenomenological precision and becomes merely mechanical. When techniques — and with them, aims and intentions — are unconsciously mixed or blurred, the result is confusion, inconsistency, and the loss or corruption of direction. This tendency reflects a broader problem of modernity, where the desire to innovate or create something 'unique' often overrides the need for depth, coherence, and continuity within an established lineage or framework.

A natural continuation from here is to look more closely at the inner dynamics of mind that distinguish *yoga-nidrā* from any psychologically-induced trance such as hypnosis.

When we talk about hypnosis, it is important primarily to detach the term from its historically-charged associations and to see it in a contemporary context. For a long time, hypnosis was considered a dubious approach because it was used by street performers and stage magicians. Even today, many still associate it with so-called 'show hypnosis'. As of the twentieth century, however, hypnosis has been able to emancipate itself as a valid psychological method in medicine, with various techniques being continuously developed on the basis of the latest science.

The term 'hypnosis' is derived from the ancient Greek *hýpnos* (ὕπνος), sleep, and is described in the *Encyclopaedia of Medical History* as a 'state of artificially induced partial sleep in connection with an altered state of consciousness'.[511] This state is also referred to as 'hypnosedation' and is often used synonymously with the term 'trance'.

---

511 Laier, Michael. (2005). *Hypnose*. (pp. 1193–1195). In Werner E. Gerabek, Bernhard D. Haage, Gundolf, pp. 648.

However, the view that hypnosis has nothing to do with sleep is becoming increasingly accepted. In the standard German work by Revenstorf, Hypnosis in *Psychotherapy, Psychosomatics and Medicine*, in this regard it states:

> *The state of hypnotic trance has nothing in common with sleep (Bass 1931), even though it has sometimes been thought to be so historically, for example by Puységur, a student of Mesmer (1734–1815), and also by Braid (1795–1860), who named hypnosis after the Greek god of sleep, Hypnos, or by Pawlow (1849–1936), who described it as a partial sleep. Rather, the hypnotic trance often resembles a relaxed waking state with increased alpha activity on the EEG. With newer imaging techniques such as SPECT or PET, von Walter (1992) demonstrated changes in the activity of the frontal lobe, but these do not allow for a simple interpretation. In addition, there were changes in the activity of the cingulate cortex, the occipital lobe, etc. Decades of research using EEG data to examine lateralisation from the left to the right hemisphere have not, however, produced any clear results [...].*[512]

Inner States During Satyananda Yoga Nidra vs. During Hypnosis (Directed Impartial Awareness vs. Trance)

Nursingh Charan Panda[513] differentiates between what he calls 'hypnotic trance' and 'yogic trance'. He makes it clear that an altered consciousness seems to be common to both techniques, but the two states are not identical. He further explains that hypnosis generally involves two people: the hypnotist and the client. The hypnotist actively participates in the patient's phenomenological field and attempts to bypass the patient's conscious mind and to induce hypnotic suggestions into the unconscious.[514] In contrast, when practising *yoga-nidrā*, only the technique itself is the object of instruction, with

---

512 Revenstorf, Dirk, Dr. & Burkhard, Peter, Dipl.-Psych. Dr. (Hsg.). (2009). *Hypnose in Psychotherapie, Psychosomatik und Medizin*. (2nd edition). Heidelberg: Springer Medizin Verlag, p.17.

513 Prof. Nursingh Charan Panda (1929–2015) was an Indian scientist, psychologist and author. He studied *yoga-nidrā* as a psychologist and compared the Western and Indian approaches in his book about *yoga-nidrā*.

514 In hypnotherapy, the term 'subconscious' is not usually used, only 'unconscious'. One exception to this are approaches that refer to the French pioneer of dynamic psychiatry, Pierre Janet. In psychoanalysis, on the other hand, only 'being unconscious' and 'the unconscious' are used. For the concept of levels of consciousness in yoga, see Part I. Chapter 9. *The Levels of Consciousness and yoga-nidrā*.

the facilitator playing a neutral role—they only provide the technique. This is why *yoga-nidrā* can also be practised independently with the help of an audio recording. Particularly advanced practitioners can also perform the basic stages of the practice independently.[515]

In her book *Yoga Nidra*[516], Kamini Desai[517] also distinguishes hypnosis, which aims to reform and optimise the body-mind complex, from *yoga-nidrā*, which aims to transform and ultimately transcend it.

According to Swāmī Satyānanda, hypnosis and *yoga-nidrā* have relaxation as a common starting point, but then lead in two different directions. Nevertheless, the mind expands much further during *yoga-nidrā* than it does during hypnosis. The aim of *yoga-nidrā* is to maintain full awareness in the deeper layers of consciousness (*jāgrat*—waking state, *svapna*—dreaming state and *suṣupti*/*nidrā*—deep sleep) in order to reach the superconscious state of *turīya*.[518] In a yogic context, the mastery of *pratyāhāra* and activating a spontaneous inner purification of the subconscious mind from stored experiences and impressions becomes essential for the individual's further development. It can therefore be assumed that *pratyāhāra-yoga-nidrā* in its initial stages is primarily a technique for purifying the subconscious mind. When practised in daily life, it can be used to maintain mental and spiritual hygiene.

Swāmī Satyānanda describes the state of consciousness during *yoga-nidrā* as 'the threshold between this and that'[519]. This is a state in which consciousness is completely detached from external sensory impressions and is in a transitional phase between wakefulness and sleeping. This phase is deliberately extended here. This so-called 'hypnagogic' state—the state of consciousness at the beginning of sleep—and the similar 'hypnopompic' state—the state of consciousness that leads out of sleep[520]—lead

---

515 Bowers, Patricia. (1978). Hypnotizability, creativity and the role of effortless experiencing. *The International journal of clinical and experimental hypnosis*. 26(3), 184–202. https://doi.org/10.1080/00207147808409320.

516 Desai, Kamini. (2017). *Yoga Nidra – The Art of Transformational Sleep*. Twin Lakes: Lotus Press, p. 133–134.

517 Kamini Desai, PhD – anthropologist, psychologist and author. She has been developing the Amrit Yoga Nidra method at the Amrit Yoga Institute – I AM Yoga Nidra™ – with her father Yogi Amrit Desai since the 2000s.

518 Saraswati, Satyananda, Swami. (2006). *Yoga Nidra*. (12th reprint). Munger: Yoga Publications Trust, p. 31–32.

519 Ibid., p. 253.

520 The term hypnopompic state (or hypnopompia) was coined by the psychological researcher Frederic Myers (1843–1901). This is contrasted with the hypnagogic state at the beginning of sleep. However,

to a qualitative broadening and deepening of sensory experiences. The aim is to keep the mind active and directed inward, without sinking into deep sleep, maintaining conscious awareness throughout.

In order to achieve this awareness during *yoga-nidrā*, the instructions from the facilitator are given in a specific, at a temperate pace, without allowing for extended periods of pausing or silence. This tendency to pay increased attention when the pace is faster rather than slower helps the practitioner to remain more aware of the various internal experiences. Awareness is maintained without interruption in order to expand it to the various levels of consciousness to the greatest extent possible. In contrast, hypnotic induction often uses contrary means such as fractionation[521] and pauses to discuss an event in order to deepen the trance feeling, bypass the patient's rational mind and influence unconscious cognitive attitudes. A similar approach is often used for propaganda purposes or as a tool for mass formation.

Direction of Awareness in Satyananada Yoga Nidra vs. Suggestion in Hypnosis

In yoga, expectations of a particular effect or result from the practice are generally not encouraged, as they can significantly alter the experience and the practice process. We should approach our practice each time as a new experience, as non-judgmentally as possible. In this sense, suggestions are generally avoided in the instructions.

One could certainly claim, in reference to Paul Watzlawick, that one cannot not suggest.[522] Explaining a method and then answering the question of why it should be practised at all and what effects it should achieve can in itself act as a strong suggestion, because it induces an expectation, but perhaps also resistance—both will influence the experience. However, the question arises whether suggestion should be used consciously to achieve a certain effect, i.e., to steer the experience of the method in a certain direction.

the term hypnagogia is also often used in a more general sense to encompass both falling asleep and waking up.

521 'Fractionated hypnosis' according to Vogt and Brodmann is achieved by briefly reawakening and re-entering the trance state.

522 'One cannot not communicate.' – Watzlawick, Paul., Beavin, Janet, H., & Jackson, Don. D. (1969). *Menschliche Kommunikation*. Stuttgart, Wien: Huber Bern Verlag, p. 53.

Nevertheless, suggestion cannot be avoided altogether. This has also been discussed in psychoanalysis. Sigmund Freud, who practised hypnosis and then turned away from it before developing his own method[523], said that in the mass application of psychotherapy, the 'pure gold of psychoanalysis' had to be mixed with the 'copper of suggestion'.[524]

In psychoanalysis, the avoidance of suggestion and the effort to 'keep the gold pure' have led to the patient being given no guidance other than to be told to freely associate (that is, to say everything that comes to mind). No questions from the patient were answered, except for those that concerned organisational matters (such as making appointments or fees). Rather, every question was examined for hidden fears and desires of the patient: for example, if the patient asked what the therapy should achieve, this was interpreted as meaning that he was afraid that the therapy might be useless or that the therapist was unable to help him, or that he wanted more certainty. Every question was answered with a counter-question or interpretation. Today, this is rarely handled in such a strict form consistently, since the view has been established that this could lead to a deterioration in the condition of mentally unstable patients and would also be less accepted by comparatively more stable patients than in earlier times.[525]

In hypnosis, on the other hand, a state of heightened suggestibility is induced through the use of special techniques and suggestions, and used by the hypnotist to guide the client towards a specific goal. In *yoga-nidrā*, on the other hand, direct suggestion is avoided as far as possible. During Stage 2, *saṃkalpa*, the personal resolve is formulated by the practitioner himself in the form of autosuggestion, to be stored by the subconscious or unconscious and subsequently implemented in actions.

When first learnt, Stage 5 of *yoga-nidrā* — Pairs of Opposites — seems like a suggestive episode. It could be used, in a slightly modified form, for hypnosis, and some psychotherapists also use this stage on its own in their

---

523 See Ranefeld, Johannes. (2012). Immer und überall. Die Suggestion. (pp. 199–210). In Peter, Geißler. *Stimme und Suggestion. Die „musikalische Dimension" und ihre suggestive Kraft im psychotherapeutischen Geschehen.* Psychosozial-Verlag, pp. 199–210.

524 Freud, Sigmund. (1925). Wege der psychoanalytischen Therapie. In Sigmund Freud, Anna Freud, & A. J. Storfer (Hgs.). *Gesammelte Schriften von Sigmund Freud.* 6. Band. Leipzig, Wien, Zürich: Internationaler Psychoanalytischer Verlag, pp. 192–194.

525 See Gerd, Rudolf. (2011). *Psychodynamische Psychotherapie. Die Arbeit an Konflikt, Struktur und Trauma.* Stuttgart. Schattauer Verlag.

therapeutic practice. During *yoga-nidrā*, the experience is consciously steered in a certain direction, and this only works because the instructions are formulated in the manner of: 'Awaken the idea of heaviness in the body.' Within the overall framework of *yoga-nidrā*, this suggests either, 'This is the result of the technique.', or, 'The method is giving you the opportunity to yourself recall this from your already stored experiences.', or, 'In this state, you can now do this with your own will.' The main difference to the control-based approach of hypnosis is that there is no suggestion here: not 'The therapist/facilitator does this to you', but rather: 'The method allows this to happen.' Instead of taking an active suggestive role, the task of the facilitator is to guide the practitioners through the practice and to let their own consciousness interact with the technique naturally, without interfering with this process.

In non-control-based hypnosis, on the other hand, suggestion is no longer used in the sense of 'the therapist causes something'—but rather formulated, for example, as 'if you pay attention to the breeze and try to feel it on your face, you will be able to perceive a coolness on your face'. The suggestion is not that the hypnotherapist causes the experience of coolness, but that the experience will inevitably arise when the patient pays attention to the breeze on his face. This has a real background—sweat on the skin cools when there is air movement—but it is only by directing attention to this aspect that the patient consciously perceives it, and through concentration, the feeling can now be intensified. As soon as the patient has acquired the knowledge of how to evoke the desired sensation of his own will—which is the goal in *yoga-nidrā*—then he has, so to speak, freed himself from suggestion. It is no longer something or someone else that is causing the effect, but rather the patient themselves who can determine it. In this sense, the clear goal of yoga is to subject such physical processes to the conscious will and thus free them from the necessity for suggestion and also from external influence.

Revenstorf writes on the subject of suggestion:

> *The term suggestion is derived from the Latin 'sub-gerere' or 'suggerere', literally translated as 'to push under'. While in English and French 'to suggest' or 'suger' is used in the positive sense of 'to propose', in German 'suggestieren' has a predominantly negative connotation in the sense of 'to blow in, to whisper' (Peter 1996d). Suggestion phenomena are by no means limited to the field of hypnosis, and not all forms of suggestibility are related to hypnotisability*

> *(Evans 1989). On the other hand, with a few exceptions, all known hypnotisability scales are based on suggestion items. Gheorghiu (1996) argues that all psychophysiological processes can be influenced by suggestion. In everyday life, processes of suggestive influence are constantly at work in the interpersonal realm, whether in direct or indirect, verbal or non-verbal forms. Suggestional processes are of great importance in resolving ambiguity and uncertainty. Often we find ourselves in situations characterised by a lack of clarity and certainty. When there is a lack of reference points for important decisions and our ability to make predictions and exercise control is limited, suggestion phenomena play an important role by influencing our behaviour and experience. To meet the criteria of a suggestion, the recipient must at least have the virtual possibility of reacting differently than in the suggested way. Furthermore, the response must be involuntary.*[526]

In the process of hypnosis, another phenomenon—a kind of temporary amnesia—may occur in some cases. An intellectual task is performed unconsciously or subconsciously, without involving superficial awareness. An unconscious process and conscious experience occur simultaneously, without the former being accessible to overt awareness. *Yoga-nidrā* differs from a hypnotic state in that, although amnesia and other hypnotic phenomena may occur, the practitioner tries as best as they can to remain an aware and neutral observer and not to become attached to images, sensations or experiences.[527]

Hypnotic induction often involves formal or informal tests in order to determine hypnotisability and the use of methods of confirmation such as arm levitation, catalepsy and time distortion. These allow the hypnotist to verify the state in which the hypnotised person is, and the hypnotised person can experience this as a confirmation of the effect of the hypnosis, which is thus simultaneously deepened again.[528] In *yoga-nidrā*, phenomena such as time distortion, catalepsy and primary process images can occur, although they are not meaningful as a confirmation of the state.

---

526 Revenstorf, Dirk, Dr. & Burkhard, Peter, Dipl.-Psych. Dr. (Hsg.). (2009). *Hypnose in Psychotherapie, Psychosomatik und Medizin*. (2nd edition). Heidelberg: Springer Medizin Verlag, p. 105.

527 Panda, Nursing, Charan. (2011). *Yoga-Nidra*. (2nd edition). New Delhi: D.K. Printworld (P) Ltd, p. 6.

528 Yapko, Michael, PhD. (2018). *Trancework: An Introduction to the Practice of Clinical Hypnosis*. (5th edition). Oxfordshire: Routledge.

The Use of Language and Voice

Another important difference lies in the use of language during hypnosis vs. during *yoga-nidrā*. Hypnotic language is specific—it is poetic, symbolic and metaphorical. The hypnotherapist also gives instructions in the first person during hypnosis, e.g.: 'Follow my voice'. In *yoga-nidrā*, on the other hand, instructions are formulated as neutral as possible, avoiding personal pronouns such as 'I', 'mine' and 'we', so that the facilitator is not present as a person, except for his voice in the background. This point is particularly important when giving instructions. Furthermore, during the introduction, 'you' and 'yours' are turned into neutral formulations. This serves to stimulate a judgement-free observer attitude. However, when guiding out of the practice, the personal pronouns 'you' and 'yours' are used again to help the practitioner return to everyday consciousness.

The voice and intonation of the facilitator are usually diametrically opposed in the two methods. Depending on the type of hypnotherapy used, the range of different vocal intonations can extend from the neutral and clear to the very soothing and suggestive during hypnosis. Some hypnotherapists generally prefer to speak with a clear and neutral voice during therapy. Hypnotherapists who follow the approach of Milton Erickson often try to speak in a deliberately 'casual' way in order to subtly insert suggestions, while some others use a particularly monotonous language. In most cases, the way of speaking is individually tailored to the client, for example, starting from the client's manner and speed of speaking and then gradually transitioning to a calmer and more relaxed tone.

Revenstorf recommends:

> *The therapist lowers their voice as they breathe out towards the end of the sentence. In particular, when addressing vague physical sensations, the voice becomes gentle, quieter and deeper. The therapist can shift the location of their voice downwards. A person with their eyes closed is able to perceive such subtle differences and use them during the trance. If the patient has their eyes open and the therapist is underlining their words with gestures, the hand movements should taper off towards the centre of the body or downwards. The therapist adjusts to the patient's baseline level and then demonstrates how to react to the suggestions for deepening by implementing them themselves. He*

> *thus takes a small step forward by audibly breathing out more deeply, visibly releasing tension, calming or completely stopping his own movements, closing his eyes briefly (suggesting that he is closing his eyelids), slowing down his speech (calming his thoughts), and so on.*[529]

By contrast, during *yoga-nidrā*, the voice and intonation should remain as consistent, clear and neutral as possible. The facilitator should avoid lowering their voice or breathing audibly with the participant. The voice and intonation should not be adapted to the participant, but should always remain the same for all practitioners.

Disidentification vs. Dissociation

A key feature common to both methods is the observer. In Yoga, this is referred to as the *draṣṭā*—the non-judgmental, neutral observer—who is disidentified from the action. In hypnosis, the observer dissociates from the everyday functioning between internal mental and external stimuli, as well as from mental functions that are normally connected.[530] Furthermore, hypnotic reactions are attributed to two dissociative mechanisms. These mechanisms are often used to process traumatic experiences and to reduce pain. In the early 1980s, Ernest Hilgard[531] developed his neo-dissociation theory, which assumes that hypnotic reactions are due to a division of consciousness into two or more simultaneous streams, separated by an amnesic barrier, which prevent access to suggestion-related executive functions, monitoring functions, or both. He recognised the existence of a 'hidden observer' who can process and reproduce the sensory impressions and knows all the hidden and overt information.[532] K.S. Bowers[533] in his theory of dissociative control,

529 Revenstorf, Dirk, Dr. & Burkhard, Peter, Dipl.-Psych. Dr. (Hsg.). (2009). Hypnose in *Psychotherapie, Psychosomatik und Medizin*. (2nd edition). Heidelberg: Springer Medizin Verlag, p. 220.

530 Kirsch, Irving & Lynn, Steven Jay. (1998). Social-cognitive alternatives to dissociation theories of hypnotic involuntariness. *Psychological Bulletin*. 2(1), pp. 66–80.

531 Hilgard, E.R. (1989). Eine Neo-Dissoziationstheorie des geteilten Bewusstseins. In *Zeitschrift Hypnose und Kognition* (HyKog). 6(2).

532 Hilgard, E. R. Neodissociation Theory. In Lynn, S. J./Rhue, J. W. (Eds.). (1994). *Dissociation: Clinical and Theoretical Perspectives*. New York: Guilford Press, pp. 32–51.

533 Bowers, K. S. (1994). Dissociated control, imagination, and the phenomenology of dissociation. In D. Spiegel (Ed.), *Dissociation: Culture, mind, and body* (pp. 21–38). Washington DC: American Psychiatric

proposed that hypnotic inductions weaken the frontal control of behavioural schemas, thereby allowing the hypnotist's suggestions to directly activate behaviour. In *yoga-nidrā*, on the other hand, *draṣṭā* causes disidentification. It is this disidentification which firstly allows for a letting go on all levels and a purification of the impressions stored in the subconscious (*saṃskāras*). Secondly, it allows that through the release of these impressions, no further re-experiencing or re-traumatisation can take place, yet these impressions do not touch the practitioner, although sometimes stronger emotions might arise as well. This makes it possible for these stored experiences to be weakened or, in other words, neutralised in a safe and controlled manner.

The Relation Between Facilitator and Practitioner

Another difference between the two methods lies in the relationship between the hypnotist and the client. It is one-sidedly personal, and both are more in tune with each other than the facilitator and the practitioner during a *yoga-nidrā* practice. The hypnotist has clear control over the client's hypnotic process, which can create a natural and temporary dependency on the part of the client. During hypnosis, verbal communication is possible, which is fundamentally not the case with *yoga-nidrā*.

Furthermore, in *yoga-nidrā* the facilitator guides the practitioner, but it is the practitioner who does the shifting and intensification of the awareness, while in hypnosis, for example, the patient relinquishes semi-complete control to the professional.

Visualisation and the Inner Images

In order to visualise, the mind should be in a relaxed state. This is the starting position for both methods.

In many tantric methods, visualisation is used as a means to various ends. Satyananda Yoga Nidra, as a method derived from the Tantras, also uses such means. In Stage 6 — Visualisation — one is immersed in the *pratyāhāra*

Association, pp. 21–40.

state, while the subconscious is being cleansed. For this, specific images and symbols are used, in order to bring to the surface and release deeply stored impressions—shapes, colours, sense impressions, ideas, associations, feelings, thoughts and experiences—which we connect with those respective images and symbols in the subconscious. They can be compared with keys which open the locks of the stored impressions, in order to go further and further in the process of purifying the mind. The point during *pratyāhāra-yoga-nidrā* is not to necessarily 'visualise' or 'see' those particular images, but to unlock and release the stored impressions. As a consequence of practicing this Stage, the general ability to visualise and creativity can develop. The purification process, however, happens immediately, and neither are the images and symbols specifically selected for the respective practitioner nor are any suggestive images used. To prevent the practitioner from brooding and losing spontaneity and impartiality in the process, the terms are said in rapid succession, but with a neutral tone. Sentences or descriptive phrases are used very rarely. The series of images are carefully selected, but are not linked to one another in any meaningful way. Generally, neutral or rather positive, universal images are chosen. As a facilitator, you can and should work with the same group of participants for a while with the same series of images.

Visualisation during *yoga-nidrā* should not be understood as an 'imaginary journey'. By releasing the impressions stored in the subconscious (*saṃskāras*), blocked mental energy (*citta-śakti*) is released, which is needed again to achieve deeper states of immersion and to be able to abide in them. If these impressions have not been released and purified, they would become an obstacle to achieving a state of deep immersion. They would keep surfacing and disrupting deeper states of immersion and absorption, ultimately tearing you away from them.

In hypnosis, on the other hand, a considerable amount of work is done with images, symbols and ideas in order to recognise and resolve internal conflicts and to reinterpret difficult situations internally. The images are individually chosen to be related to the patient and deliberately focused on specific problem areas. For example, the patient may visualise a stressful situation from their childhood and then imagine how a helping person, for example the adult self or a trusted person who was missing at the time, helps, comforts or encourages him as a child. Or, conversely, a situation in the future is imagined, and the hypnotic trance is used to search for what could be helpful in it. The therapist works with suggestive images and concepts which can be both supportive and stabilising, but also fundamentally confronting. The visualisation during hypnotherapy is also intended to generally promote the ability to imagine.

In hypnosis, imagination can work with both dissociation and association. For example, a pain in one part of the body can be associated with a colour, such as red, and a pain-free state with another, such as blue (after the patient has been asked to associate colours themselves while in a trance). Then, a painful body part is first imagined in red, and after that a slow colour change to bluish occurs. Distantly related, albeit much more elaborate techniques have been used in Tibetan Buddhist meditation practices.[534]

An example of the use of dissociation would be if the patient imagines that they are sitting in front of a screen and watching a video recording of a stressful situation that they actually experienced in the past, but which can now be paused or fast-forwarded or rewound at any time. In the first step, this results in a partial dissociation of the remembered images from the emotions experienced at the time, and thus also control over the memories previously experienced as uncontrollable and anxiety-inducing.[535]

Effects on the Brain

Although we now know a lot more about the measurable effects of hypnosis and *yoga-nidrā* than we did in the days before brain scans, our current knowledge is by no means definitive or complete.

So far, PET/CT[536]-scans indicate that, in hypnosis, the left frontal, executive brain functions are suspended, while the right posterior part of the brain is activated. It seems that the changes occur because one aspect of the brain is covered over, allowing another to function more optimally, by reducing the left brain hemisphere's activities which normally dominate, to access

---

534 Vgl. WWalter, Michael. (1996). Jabir, the buddhist Yogi, Part Two: Winds and Immortality. In *Journal of Indian Philosophy* 24. Amsterdam: Kluwer Academic Publishers, p. 145–164.

535 So-called 'screen technique', which is used both in and outside of hypnotherapy. Cf. Sternek, Katharina. (2014). Über den Einsatz und die Wirkungsweise von 'Bildschirm-Techniken'. Österreich: *Zeitschrift für Gestalttheoretische Psychotherapie*. 6(1). 20–29. /https://www.oeagp.at/cms/uploads/pdf/Fachartikel/Sternek2014Bildschirmtechniken.pdf (accessed on 02.03.2022).

536 PET: positron emission tomography; CT: computed tomography.

the right.[537] In contrast, the PET scans of *yoga-nidrā* practitioners show that distinct centres in the brain were activated in turn during each Stage of the practice. All the active areas in both hemispheres of the brain were fundamentally congruent.[538]

Extended EEG measurements of brain waves during *yoga-nidrā* have shown a homogeneous distribution of alpha and theta brain activity.[539] Hypnotic states are mostly associated with increased theta wave activity. However, they show an asymmetry of wave patterns across the two hemispheres, unlike some studies involving *yoga-nidrā*. Studies taking into account the sensitivity to hypnosis showed that highly-receptive individuals showed an asymmetry with stronger beta wave activity in the left hemisphere, while less-receptive individuals showed only weak asymmetry.[540] However, the results regarding brain waves are not a definitive indicator of how the mind works. During *yoga-nidrā*, certain physiological changes—such as heart rate, respiration, and EEG activity—can be measured, but these metrics do not capture the practitioner's qualitative expansion of awareness. This is an area which requires further research, whereby it would be interesting to take into account the divergence between the different hypnosis and *yoga-nidrā* techniques and their specific effects.

Swāmī Satyānanda further distinguishes between hypnosis and *yoga-nidrā* in terms of what he refers to as the energetic effect on the brain and the modes of perception:

> *Scientifically speaking, when the central nervous system and the master cortex do not supply the needed stimuli to the brain, and when the brain is isolated, it enters into a state which is called hypnosis. It is a momentary happening, a very small range of experience where the brain and cerebral cortex are dissociated from the energy channels. [...] If you close off* iḍā *and* piṅgalā *by means of* pratyāhāra, *then the brain is isolated. That is hypnosis. But, if*

537 Gruzelier, J. (1998). A working model of the neurophysiology of hypnosis: a review of evidence. *Contemporary Hypnosis*. 15(1), 3–21. https://doi.org/10.1002/CH.112 (accessed on 22.02.2022), pp. 3–21.

538 Saraswati, Satyananda, Swami. (2006). *Yoga Nidra*. (12th reprint). Munger: Yoga Publications Trust, pp. 240–244.

539 Ibid., p. 252–253.

540 Sabourin, M. E., Cutcomb, S. D., Crawford, H. J., & Pribram, K. (1990). EEG correlates of hypnotic susceptibility and hypnotic trance: spectral analysis and coherence. *International journal of psychophysiology : official journal of the International Organization of Psychophysiology*. 10(2), 125–142. https://doi.org/10.1016/0167-8760(90)90027-b (accessed on 20.04.2021).

> *at the same time, you can awaken* suṣumṇā *(which is closed in most people), then, although you have dissociated the two channels of communication* (iḍā *and* piṅgalā) *from the brain, the central nervous system is awakened, and in place* iḍā *and* piṅgalā, suṣumṇā *will supply the necessary energy and stimuli to the brain.*[541]

The main energy channels referred to here are *iḍā*, *piṅgalā* and *suṣumṇā*, which cannot necessarily be measured using modern scientific instruments, but are, in a modern yogic context, nevertheless associated with energy distribution and the functioning and control of the parasympathetic, sympathetic and central nervous systems respectively.

For further detailed information regarding the effects of Satyananda Yoga Nidra on brain activity and neuroplasticity, see Part I. Chapter 10. *Brain activity and states of consciousness during yoga-nidrā; Results of Brain Research on Satyananda Yoga Nidra* and Part V. Appendix 2. *Effects of yoga-nidrā on brain activity and neuroplasticity*.

Further Considerations

Individuals come to psychotherapy with a specific problem and expect help and a solution. However, in order to go beyond the one-sidedness of symptomatic treatments, personal and spiritual growth may also be considered as a complementary aspect of healing in long-term psychotherapy.

In a holistic approach, one could distinguish three areas which are equally important:

- Firstly, the goal- and solution-oriented treatment of psychological problems, as practised primarily in psychological counselling, behavioural therapy, systemic therapy and hypnotherapy.

---

541 Saraswati, Satyananda, Swami. (2006). *Yoga Nidra*. (12th reprint). Munger: Yoga Publications Trust, p. 32–33.

- Secondly, a general self-reflection encompassing aspects of the entire personality and individual history, as more commonly sought in psychodynamic and humanistic therapies, most comprehensively in 'non-ideological' psychoanalysis.
- Thirdly, setting spiritual goals aimed at leading the person beyond the boundaries of their own individuality. There are certainly fluid transitions between the first and second approaches, as well as between the second and third approach, but a certain division of tasks makes sense, since all three approaches each have their own justification.

However, spiritual goals are intended to go beyond the scope of therapy. There is a danger that in the attempts to pursue spiritual goals in this context, however, — as in the so-called 'transpersonal' psychotherapy methods[542], these spiritual goals — taken out of their original context — are then treated superficially. Thus, spiritual goals as the aim of a practice should be pursued through methods which were originally designed for that purpose, such as those developed in Yoga. While therapy is generally a time- and goal-limited process, yoga can and usually is a lifee-long practice.

It is now clear that a direct comparison between hypnosis or hypnotherapy and *yoga-nidrā* is not straightforward to make. In contemporary psychotherapy, as in hypnosis, there are many different schools of thought and approaches, which makes it almost impossible to do equal justice to all positions in a single publication.

> It should not be forgotten that, although *yoga-nidrā* can be and is used as a deep relaxation technique in its own right, it is primarily a method for spiritual growth. To achieve its full benefits, it should be integrated into a holistic *sādhana*. Therefore, it is important to overcome the reductionist approach which is often found in the transfer of Eastern methods into a Western paradigm.[543]

---

542 For example, following Grof, Dürckheim or Assagioli.

543 Compare Goldberg, Philip. (2013). *American Veda: From Emerson and the Beatles to Yoga and Meditation – How Indian Spirituality Changed the West.* New York: Random House Verlag.

CHAPTER 18

Overview of Clinical Studies and Scientific Findings on Satyananda Yoga Nidra

BIHAR YOGA HAS BEEN SUCCESSFULLY implemented in various social, professional and health-related areas since the 1970s. Its integral approach, which also includes Satyananda Yoga Nidra, has been used in schools, hospitals, by the police and military, in prisons and also in business in numerous countries on all continents. In addition, positive effects have been observed in people suffering from various physical and mental health conditions, such as the effects of stress, anxiety, migraines, sleep disorders, the effects of cancer, coronary heart disease, diabetes, asthma, trauma-related disorders, PTSD, etc.

The many and extensive preventive and therapeutic effects of the Bihar Yoga system, especially of the Satyananda Yoga Nidra method, on the physical and psychological level have been proven by clinical studies since the 1970s, but these have yet not covered all areas of application and further research is needed. The results of the first scientific studies of Satyananda Yoga Nidra conducted between 1974 and 1989 were presented in Svāmī Satyānanda's book

Yoga Nidra[544]. More recent research has been published by the Yoga Research Foundation and in the collected volumes commemorating the 50th anniversary of the Bihar School of Yoga. A summary of the most important studies conducted up to 2012 can be found in Kamakhya Kumar's *A Handbook of Yoga-Nidrā*[545]. Two other publications presenting research on Satyananda Yoga Nidra are Svāmī Prakāśānanda's[546] book *Yoga Nidra — Neue Erkenntnisse*[547] in German and Svāmī Janakānanda's[548] E-Book *A Deeper Yoga and Yoga Nidra*[549]. Most of the research results are also available in scientific journals and in databases on the internet. As including all information from the available sources lies beyond the scope and purpose of this book, readers are encouraged to consult the original publications for detailed accounts of the studies on Satyananda Yoga Nidra referenced herein. Nevertheless, a summary is provided below.

Particularly noteworthy is the work of scientists Kamakhya Kumar[550] and Maarten Immnik[551] who have devoted a substantial part of their research to the effects of integral yoga (Bihar Yoga), especially Satyananda Yoga Nidra, across various areas of health. Their numerous studies are, firstly, enhanced by their own yoga background, especially since much of this research was conducted together with yoga practitioners. Due to his work in the university sector, Kumar had the opportunity to recruit a larger number of student subjects who regularly practised yoga (*āsana*, *prāṇāyāma* and *ṣaṭkarman*) for several of his studies and thus to conduct research on various aspects of *yoga-nidrā* in an integral yoga context. Immnik examined the neurocognitive processes underlying the learning and execution of complex motor sequences,

---

544 Satyananda, Swami. (2006). *Yoga Nidra*. (12th reprint). Munger: Yoga Publications Trust, pp. 179–253.

545 Kumar, Kamakhya. (2013). *A Handbook of Yoga-Nidrā*. New Delhi: D. K. Printworld Ltd.

546 Svāmī Prakāśānanda (1938–2020) was a disciple of Svāmī Satyānanda and founder of the Satyananda Yoga Centre in Germany and founder of Ananda Verlag, Germany.

547 Saraswati, Prakashananda, Swami. (2003). *Yoga Nidra – Neue Erkenntnisse*. Tettnang: Ananda Verlag.

548 Svāmī Janakānanda (born 1939) is a disciple of Svāmī Satyānanda and founder of the renowned Scandinavian Yoga and Meditation School in Denmark and the renowned Håå International Retreat Center in Sweden, where he currently lives.

549 Janakānanda, Swami. (2022). *A deeper yoga and Yoga Nidra*. [eBook edition]. Hamneda: Bindu.

550 Dr Kamakhya Kumar completed his postgraduate studies in Yogic Science at Bihar Yoga Bharati, Munger, India, in 2001 and is, among other things, the founder and head of the Department of Yoga Science at Uttarakhand Sanskrit University in Haridwar, India.

551 Dr Maarten Immink is Senior Lecturer in Motor Behaviour at the School of Health Sciences, Flinders University, Adelaide, Australia, and Editor-in-Chief of the *Journal of Motor Learning and Development*. He is also an accredited Satyananda Yoga and Meditation teacher with experience in the application of yoga and meditation practices for neurological disorders.

in particular the significance of integral yoga, including Satyananda Yoga Nidra, for the long-term treatment of neurological disorders and stroke patients with neuropsychiatric symptoms. The studies conducted by Gosh, Kjær and Lou are of considerable interest, as they employ neuroimaging techniques to examine changes in brain activity among equally experienced yoga practitioners during the individual Stages of *yoga-nidrā*. These research results are also presented in this book.

The effects of Satyananda Yoga Nidra, referred to in this chapter simply as *yoga-nidrā* for brevity, have been the subject of numerous clinical studies to date, which have shown that Svāmī Satyānanda's method is associated with positive physiological changes, including improvements in several haematological variables, such as the red blood cell count (RCB), as well as in blood sugar levels in non-insulin-dependent patients and hormonal status. Neuroimaging studies showed that the method positively influences the endogenous production of dopamine and cerebral blood flow (CBF), which is further confirmation that its effects on the central nervous system can be objectively measured. Furthermore, it has been shown that *yoga-nidrā* can also significantly reduce psychometrically measurable indices of stress and anxiety.[552]

The following sections contain a general overview of scientific research papers dealing exclusively with Satyananda Yoga Nidra, including a large amount of peer-reviewed studies. You can find summaries of those studies and their results, grouped thematically and chronologically in Part V. *Appendix 2*.

This overview does not claim to be complete. During the research for this book, it was noted that those studies conducted in India were mainly devoted to the Satyananda Yoga Nidra method, whereas in the West, Richard Miller's[553] method—iRest—has been examined in numerous studies. Miller himself worked as a clinician and spent decades studying the effects of his own method in the clinical-therapeutic field, specifically with war veterans and PTSD patients.

552 Kumar, Kamakhya, Pandi-Perumal, S. R., Spence, D. W., Srivastava, N., Kanchibhotla, D., Sharma, G. S., Gupta, R., & Batmanabane, G. (2022). The Origin and Clinical Relevance of Yoga Nidra. *Sleep and vigilance*. 6(1), pp. 61–84. https://doi.org/10.1007/s41782-022-00202-7 (accessed on 13.09.2023).

553 Dr Richard Miller (b. 1948), USA, is a clinical psychologist, author, researcher and spiritual and yoga teacher. He developed his own *yoga-nidrā* method, which he called iRest. See reference to thos method in Part 4. Chapter 19. *The Contemporary Yoga-Nidrā Approach – Origin and Development*.

However, some Western research reports on *yoga-nidrā* are not transparent, as they do not state which *yoga-nidrā* technique was used or which Stages were examined, also leaving open the type of instruction used. It is also not known whether the respective Western researchers were informed about the large number of *yoga-nidrā* techniques and their differences, nor how they selected the particular technique they studied.[554]

Main Areas of Research

It is generally assumed in both scientific research and among practitioners that the process of the various immersive methods is associated with a comprehensive relaxation reaction, which is mediated by the parasympathetic nervous system and includes the following measurable effects:

- reduction in oxygen consumption;
- reduction in heart and respiratory rates, blood pressure, blood lactate levels (an indication of reduced muscle activity) and muscle tone (similar to REM sleep);
- increase in blood flow to the internal organs;
- increase in skin resistance (as measured using electrodermal activity (EDA)).[555]

Four elements promote this relaxation response during the immersive practice:

- a mental process (method) for switching the mind from logical and outward-oriented thinking (left hemisphere) towards intuitive and inward-oriented thinking (right hemisphere);

554 It would certainly be possible to compare the results of studies that used either the Satyananda Yoga Nidra method or other methods. However, this would go well beyond the scope of this book.

555 Nataraja, Shanida. (2008). *The Blissful Brain – Neuroscience and proof of the power of meditation*. London: Octopus Publishing Group Ltd, p. 102–103.

- the cultivation of a neutral observer attitude which does not evaluate the process of immersion nor allow itself to be distracted by the flow of thoughts;
- a comfortable position which requires only minimal muscle effort but is not too comfortable (to prevent the practitioner from falling asleep);
- a quiet environment, which is especially important for beginners.[556]

As already discussed in this book, *yoga-nidrā* is embedded in the integral yoga system of Svāmī Satyānanda and is categorised as a *pratyāhāra*-focused technique in the context of *rāja-yoga*. Thus, *yoga-nidrā* serves to prepare the mind for yogic discipline. In this original sense, the effect of the method unfolds and increases in interaction with the other chosen yoga techniques, as well as through the practitioner's engagement with Yoga philosophy and psychology. Consequently, the question arises as to whether scientific studies should take this starting point into account and examine *yoga-nidrā* in its integral context, rather than looking at the technique in isolation. Fortunately, there are many studies which do include the integral context. The yoga background of the researchers or their collaboration with yoga experts can be generally seen as an advantage, particularly in the process of preparing for such studies.

It should be recalled here that these studies aim to examine the clinical effects of Satyananda Yoga Nidra using the means, questions and insights available to research at the respective time of their implementation. This means a strong reduction of the method to its physical and psychological effects and could lead to confusing the effects with the goal of the method. Even if research into the effects of *yoga-nidrā* is justified and can contribute to a more targeted use of *yoga-nidrā* or to the alleviation of physical and psychological suffering, the actual goal of the method should not be overlooked.

556 Ibid.

Yoga-nidrā as reducer of physical and mental tension, stress and anxiety

Stress is a cognitive and/or emotional reaction of an individual to a situation that requires adaptation. If the demands of the situation exceed the individual's ability to cope with them, stress arises, which can manifest itself in psychological and physical symptoms.

Over the past decades, numerous studies have investigated the physiological and psychological effects of Satyananda Yoga Nidra and related relaxation techniques. In his book *Yoga-Nidra*, Svāmī Satyānanda cites the work of Kodethur Udupa (1979), who identified four stages in the development of stress disorders and demonstrated that regular yoga practice was significantly more effective in reducing stress and hypertension than the contemporary pharmacological antihypertensive treatments. His findings also showed that strenuous physical exercise or intense *āsana* practice could elevate stress hormones, whereas *śavāsana* served as an effective preventive measure against stress.

Further studies reinforced these findings. Bahrke (1979) concluded that 'yogic relaxation', understood as *yoga-nidrā*, effectively reduces psychological tension and enhances psychological well-being in individuals with anxiety. Carrington et al. (1980) observed that *yoga-nidrā* functions as a preventive method suitable for healthy, active individuals to alleviate psychosomatic illnesses and increase stress resistance. Similarly, Seith et al. (1981) compared *śavāsana* with contemporary medical treatments for tension headaches and found it to be equally effective, particularly in younger participants. Supporting this, Chesney and Shelton (1976) reported that *śavāsana* alone or combined with EMG biofeedback produced better outcomes than biofeedback alone — a finding echoed by Masur (1976) and White and Alexander (1976), who found no significant difference between biofeedback and placebo.

More recent studies have continued to substantiate the therapeutic potential of *yoga-nidrā*. Kumar (2004, 2008) documented significant reductions in stress levels and improvements in general well-being among practitioners, with later results showing decreased anxiety levels, particularly in male participants. Kumari and Tripathi (2020), studying patients with stress syndrome at Sir Sundar Lal Hospital (BHU, Varanasi), reported that *yoga-nidrā* significantly reduced stress and anxiety levels compared to herbal treatments, a conclusion further supported by their follow-up study in 2023. Jayshree and Choudhury (2022) extended these findings in a clinical context, demonstrating that a *yoga-nidrā* programme effectively reduced stress, anxiety, and depression in haemodialysis patients, while no improvement was observed in a non-intervention control group.

These studies highlight Satyananda Yoga Nidra's effectiveness as a scientifically supported method that fosters deep psychophysiological balance, addressing both the physiological and psychological dimensions of stress and anxiety while promoting stress management and self-regulation. The practice relaxes the entire nervous system and interrupts the 'fight or flight' mechanism, which often remains chronically activated in everyday life, while re-engaging the vagal system in a balanced way. In this way, *yoga-nidrā* helps to release both physical and mental stress and enhances the capacity for conscious response.

Yoga-nidrā with adolescents in the education system — anxiety and stress reduction, improvement of emotional intelligence, increased learning ability and memory, well-being and creativity, reduction of cortisol levels

A substantial body of research has explored the effects of Satyananda Yoga Nidra in educational settings, particularly among adolescents and young adults, revealing benefits across multiple domains.

- **Stress and anxiety reduction.**

Several studies demonstrate that *yoga-nidrā* significantly reduces stress and anxiety levels. Kumar (2004) found that university students practicing *yoga-nidrā* experienced lower anxiety and improved well-being, leading to recommendations for its integration into university curricula. Rani et al. (2013) reported decreased stress levels in first-year nursing students, while Singh et al. (2015) observed reductions in stress and anxiety among medical students, alongside improved regulation of the sympathetic and parasympathetic nervous systems. Sachdeva (2016) and Graham (2021–2022) found that weekly *yoga-nidrā* practice at school reduced stress and improved behavioral responses in students. Tiwary et al. (2020) showed decreased cortisol levels in medical students, confirming its stress-regulating effects. D'souza et al. (2021) reported reductions in psychosocial stress, including stress related to home, school performance, teacher interactions, future uncertainty, and social conflicts.

- **Cognitive performance, learning and memory**

Satyananda Yoga Nidra also positively influences memory, learning, and creative abilities. Verma (2004) observed improved memory performance in students aged 13 to 15 following *yoga-nidrā* practice, while Gupta (2004) found significant increases in creativity in schoolchildren aged 10 to 12. Kanchibhotla et al. (2021) reported enhanced verbal memory in visually impaired children, indicating potential benefits for academic achievement. These findings suggest that even brief daily or weekly practice can support cognitive development and enhance learning capacity.

- **Emotional intelligence, self-confidence, and well-being**

Yoga-nidrā improves emotional and psychological functioning. Bhushan (2006a, 2006b) documented enhanced personality traits and self-confidence in teenagers. Vaishnav et al. (2018) found increased happiness, calmness, inspiration, alertness, self-confidence, and emotional regulation in adolescents aged 13 to 15. Ganpat (2020) reported improvements in emotional intelligence, including emotional sensitivity, maturity, and competence in university students. Gupta and Singh (2022) observed improvements in psychological well-being among adolescent girls, demonstrating benefits for self-awareness and mental health during puberty.

- **Behavioral and physiological regulation**

Satyananda Yoga Nidra supports changes in behavior and physiological patterns. Bhushan and Sinha (2001) found that school students showed improved concentration, reduced stress, positive behavioral changes, and enhanced happiness. Jensen et al. (2012) observed more stable breathing patterns in boys with disruptive behavior disorders during *yoga-nidrā*. Chowdhary (2019) reported improvements in resting heart rate, breathing rate, and vital capacity in adolescents practicing *yoga-nidrā* and *prāṇāyāma*. Pandey and Dalal (2020) noted increases in emotional maturity and mental health in young adults. Jaiganesh et al. (2022) showed that combining *sūrya-namaskāra* with *yoga-nidrā* reduced stress in high school students more effectively than exercise alone.

Across these studies, Satyananda Yoga Nidra demonstrates a wide-ranging impact on adolescents and young adults. It reduces stress and anxiety, enhances cognitive performance, promotes emotional intelligence and self-confidence, and improves behavioral and physiological regulation. These findings support the integration of this method into educational curricula and developmental programmes to foster mental, emotional, and physical well-being.

Yoga-nidrā as a reducer of symptoms of fatigue and its beneficial effects on mental and psychosomatic disorders

Research indicates that Satyananda Yoga Nidra has significant therapeutic potential for alleviating symptoms of fatigue and addressing a range of mental and psychosomatic conditions.

Gersten (1978) demonstrated that this method can enhance a practitioner's sense of self-efficacy, enabling individuals to recognise and systematically address personal challenges and interpersonal conflicts. Similarly, Mathew (1981) reported that *yoga-nidrā* is an effective intervention for both acute and chronic mental disorders, particularly in cases of excessive anxiety and neurotic behavioural patterns. Participants in the yoga group exhibited significant improvements in regressive responsiveness, along with reductions in feelings of guilt, physiological arousal, and fatigue.

These findings were further corroborated by Kumar (2010), who observed statistically significant differences in measures of stress, as well as the perceived severity and impact of tinnitus. The results suggest that *yoga-nidrā* can mitigate everyday stress associated with tinnitus and reduce the subjective experience of its symptoms.

Collectively, these studies support the role of Satyananda Yoga Nidra as a practical and effective method for enhancing self-regulation, reducing fatigue, and alleviating both mental and psychosomatic symptoms. Its incorporation into therapeutic or preventive programmes may offer meaningful benefits for individuals experiencing stress-related or neurotic conditions.

Yoga-nidrā as an effective aid for sleep disorders, chronic insomnia, and improved sleep quality

The state achieved through *yoga-nidrā* is related to both sleep and relaxation, but has unique qualities. During deep sleep, consciousness is largely absent, and unresolved cognitive or emotional activity is not actively processed. In the relaxation state, parasympathetic activity in the autonomic nervous system is increased, and dream-like experiences may occur. However, Satyananda Yoga Nidra is distinct in that routine mental activities of daily cognition are largely suspended, yet awareness of environmental stimuli remains intact. In both Satyananda Yoga Nidra and sleep, there is a mental disconnection from external stimuli. In *yoga-nidrā* this is due to the state of *pratyāhāra*. According to Hobson and Pace-Schott, one of the mechanisms in the brain that 'switches off' the awareness of external stimuli during sleep is the inhibition of the transmission of sensory signals from the thalamus to the cerebral cortex.[557] This inhibition enables the cerebral cortex to switch from external sensory impressions, which occur via the thalamus, to the 'offline' mode of the internalised state.[558]

Svāmī Satyānanda states in his book *Yoga Nidra* that one hour of *yoga-nidrā* practice is equivalent to about four hours of sleep.[559] This statement has been repeated by everyone who has dealt with this method in any way, without consulting further sources. Although it can be assumed that Svāmī Satyānanda, as the inventor of the technique, was able to substantiate this statement through his extensive experience as both practitioner and facilitator, the author is not yet aware of any clinical studies that would confirm

557 Hobson, J. A., & Pace-Schott, E. F. (2002). *The cognitive neuroscience of sleep: neuronal systems, consciousness and learning*. Nature reviews. Neuroscience, 3(9), 679–693. https://doi.org/10.1038/nrn915 (accessed on 28.10.2022).

558 Immnik, M.A. (2013). Scientific Exploration into Satyananda Yoga Nidra™. In Collection volume (2013). *Experience of Yoga, Golden Jubilee of Bihar School of Yoga*. Bihar: Yoga Publication Trust. p. 170.

559 Saraswati, Satyananda, Swami. (2006). *Yoga Nidra*. (12th reprint). Munger: Yoga Publications Trust, p. 14.

or disprove this claim. In the meantime, however, a number of studies have shown that Satyananda Yoga Nidra is, indeed, a promising treatment for insomnia and significantly improves sleep quality[560], attention after lack of sleep (Kohler et at., 2017), and neuroplasticity (Immnik, 2012).

Multiple studies have investigated the effects of *yoga-nidrā* on sleep, stress, and cognitive functioning.

Datta et al. (2012–2016) compared guided Satyananda Yoga Nidra with cognitive behavioural therapy (CBT) in chronic insomnia patients. Both interventions improved sleep duration and efficiency, but only *yoga-nidrā* significantly reduced salivary cortisol, indicating stress reduction. Datta et al. (2017) confirmed these effects in two older patients, with improvements in sleep, anxiety, depression, and stress persisting three months post-intervention.

Kohler et al. (2017) found that a single *yoga-nidrā* session improved attention and reduced drowsiness after sleep deprivation. Sharpe et al. (2021) reported enhanced relaxation, easier sleep onset, and reduced anxiety and pain. Verma et al. (2021) demonstrated improved sleep, stress reduction, and quality of life in patients with acute insomnia. Datta et al. (2021) reinforced these findings, showing significant cortisol reduction and improved sleep metrics. Sharpe et al. (2023) observed lower breathing rates and enhanced mood in adults with insomnia. Datta et al. (2023) reported faster reaction times, improved deep sleep activity, and better emotional recognition after two weeks of practice.

These studies show that Satyananda Yoga Nidra effectively improves sleep quality, reduces stress, and enhances cognitive performance, making it a practical intervention for both clinical and everyday applications.

Yoga-nidrā and migraine relief

Migraine is an episodic, debilitating headache and requires both long-term treatment and prevention. The treatment of migraine includes both medication for the acute cases of the condition and preventive preparations, as well

560 Shealy R. C. (1979). The effectiveness of various treatment techniques on different degrees and durations of sleep-onset insomnia. *Behaviour research and therapy*. 17(6), 541–546. https://doi.org/10.1016/0005-7967(79)90097-4 (accessed on 12.09.2023).

as non-pharmacological strategies. Although great progress has been made in migraine research in recent decades, treatment does not provide complete relief for many patients. Biofeedback and relaxation have been shown to be useful alternatives to standard medical therapy for both migraine and tension-type headaches. Treating migraine with yoga therapy can reduce the cost of medication and have a positive effect on overall health. Yoga has been shown to improve quality of life and reduce the number of headache episodes as well as the frequency of medication use.[561]

Satyananda Yoga Nidra has demonstrated significant potential as an adjunct therapy for migraine management. Clinical findings indicate that patients practising *yoga-nidrā* in combination with conventional therapy experience a greater reduction in both the frequency and intensity of migraine attacks compared to those receiving standard treatment alone (Kisan et al., 2014). These improvements are accompanied by enhanced vagal tone and a reduction in sympathetic activity, suggesting a restoration of autonomic balance.

Neurophysiological evidence further supports these findings: Satyananda Yoga Nidra practice has been associated with increased alpha wave activity, indicative of a relaxed yet alert state and dominance of the parasympathetic nervous system (Shashikiran et al., 2022). This shift towards parasympathetic activation contributes to the reduction of stress-related triggers and neuropsychological symptoms commonly associated with migraine. Overall, *yoga-nidrā* appears to be a promising, non-pharmacological intervention for alleviating migraine symptoms and promoting autonomic regulation.

Yoga-nidrā as a promoter of physical, mental and psychological health, general well-being and self-confidence

Siddhartha Bhushan (2001), former lecturer at the Department of Yoga Psychology, in the former Bihar Yoga Bharati University, Munger, ascribes preventive, health-promoting and healing effects to the Satyananda Yoga

561 See also, for example: Kisan, R., Sujan, M., Adoor, M., Rao, R., Nalini, A., Kutty, B. M., Chindanda Murthy, B., Raju, T., & Sathyaprabha, T. (2014). Effect of Yoga on migraine: A comprehensive study using clinical profile and cardiac autonomic functions. *International journal of yoga*. 7(2), 126–132. https://doi.org/10.4103/0973-6131.133891 (accessed on 12.09.2023).

Nidra technique based on his research. It helps to prevent stress susceptibility and stress-related disorders by inducing deep physical, emotional and mental relaxation, training the mind to remain calm and composed, and releasing suppressed desires and thoughts from the deeper areas of the mind. The research suggests that *yoga-nidrā* can be used as a therapeutic technique for treating mental disorders such as anxiety, aggression, insomnia, etc. and illnesses such as asthma, coronary disease, cancer, high blood pressure, etc.[562]

The scientific evidence suggests that Satyananda Yoga Nidra can significantly enhance physical, mental, and emotional well-being, supporting resilience, psychological stability, and a more positive self-concept (Dwivedi, 2020). Its applicability across different populations highlights its versatility as a tool for promoting holistic health and personal development.

Kumar (2006) found that Satyananda Yoga Nidra is an effective intervention for enhancing overall well-being, self-confidence, and mental health. His study indicates that regular practice reduces stress and anxiety, induces deep relaxation, and produces measurable physiological changes, including increased alpha-wave activity in the brain and improved electrodermal responses, reflecting enhanced autonomic regulation.

Satyananda Yoga Nidra has also been shown to improve self-esteem and statistically significant gains in self-perception among burn patients. *Yoga-nidrā* was particularly effective in boosting self-confidence and body image, demonstrating its therapeutic potential (Ozdemir and Saritas, 2019).

Yoga-nidrā for excessive weight/obesity

Regular practice of Satyananda Yoga Nidra, particularly when combined with physical activity, has been shown to reduce anxiety, enhance emotional maturity, and support overall psychological well-being in individuals who are overweight or obese (Selvam and Elangovan, 2018).

562 Bushan, Siddhartha. (2001). Yoga Nidra: Its Advantages and Applications. *Yoga Magazine*. http://www.yogamag.net/archives/2000s/2001/0103/0103ygnd.html (accessed on 14.09.2023).

Yoga-nidrā supporting and strengthening the immune system and affecting Complete Blood Count (CBC)

There is a direct link between the nervous and immune systems.[563] For example, stress causes increased secretion of the stress hormone cortisol, which acts as a natural immunosuppresor, reducing the body's ability to fight off bacteria and viruses. Stress hormones of the corticosteroid group also inhibit or suppress the immune system by reducing the number of lymphocytes (white blood cells needed to fight disease) in our body.[564] This interaction between the psyche, nervous system and immune system is the subject of the interdisciplinary field of psychoneuroimmunology and its neighbouring field, psychoneuroendocrinology, which studies the interactions between the psyche, nervous and endocrine systems.

This networked thinking in biomedical research has already shown that the nervous system and hormones influence the immune system and vice versa.

It can therefore be assumed that there is a close connection between our immunity and the degree of our relaxation. A relaxed state promotes the reduction of stress hormones that affect the immune system, while also stimulating the lymphatic system to flush toxins from the body, as well as affecting the supply of the various organs with oxygen-rich blood to help them function optimally.

Evidence from multiple studies suggests that Satyananda Yoga Nidra can enhance autonomic function by modulating reflex control of the sympathetic and parasympathetic branches, thereby improving physiological responses to stress. The deep relaxation that occurs on a physical, mental and emotional level during *yoga-nidrā* has been shown to make this method a very effective immune system booster. Kumar (2007) states, 'We all know that sleep is good for us, but the latest research shows that practising *yoga-nidrā* [Satyananda

---

563 See, for example, Macey, Jennifer. (2005). Stress in relation to immunity. *Journal of Experimental Medicine*. 02(11), pp. 1456–1482. https://www.researchgate.net/profile/Kamakhya-Kumar/publication/215451321_A_study_of_the_improvement_of_Physical_and_Mental_Health_through_Yoga_nidra/links/0c9605390532ac1002000000/A-study-of-the-improvement-of-Physical-and-Mental-Health-through-Yoga-nidra.pdf (accessed on 13.09.2023).

564 Kumar, Kamakhya. (2020). Role of Yoga-nidra in Immunity Development. *International Journal of Yoga and Allied Science*. 11(2), 358–61. https://www.researchgate.net/publication/350965226_Role_of_Yoga-nidra_in_Immunity_Development (accessed on 13.09.2023).

Yoga Nidra] can not only help us fight infection but also lower our stress levels.'[565] Pandya and Kumar (2007) found that 30 minutes of daily practice increased alpha brain waves and electrodermal activity, while lowering pulse, respiratory rate, and blood pressure. Kumar (2007) and Kumar & Joshi (2009) observed improvements in haemoglobin, leukocyte count, and galvanic skin response, supporting enhanced immune function. Kumar & Pandya (2012) reported reduced erythrocyte sedimentation rate (ESR), further indicating strengthened immunity.

Satyananda Yoga Nidra can be used as a method to support physiological balance and immune health, with potential benefits for individuals with weakened immunity.

Yoga-nidrā regulating high blood pressure and helping with heart disease

The various yoga 'relaxation techniques' cause a series of physical and mental changes known as the relaxation response. Situations that require constant behavioural adaptation activate an integrated hypothalamic response — the emergency response. Chronic stress response is believed to be one of the main factors causing hypertension. Both prevention and treatment of these diseases can be done by using the relaxation response — an integrated hypothalamic response, the physiological changes induced by which appear to be the opposite to those caused by the fight-or-flight response.[566]

Chronic high blood pressure has several causes that usually remain undetected. Numerous clinical studies have shown that Satyananda Yoga Nidra is recognised as a highly effective intervention for lowering blood pressure in chronically hypertensive patients. During *yoga-nidrā*, the heart rate, breathing, stress, anxiety and irritability of hypertensive patients are reduced. Through the interaction of body and mind, relaxation of the body brings about relaxation of the entire nervous system and a calming of physical and

565 Kumar, Kamakhya. (2007). The Healing Sleep, Yoga Magazine Mind Body Spirit. 3(50), 42–44. In Kumakhya, Kumar. (2013). *A Handbook of Yoga Nidra*. New Delhi: D. K. Printworld (P) Ltd., p. 64.

566 See for example: Benson, H., Greenwood, M. M., & Klemchuk, H. (1975). The relaxation response: psychophysiologic aspects and clinical applications. *International journal of psychiatry in medicine*. 6(1–2), 87–98. https://doi.org/10.2190/376W-E4MT-QM6Q-H0UM (accessed on 13.09.2023).

mental activities. The reduction in muscular and alteration in neuronal activity slows down the resting metabolic rate, and the blood vessels dilate. This can reduce cardiac output and stress on the heart. Systolic and diastolic blood pressure and the pulse rate fall, as the relaxed organism requires less oxygen and, accordingly, less metabolic activity.[567]

Research demonstrates that Satyananda Yoga Nidra effectively reduces blood pressure, improves autonomic function, and alleviates stress. Early studies showed that extended *śavāsana* (Datey & Bhagat, 1977) and long-term *yoga-nidrā* practice (Bali, 1979; Agras, 1980) significantly lowered blood pressure and anxiety, with lasting effects.

Controlled studies confirmed these benefits: *yoga-nidrā* reduced systolic and diastolic pressure, pulse rate, respiratory rate, and anxiety, improved immunity, and decreased medication use in hypertensive patients (Nirmalānanda & Choudhary, 2006–2007; Kumar, 2005; Pandya & Kumar, 2007). HRV studies indicated enhanced parasympathetic activity, whether *yoga-nidrā* was practiced alone or combined with *haṭha-yoga* (Markil et al., 2012; Chhetri et al., 2020). Additional interventions, such as *śiro-dhāra* or *bhrāmarī-prāṇāyāma*, further improved cardiovascular and autonomic outcomes (Devi & Kala, 2015; Bajpai, 2015).

Recent studies confirm its effectiveness across age groups: older adults experienced lower blood pressure (Thangam & Bharati, 2019), and *ōṃ*-repetition combined with *yoga-nidrā* reduced stress and improved sleep and autonomic function in hypertensive patients (Rajagopalan et al., 2022; Anjana et al., 2022).

Satyananda Yoga Nidra proves to be a safe, evidence-based intervention for lowering blood pressure, enhancing autonomic balance, and reducing stress and anxiety.

Yoga-nidrā and asthma

According to Svāmī Nirmalānanda, in modern yoga, the root cause of asthma — a chronic lung disease that causes inflammation and narrowing of the airways — is considered to be the disruption of a mechanism in the higher

567 Kumar, Kamakhya. (2013). *A Handbook of Yoga-Nidrā*. New Delhi: D. K. Printworld (P) Ltd, p. 122–123.

brain centres, which is reflected in the respiratory system, although it seems that it is a respiratory disease. According to Svāmī Satyānanda, asthma can be completely managed through specific techniques of integral yoga and *haṭha-yoga*. Some yoga techniques can be used to prevent asthma attacks, while others can be used during an acute asthma attack.[568] According to modern allopathic medicine, asthma can affect the brain through the 'lung-brain axis', leading to cognitive impairment, mood disorders like anxiety and depression, and structural brain changes. Chronic inflammation in asthma can cause neuroinflammation and structural alterations, such as hippocampal atrophy and reduced overall brain volume. Additionally, hypoxia from poor asthma control can damage the hippocampus, further impacting cognitive function. Despite the disagreement in approach, both views concur on the fact that asthma and brain health are intricately connected and as such that connection provides an avenue for intervention by means of Satyananda Yoga Nidra.

Research indicates that the integral Bihar Yoga system, which includes Satyananda Yoga Nidra, can be an effective complementary therapy for individuals with chronic respiratory conditions such as asthma and chronic obstructive pulmonary disease (COPD) (Nirmalānanda & Tiwari, 2006–2007). Participants experienced notable relief from respiratory symptoms, improved breathing efficiency, and a reduced dependence on medication following regular practice. These findings suggest that *yoga-nidrā*, as part of a comprehensive yogic approach, may support respiratory function, enhance lung capacity, and improve overall quality of life in individuals with long-standing pulmonary disorders.

Yoga-nidrā alleviating physical and psychological menstrual disorders and having a positive effect on the endocrine system and hormonal status

Satyananda Yoga Nidra can be an effective complementary therapy for alleviating physical and psychological symptoms associated with menstrual disorders and for supporting hormonal regulation. Regular practice has been

568 Nirmalananda, Swami. (n.d.). Research IV: Effect of Yoga on Satyananda Yoga on Asthma and COPD. In Yoga Research Foundation: Volume two. (2017). *Promotion of Health 1988–2007*. Bihar: Yoga Publication Trust, p. 83.

shown to reduce anxiety and depression, enhance psychological well-being, vitality, and general health, and improve overall mental and emotional stability (Rani et al., 2011; 2012; 2016).

In women with menstrual disorders, Satyananda Yoga Nidra led to significant improvements in pain symptoms as well as in gastrointestinal, cardiovascular, and urogenital function. Regular practice (35–40 minutes, five days per week over six months) also resulted in enhanced autonomic regulation, including reductions in heart rate, systolic and diastolic blood pressure, improved postural hypotension, and better control of breathing and handgrip strength.

Hormonal analyses demonstrated significant reductions in thyroid-stimulating hormone (TSH), follicle-stimulating hormone (FSH), luteinising hormone (LH), and prolactin following consistent *yoga-nidrā* practice. Moreover, complementary interventions combining *sūrya-namaskāra* and Satyananda Yoga Nidra further alleviated physical discomfort during menstruation, lowered anxiety, and improved self-concept over a 24-week period.

Overall, these findings suggest that Satyananda Yoga Nidra is a promising non-pharmacological intervention for managing both acute and chronic menstrual, hormonal, and psychosomatic disorders, supporting mental health, physiological regulation, and quality of life.

Yoga-nidrā and pain management

Evidence suggests that Yoga Nidra can be an effective adjunct for pain management across different clinical contexts. In their study Li et al. (2018) results indicate significant reductions in perceived pain and procedural difficulty, as observed during colonoscopy procedures, where patients receiving Satyananda Yoga Nidra reported improved willingness to repeat the procedure and a shorter procedure duration compared to control groups. Although reductions in blood pressure were not statistically significant, *yoga-nidrā* outperformed relaxation music in reducing subjective pain levels.

Further investigations demonstrated that both short-term and long-term Satyananda Yoga Nidra practice can lead to meaningful reductions in pain intensity, including in conditions such as lumbar spondylitis, highlighting its potential as a non-pharmacological intervention for managing acute and chronic pain (Manik et al., 2017).

Overall, these findings support Satyananda Yoga Nidra as a safe, accessible, and effective method for alleviating pain and enhancing patient comfort and satisfaction in both procedural and chronic pain settings.

Yoga-nidrā and its effect on diabetes patients

Diabetes is a metabolic disorder that has become a major public health challenge worldwide. The burden of diabetes is highest in Southeast Asian countries. The prevalence of diabetes is rapidly increasing, especially among urban populations, in part due to rising obesity and insufficient physical activity.[569] The standard treatment of substituting insulin permanently blocks the body's natural ability to produce the hormone, making the patient entirely dependent on an external supply. Svāmī Nirañjanānanda pointed out that yoga is helpful in managing non-insulin-dependent diabetes mellitus.[570]

Research indicates that Satyananda Yoga Nidra can have a beneficial impact on glycaemic control and related risk factors in patients with type 2 diabetes mellitus. Nirmalānanda (1998) reported significant improvements in blood glucose levels among non-insulin-dependent diabetic patients practising the Bihar Yoga Integral Yoga system, including *yoga-nidrā*. Subsequent studies (Nirmalānanda, 2002, 2003) demonstrated improvements in fasting and mid-morning blood glucose levels, as well as secondary indicators such as body mass index (BMI), waist-to-hip ratio, and lipid profile, with some participants able to reduce their medication dosage.

Further evidence from Amita et al. (2009) showed that three months of regular Satyananda Yoga Nidra practice significantly decreased mean blood glucose levels and improved diabetes-related symptoms. Participants practising *yoga-nidrā* alongside conventional hypoglycaemic medication exhibited

569 Amita, S., Prabhakar, S., Manoj, I., Harminder, S. & Pavan, T. (2009). Effect of yoga-nidra on blood glucose level in diabetic patients. *Indian journal of physiology and pharmacology*. 53(1), 97–101. https://pubmed.ncbi.nlm.nih.gov/19810584/ (accessed on 13.09.2023).

570 Nirmalananda, Swami. (2017). In Yoga Research Foundation: Volume Two. *Promotion of Health 1988–2007*. Bihar: Yoga Publication Trust, p. 26.

better control of fluctuating blood glucose and associated symptoms than those receiving medication alone.

These findings suggest that Satyananda Yoga Nidra can serve as a valuable adjunctive therapy for type 2 diabetes, contributing to improved glycaemic stability, symptom management, and overall metabolic health.

Yoga-nidrā promoting the mental health of people who have suffered physical or emotional abuse

Lata and Singh (2014) investigated the effects of Satyananda Yoga Nidra on individuals who had experienced physical or emotional abuse. In a before-and-after comparison, participants showed a significant reduction in scores on the Mental Health Battery, indicating improvements in overall mental well-being. Participants reported acquiring skills through *yoga-nidrā* that enabled them to manage stress and anxiety more effectively in challenging situations. The programme was associated with reductions in nervousness, tension, depression, dejection, hopelessness, physical discomfort, and illness, while enhancing feelings of happiness, contentment, cheerfulness, and a sense of freedom. Participants also reported gaining a new perspective on life. This study suggests that Satyananda Yoga Nidra may exert a positive influence on both the mental and physical well-being of adolescents who have experienced emotional or physical abuse.

Yoga-nidrā strengthening the immune system of HIV/AIDS patients

Regular practice of Satyananda Yoga Nidra in HIV/AIDS patients was associated with a notable increase in CD4 cell counts and significant improvements in clinical symptoms, including weight loss, fatigue, memory impairment, depression, recurrent fever, and skin conditions. Moderate improvements were observed in respiratory and gastrointestinal symptoms, and slight improvements in pulmonary tuberculosis. Overall, half of the patients experienced significant improvement, with additional moderate or slight improvements in others (Mishra, 2013).

Satyananda Yoga Nidra may serve as an effective complementary approach to enhance immune function and support overall well-being in HIV-positive patients.

Yoga-nidrā as a method of promoting self-efficacy and self-care in a professional context

Practice of Satyananda Yoga Nidra was associated with significant reductions in stress levels among nurses and nursing students (Rani et al., 2013; Christine, 2017). Participants reported feelings of relaxation, calmness, and peace (Rani et al., 2013). Improvements were also observed in postprandial blood glucose (Kim, 2014), muscle fatigue (Anderson et al., 2017), and positive attitudes toward career decisions (Reddy et al., 2018). These findings suggest that Satyananda Yoga Nidra can enhance self-efficacy, self-care, and professional resilience, and may be a cost-effective adjunct for training programmes aimed at healthcare providers.

Yoga-nidrā having a positive effect on athletic performance

Satyananda Yoga Nidra has been shown to enhance concentration and attention in athletes, as evidenced by improved performance in archers (Deuskar et al., 2006; Sethi & Singh, 2016). Wrestlers who practised Satyananda Yoga Nidra demonstrated faster simple visual reaction and anticipation times compared to controls (Sethi & Singh, 2016). Anxiety levels, particularly in athletes with mild to moderate symptoms, were significantly reduced following Satyananda Yoga Nidra training (Mahesh & Sanjit, 2016), highlighting its potential to address psychological barriers such as fear of failure. Satyananda Yoga Nidra was also found to be more effective than audiovisual biofeedback for faster recovery from exertion, increasing alpha wave activity and activating the parasympathetic nervous system, thereby reducing psychophysiological stress and muscle tension (Das & Pandey, 2020). Improvements in sleep quality were observed, with shorter sleep onset latency, increased sleep efficiency, and better overall rest compared to progressive muscle relaxation (Datta et al., 2022).

The use of *yoga-nidrā* for stroke patients

At the University of Western Australia, several clinical trials (Immnik and Hiller, 2011; Garett, Immnik and Hiller, 2011; Immnik, Chan and Hiller, 2012; Chan, Immnik and Hiller, 2012) were conducted with patients suffering from stroke-related movement restrictions to examine the effect of Satyananda Yoga Nidra, which was used as a key element of the intervention programme. The results of these studies showed that the mental health of the participants, their sense of the affected body regions and their mobility had improved significantly.

Effects of yoga-nidrā on brain activity and neuroplasticity

Neuroimaging studies have shown that the states of consciousness during or after practising Satyananda Yoga Nidra are associated with measurable changes in brain activity. Brainwave activity during this practice follows the changes in the brain that occur when we transition from wakefulness to sleep and brain activity moves from beta and alpha to theta and delta waves, respectively, while consciousness is maintained. Consequently, the *yoga-nidrā* state could be crucial for processes involved in neuroplasticity.

Immnik[571] provides an overview of the neuronal effect of Satyananda Yoga Nidra, particularly in connection with complex movement sequences. For this, he drew, among other things, on the study by Toma et al. (1999) which showed that muscle relaxation (measured using electromyography) occurs after activation of associated somatosensory and motor cortex areas. This effect probably occurs in the process of perceiving and visualising body regions in Stage 3 — Rotation of Awareness Throughout the Body. Furthermore, Immnik explains that research (e.g. Gosschalk and Gregg, 1996; Esmeralda et al. 2004) has sufficiently demonstrated that active muscle relaxation promotes performance in memory recall tasks. It was concluded that the process of active relaxation could also be an important factor in promoting neuroplasticity. Based on this scientific knowledge, Immnik hypothesised

571 Immnik, Maarten, A. Scientific Explorations into Satyananda Yoga. In Collection volume. (2013). *Experience of Yoga*. Golden Jubilee 1963–2013. Bihar: Yoga Publikation Trust, p. 170–171.

that Stage 3 of *yoga-nidrā* in particular could be an effective means of establishing changes in movement generation (mind-body connection), which could then be further deepened in the final and more subtle stages of *yoga-nidrā* practice. This hypothesis was confirmed by a prior study (Immnik 2012).

Two studies that used neuroimaging techniques provided evidence that Satyananda Yoga Nidra can promote movement-related neuroplasticity. Lou et al. (1999) found increased cerebral blood flow — a parameter for brain activity — in the parietal cortex (sensory processing), the hippocampus (formation of long-term memory) and in the frontal lobes, which are associated with focusing attention and executive functions (goals, motivation, strategy). The activity in these areas of the brain is also high when we learn or perform a difficult movement. Hobson and Pace-Schott (2002) found in a study that the level of the neurotransmitter dopamine[572] increases during sleep. Flöel et al. (2005) later demonstrated that an increased release of dopamine is directly related to learning and executing movements. In particular, the study by Kjaer et al. (2002) showed that subjects who practised Satyananda Yoga Nidra were able to achieve theta states and that their dopamine levels rose significantly during the practice.

Immnik concludes that if Satyananda Yoga Nidra does facilitate sleep-like processes important for neuroplasticity, then this technique could be used after motor learning sessions to promote the brain changes necessary for improving motor performance and efficiency. This concept would have far-reaching implications for areas such as physical education (e.g. for children learning new movement patterns), industry (e.g. for operating machines), health sciences (e.g. movement rehabilitation) and sports or high-performance sports sciences.

For a more detailed discussion of the effects of Satyananda Yoga Nidra on brain activity and neuroplasticity, see Part I. Chapter 10. *Brain activity and states of consciousness during yoga-nidrā; Results of Brain Research on Satyananda Yoga Nidra* and Part V. Appendix 2. *Effects of yoga-nidrā on brain activity and neuroplasticity*.

---

572 Dopamine is produced in the basal ganglia, which consists of a neuronal structure that is also activated during sleep. The neurotransmitter dopamine controls emotional, mental and motor reactions.

Yoga-nidrā and distance learning during the COVID-19 lockdowns

Satyananda Yoga Nidra delivered through online or digital platforms during the COVID-19 lockdowns was shown to improve multiple aspects of mental and physical well-being. Mood and daytime emotional state significantly improved in participants (Gulia & Sreedharan, 2021). Sleep quality increased, including reductions in insomnia and associated symptoms such as headaches (Sharpe et al., 2021). Anxiety and depression levels decreased, with online *yoga-nidrā* practice proving more effective than standard relaxation exercises in healthcare workers (Gunjiganvi et al., 2021). Physical well-being indicators, including body mass index and daily activity patterns, also improved (Gulia & Sreedharan, 2021; Sharpe et al., 2021). These findings demonstrate that Satyananda Yoga Nidra is a feasible and effective complementary practice for promoting mental health, enhancing sleep, and supporting overall well-being during periods of remote learning or restricted access to in-person classes.

Part Four

Overview of the Contemporary Developments of yoga-nidrā in the Western Context

CHAPTER 19

The Contemporary Approach to *yoga-nidrā* — Origins and Development

We might note in this context that the term yoga-nidrā (yogic sleep) is used as a synonym of the 'fourth state' of samādhi (turīya) in some 12th century yogic texts. It does not appear to refer to a specific technique of yoga until the 20th century Satyananda Yoga Nidra, as taught by modern yoga guru Satyananda Saraswati (1923–2009).[573]

THE ROOTS OF *YOGA-NIDRĀ*, AS previously discussed, go back millennia.[574] The oldest sources, as well as later texts that mention the term, describe a state called *yoga-nidrā*, but do not provide a specific technique for entering or experiencing that state. In the 1960s, two masters in North India developed their own approaches of achieving *yoga-nidrā* — each with

573 Mallinson, J. and Singelton, M. (2017). *Roots of Yoga*. London: Penguin Classics. p. 326–327.

574 See Part I. Chapter 4. *History and origin of yoga-nidrā*.

their own method — and made them available to people of the present day — Svāmī Satyānanda Sarasvatī of the Bihar School of Yoga and Svāmī Rāma Bhāratī of the Himalayan Institute. Svāmī Satyānanda was the first one to publish a book on his method and on *yoga-nidrā* as such. Svāmī Rāma briefly explains his *yoga-nidrā* method in two of his books, which will be introduced in the following pages.

These 20th century masters developed the first two *yoga-nidrā* methods as integral parts of the holistic yoga approach within their respective yoga systems. The methods were seen as having the primary goal of spiritual growth and development, and not merely as a means of mundane mental hygiene, serving only to relax, provide therapy to or aid oneself in learning new skills. Or, to let oneself be manipulated through mechanisms such as suggestion and hypnotic elements — trends visible in subsequent developments. Namely, a series of *yoga-nidrā* techniques were extracted from these two original methods in the West and are now used as stand-alone, secular techniques. However, their goals and methods sometimes differ greatly from the original methods of the two masters. Some of these diverse approaches are explained in the following chapter.

Why and How Do *Yoga-nidrā* Techniques Differ?

The term *yoga-nidrā* originally referred to a particular higher state of consciousness — be that one experienced by Viṣṇu or an individual *yogin*. In modern times, the name of this state was often used to also refer to the technique which was supposed to lead to it, thus falsely equating technique and state. When someone says, for example, 'I meditate', what is meant is, 'I practice a technique whereby my awareness can be sharpened and, over time, immersed in a 'meditative' state.' Higher states of absorption (such as *samādhi*), which are also often referred to as 'meditation' in the West, cannot be practiced — they are experienced. Therefore, the state of *yoga-nidrā* should also not be confused with the technique for achieving it, since the technique is only intended as a preparation for the state and as a way to achieve it. It is not uncommon that, in Sanskrit, the same noun denotes both a process and a state. Svāmī Satyānanda and Svāmī Rāma called their methods for ultimately reaching the state of *yoga-nidrā* by the same name with full awareness of this. However, this is something which has led to the false understanding in the West that the mere participation in a process equals the achievement of the complete state to which that process is supposed to lead.

Similarly, other practices or modern yoga 'styles' have been named after terms from the scriptures. For example, Kṛṣṇa Pattabhi Jois used the term *aṣṭāṅga-yoga* for his yoga system, following Patañjali's eight-limbed path, which forms the spiritual and ethical background of his system of *āsana* and *prāṇāyāma*. Paramahaṃsa Yogānanda described a series of practices as '*kriyā-yoga*', after the term mentioned in Patañjali's *Yoga-sūtras* 2.1, where '*kriyā-yoga*' is described as 'austerity (*tapas*), self-study of scriptures (*svādhyāya*) and surrender to the Godhead (*īśvarapraṇidhāna*)'.[575] Yogi Bhajan called his particular yoga system 'Kuṇḍalinī Yoga', although awakening the *kuṇḍalinī-śakti* and its ascent through the *cakras* towards the *sahasrāra-cakra*, which promises liberation, is a well-known goal in systems of yoga such as that described in the famous 17th century Ṣaṭcakranirūpaṇa. Likewise, Svāmī Satyānanda and Svāmī Rāma used the term *yoga-nidrā*—'yogic sleep' or 'sleep with awareness'—as a name for their methods.

> Currently, numerous practices can be found in Western yoga that are misleadingly referred to as *yoga-nidrā*[576]. A large proportion of these are used in isolation, without being placed in the holistic yoga context. The instructions are often spoken in a slow, storyteller-like voice, and suggestions, affirmations and background music or sounds are used to guide the practitioners on imaginary journeys, etc. As a rule, these relaxation-focused practices are marketed as new *yoga-nidrā* 'styles' or under their own brand names. Such techniques can certainly be helpful in letting thoughts wander and letting go, but it is doubtful that they lead to the *yoga-nidrā* state. Unfortunately, the viral use of the term *yoga-nidrā* to describe such practices has reduced the term in its general use to meaning mere relaxation, which has little to do with its original meaning and purpose.

575 See Part I. Chapter 2. *Introduction to the Integral Approach to Yoga*.

576 *Yoga-nidrā* is sometimes incorrectly translated as 'sleep yoga'.

In the West, we often encounter the approach that one should practice and teach not according to a prescribed ruleset, i.e. not 'by the book', but rather 'by feeling'. This is often based on short-term training courses (usually anywhere between a weekend and three months), which are nowadays often held online, and a lack of personal experience. This reflects the cultural misunderstandings, pace, superficiality and the pervasive commercialisation of our time. There is no doubt that it is of great importance that we allow our intuition and our 'feeling' for our own *sādhana* to guide us – we are only responsible for ourselves in this. However, if we begin teaching others and want to accompany them on their spiritual path, this brings with it a special responsibility, because *yoga-nidrā* is primarily about accessing the subconscious and thus a very sensitive state of the practitioner who is entrusting themselves to us.

For this reason, the school founded by Svāmī Satyānanda was eventually forced to clearly distinguish its own method from secular variants by trademark protection. This protected trademark can serve as an orientation for the practitioner with regard to the goals of the chosen method and the quality standards that teachers must meet. The trademark protection is not intended to monopolise the term *yoga-nidrā* itself, nor does it represent an attack on other methods. Rather, it is intended as a guide and a clear demarcation from newly emerged branches, with regard to the content and origin of the original intention, as well as the preservation of traditional and proven methodologies.

The Two Main Traditions of Contemporary *Yoga-nidrā* Methodology

The Himalayas and all of India have been home to seers and sages, who have passed on their knowledge and teachings in long lines of tradition. Yoga-like approaches date back to the late Vedic period[577] (approx. 500 BCE) and probably even further back. Such a long continuous line of tradition is called

577 See Part I. Chapter 1. *The Schools of Thought – darśanas – of India*.

paramparā. About twelve hundred years ago, Śaṅkara (c. 788 — c. 820 CE), an Indian master, philosopher and theologian, consolidated the teaching of Advaita Vedānta and founded the Daśanāmi Saṃpradāya — the 'Tradition of Ten Names' — a major ascetic order with ten branches. Śaṅkara organised his disciples, the 'renunciants'[578], into ten monastic orders and distributed them across the various regions of India. Their teachings were focused on specific topics and were passed down from master to disciple in a lineage (*paramparā*) over the millennia.

Two of these Daśanāmi lineages based in North India are the Sarasvatī and Bhāratī lineages. Sarasvatī is the goddess of knowledge, music, art, wisdom and learning. The teachings of Svāmī Satyānanda Sarasvatī come from this lineage. Bhāratī is interpreted as *bhā-* — 'the light of knowledge' — and *-ratī* — 'a lover who is absorbed in it'.[579] Bhāratī thus refers to someone who, as a lover of knowledge, is completely absorbed in the light of knowledge. Svāmī Rāma Bhāratī's teaching comes from this very branch. The focus of these two orders was on the preservation of ancient knowledge. Their systems are now characterised by an integral awareness-based yoga and immersion practices. The *yoga-nidrā* methods that have emerged from these two traditions should be understood in the context of their teachings.

Svāmī Satyānanda's teaching and method of *yoga-nidrā* have already been presented in detail.[580] In the following, Svāmī Rāma's approach to *yoga-nidrā* will be examined in more detail.[581]

Svāmī Rāma Bhāratī and the Himalayan Tradition

Svāmī Rāma Bhāratī (1925–1996) was born in northern India into a family of Brahmins. From an early age, he travelled throughout India and Tibet with mendicant monks, yogis, and *sādhus*. His teachers included Ramaṇa Maharṣi,

578 They are referred to as '*svāmīs*' – 'those who set out to master themselves'.

579 Translation: Himalayan Tradition Website, https://www.himalayatradition.ch/home/die-himalaya-tradition/ (accessed on 10.12.2022).

580 See Part II. Chapter 13. *Svāmī Satyānanda's yoga-nidrā method*.

581 The author has taken this information from the existing sources of the Himalayan Institute and the books of Svāmī Rāma. She has no personal experience of this method and has not been trained in it.

Śrī Aurobindo, Ānandamayī Mā and Rabindranath Tagore. He completed his studies with his grandmaster in Tibet.

Svāmī Rāma received a higher education in both India and Europe and was one of the first yogis to allow Western scientists to examine him while he was reaching certain stages of consciousness. In 1969, he travelled to the United States for the first time, where he founded the Himalayan Institute of Yoga Science and Philosophy in Pennsylvania. Further centres were established worldwide. Svāmī Rāma was the founder of various organisations and spread his teachings in the spirit of the Himalayan masters through publications and lectures.[582]

Svāmī Rāma's successor and current spiritual head of the Himalayan Institute is Dr Paṇḍit Rājamaṇi Ṭigunāyat. Another disciple of Svāmī Rāma, Svāmī Veda Bhāratī (1933–2015), founded the Association of Himalayan Yoga Meditation Societies International (AHYMSIN), which taught the teachings of the master until his death. Rod Stryker (born 1957), a student of Dr Paṇḍit Rājamaṇi Ṭigunāyat, founded *ParaYoga®* and *ParaYoga Nidra® — Enlightened Sleep®* in the USA.

Swāmī Rāma's Approach — an Overview

Swāmī Rāma's *yoga-nidrā* approach is based on ancient Sāṃkhya philosophy[583] and the late Vedic text *Māṇḍukya Upaniṣad*[584]. When Swāmī Rāma uses the term, he explicitly refers to the state of *yoga-nidrā* and not to the technique named after the state. The aim of his method is to purify the conscious and unconscious mind of disturbing impressions, as well as of emotions, thoughts and desires which hinder spiritual development; it is about mastering the journey from wakefulness to dream to deep sleep and then introducing the practitioner to the fourth state of consciousness — *turīya* or *yoga-nidrā*. When *turīya* is attained, the task is to establish awareness in that state.

---

582 Rama, Swami. (2018). *Mein Leben mit den Meistern des Himalayas – Erfahrungen eines modernen Weisen und Yogi*. Stuttgart: Agni Verlag. p. 416.

583 Rama, Swami. (2018). *Path of Fire and Light*. Vol. 2. Honesdale: Himalayan Institute Press. p. 176.

584 See Part I. Chapter 4. *The History and Origin of yoga-nidrā* and Part I. Chapter 9. *The Levels of Consciousness and yoga-nidrā*.

In addition, serious practitioners are encouraged to master conscious sleep and understand the relationship between consciousness, mind and body, while the mind is directed inwards and consciously placed in a deep state of rest. The practitioner should be able to consciously invoke all three states at will, perceiving them simultaneously and experiencing their unity on a personal and universal level.

In this state, wisdom is attained by recalling, observing and analysing all the *saṃskāras*, discarding disturbing thought patterns and strengthening the helpful ones. Then the practitioner gradually enters what this tradition refers to as the 'cave of the heart centre' — *anāhata-cakra* — the state of 'absence of all impressions' — the stillness of the mind. In this state, the clarity of mind is said to be more profound than in the waking state.

Furthermore, *yoga-nidrā* is also seen as a revitalising state and a way to activate and gain control over the autonomic nervous system, as well as a method for releasing all kinds of internal tension and increasing the self-healing powers of body and mind. However, all of this is an additional result of the practice and not its goal.[585]

Svāmī Rāma recommended to not modify the technique he presented, but rather to learn to gain control over one's own body and to master the autonomic nervous system. He also pointed out that the technique of *yoga-nidrā* could lead very deeply into the subtleties of one's own inner life.[586]

The Steps of Swāmī Rāma's *yoga-nidrā* Technique[587]

The ultimate goal of the *yoga-nidrā* method could be said to be the achievement of *turīya*. However, Svāmī Rāma uses the term *yoga-nidrā* as a synonym for *turīya* in his commentary on the *Māṇḍūkya-upaniṣad*. He expands upon the process of moving from the waking, through the dreaming to the state of deep sleep and then finally *turīya* by linking the steps of that process with the energy nexuses of the subtle body — the *cakras*. The waking state — *jāgrat* — he

585 Sovik, Rolf PsyD. (2013). What is Yoga Nidra? [Video] *Yoga International*. https://www.youtube.com/watch?v=4NBImrP0aPk (accessed on 20.01.2022).

586 Ibid.

587 Rama, Swami. (1982) *Enlightenment without God – Mandukya Upanishad*. Honesdale: Himalayan Institute Press and Rama, Swami. (2007) *Path of Fire and Light*. Vol. 2. Honesdale: Himalayan Institute Press.

linked to *ājñā-cakra* (regarded as being associated with the eyebrow centre; dreaming—*svapna*—he linked to *viśuddhi-cakra* (associated with the throat); deep sleep—*suṣupti*—he linked to *anāhata-cakra* (associated with the heart centre). By progressing through the stages of the practice in this way, the practitioner gradually enters the 'hollow of the heart centre'—the *anāhata-cakra*, a state of 'absence of all impressions' and stillness of the mind.

The Three-Step *yoga-nidrā* Method

Svāmī Rāma's disciple Rolf Sovik[588] describes the underlying structure of Svāmī Rāma's technique as a core practice consisting of three steps, practised in *śavāsana*:

Step 1: 61 Points—*śava-yatra*

Step 2: 57 Breaths—*śithilī-kāraṇa* and

Step 3: *yoga-nidrā*—one lets one's awareness move from the eyebrow centre (*ājñā-cakra* in Svāmī Rāma's system) to the throat centre (*viśuddhi-cakra*). Finally, one lets one's awareness rest in the heart centre (*anāhata-cakra*).

Svāmī Rāma advises practitioners not to stay in Step 3 for more than ten minutes at the beginning, because the mind does not yet have the ability to remain conscious for longer. Otherwise, there is a risk of falling asleep. The ability to remain conscious for longer periods of time can only be developed gradually.

The core practice has been expanded over time to include two further preparatory steps and currently consists of five Steps.[589] The entire practice can take up to 1.5 hours and consists of a series of preparation and relaxation steps until the actual *yoga-nidrā* begins. These preparatory steps can take about 45 minutes. They support the practice and help the body and mind to relax and

588 Rolf Sovik is a disciple of Svāmī Rāma, psychologist and president of the Himalaya-Institute in Honesdale, Pennsylvania, USA.

589 Sovik, Rolf PsyD. (2013). Yoga Nidra: Introduction to the Complete Practice. [Video]. *Yoga International*. https://www.youtube.com/watch?v=6usuqKQOiqM (accessed on 01.04.2019).

prepare the way for *yoga-nidrā*. Beginners should first systematically master these steps until they are able to consciously remain in each stage throughout. Only then can they progress to the full practice. Another goal is to remain in the desired state of *turīya* for as long as possible — and some *yogins* are even able to do this for up to 3.5 hours. Gradually, the ability to sleep consciously develops, which can replace the usual night's sleep for experienced *yogins*.[590]

Rolf Sovik explains that the state of deep relaxation is achieved during the various preparatory exercises. Initially, the brain produces alpha waves and activates the body's self-healing powers. In the final steps of the practice, theta waves multiply. They can deepen into delta waves until brain activity enters a state of non-REM sleep. When these steps are mastered, *turīya* or *yoga-nidrā* is considered achieved.

The Five Steps of the *yoga-nidrā* Method According to Svāmī Rāma

The five steps are described below according to the tradition of the Himalayan Institute and include the assertions and characteristics mentioned in the sources of that tradition.

STEP 1 — Movement with Awareness

To start with, it is important to prepare the body. The body accumulates tension throughout the day. Releasing this tension with gentle movements such as stretching the shoulders, arms, hips, legs and twisting the back opens the way for more subtle inner exercises.

STEP 2 — Exercises Without Movement

More subtle movements performed in *śavasāna* lead to a deeper and more refined perception of one's own muscles and joint systems. By concentrating on the different parts of the body, isolating, tensing up and relaxing them, the next step towards entering *yoga-nidrā* is taken.

590 Ibid.

These exercises are based on the idea that you consciously signal your body to move from your brain. In the brain, an impulse is sent to the nerve that ends in the respective body part, for example on the sole of the foot or in the fingers, in the lower back or in the chest. In this way, it is observed how the mind can control the body and how the mind is able to create tension and then release that tension in the body, while at the same time keeping the other parts of the body completely isolated and relaxed. The awareness shifts from the right to the left side of the body during the exercise, thus balancing and connecting mind and body.[591]

After completing this sequence of movement exercises, two forms of deep relaxation follow, which are performed one after the other and build on the initial technique described in Svāmī Rāma's books.

Step 3—*śava-yatra* or 'Journey Through the Corpse'

Systematic relaxation to sharpen concentration by guiding the consciousness to 61 points thoughout the body. This exercise strengthens the ability to maintain focus in the physical body (*sthūla-śarīra* or *annamaya-kośa*). Moving beyond this sense of the body, awareness is then absorbed into the subtle body (*sūkṣma-śarīra* or *prāṇamaya-kośa*). The first phase of this practice is a 31-point relaxation—from the centre of the forehead to the centre of the heart. You stay at each point for one to three breaths and then move on to the next point. The rhythm should be neither too slow, as it is easier to let your attention drift, nor too fast, as it would then be difficult to follow the instructions and stay present. Once you have mastered the first phase, you should proceed to the complete exercise of the 61 points.

This step can be deepened by visualising and perceiving these focus points as white points of light or stars, and later as a blue star. In this way, blockages in the energy flow of the *prāṇas*, caused by stress and strain, can be released. In even more advanced variations, each of the 61 points is associated with certain mantras.[592]

---

591 This step was probably influenced by the practice of progressive muscle relaxation developed by the American physician Edmund Jacobson in the 1920s and 1930s. See Jacobson, Edmund. (1978). *You must relax: Practical Methods for Reducing the Tensions of Modern Living*. New York: McGraw-Hill.

592 Possibly a technique similar to *nyāsa*.

The origin of the 61-point exercises suggests a connection with the *Vaśiṣṭha-saṃhitā* and the āyurvedic text *Suśruta-saṃhitā*, where originally 108 *marma* points (energy points) are mentioned.[593]

STEP 4—Breathing Relaxation Exercise or *śithilī-kāraṇa*

In these breathing techniques, the breath is guided through the various parts of the body and the *cakras* one after the other. As you exhale, the body relaxes and expels all toxins, while the mind is freed from fatigue, stress and tension. During inhalation, you fill your entire being with energy. This practice is said to have a deeply relaxing effect even when done on its own and to alleviate insomnia. It is said to have a supportive effect on diabetes, high blood pressure and depression. This level can also be practised as preparation for meditation.

STEP 5—Sleep with Awareness (*yoga-nidrā*)

This is the actual *yoga-nidrā* stage, in which awareness is directed to the eyebrow centre—*ājñā-cakra*—while taking three breaths using controlled diaphragmatic breathing (abdominal breathing), letting go of all thoughts, even one's mantra if one has one. Awareness is then directed to the throat centre—*viśuddhi-cakra*—where the moon is visualised. The breath flows naturally for a few breaths. This step is concluded with diaphragmatic breathing. Finally, awareness rests in the heart centre—*anāhata-cakra*—in a state of *yoga-nidrā*. Here you instruct the body and mind to sleep while consciousness is still active in the *yoga-nidrā* state. The recommended time to stay in this state is five to ten minutes to start with. You therefore consciously decide to awaken after ten minutes and then gradually move back outwards.

---

593 Parker, S., Bharati, S. V., & Fernandez, M. (2013). Defining yoga-nidra: traditional accounts, physiological research, and future directions. *International journal of yoga therapy*. 23(1), 11–16.

General Considerations

> In contrast to the Svāmī Satyānanda method, Svāmī Rāma initially directs awareness to physical movements and then, via controlled breathing, to the more subtle stages of the practice.

According to Svāmī Satyānanda, and in line with the Tantric view of sleep and dreams, most people's *prāṇas* are active in the *maṇipūra* , *svādhiṣṭhāna-*, and *mūlādhāra-cakras* with general patterns of consciousness during the sleeping state. In persons with a more sattvic temperament, the *pranas* primarily move in the *viśuddhi-cakra* and sometimes in the *anāhata-cakra*. *Viśuddhi* contains the experience of a complete lack of awareness, while dreams can occur in *anāhata*. In highly developed awareness, the *prāṇas* do not rest in *viśuddhi* or *anāhata*, but in *sahasrāra* during deep sleep and in *ājñā* during the experience of dreams and visions.[594]

According to Svāmī Rāma's method, wakefulness is attributed to the *ājñā-cakra*, dreaming to the *viśuddhi-cakra* and sleeping to the *anāhata-cakra*. *Turīya* is achieved by resting one's awareness in the heart centre — the *anāhata-cakra*.

However, while every Stage of either of the two *yoga-nidrā* methods can and does have some relation to the *cakra* system and subtle yogic physiology in general, the method of Svāmī Satyānanda does not foresee the inclusion of the *cakras* in the *pratyāhāra* practice of *yoga-nidrā* — they only become directly relevant for the *dhāraṇā* stage of the practice. Furthermore, *dhāraṇā-yoga-nidrā* does not necessarily include utilising the *cakras* either — a *dhāraṇā-yoga-nidrā* practice mentioning and using the *cakras* primarily makes sense as a part of an integral *sādhana* complemented by *āsana*, *prāṇāyāma*, *mudrā* and bhandha focusing on and working with the *cakras* specifically.

---

594 Saraswati, Satyananda Swami. (2006). *Yoga Nidra*. Munger: Yoga Publication Trust. (12th reprint), p. 61

Secular *Yoga-nidrā* Techniques

The Problem of Adaptation

As already discussed,[595] *yoga-nidrā* has attracted increased interest in psychotherapy in the West since the 1970s. The many secular *yoga-nidrā* techniques that have emerged, especially in the West, have been developed by psycho- or hypnotherapists, mainly in the English-speaking world, and are frequently used in a therapeutic context. In this way, *yoga-nidrā* was extracted from the integral yoga context and heavily adapted to the needs of Western psychotherapy and the commercialism of Western society. The goal was now neither *pratyāhāra* nor the exploration of different states of consciousness, but an increase in the observed phenomenon of deep relaxation and mental, psychological and general well-being. This effect is, of course, increasingly necessary and important in our time, is highly valued by most people and can be put to good use in various social areas. Nevertheless, it is important to be aware of the differences between the various techniques and their objectives in order to choose the method that is right for the individual.

However, it is also debatable whether such heavily modified methods should continue to be called *yoga-nidrā* if they no longer have the goal of achieving the *yoga-nidrā* state. As mentioned earlier, the concept of 'relaxation' and increased well-being originated in the late 19th and early 20th century[596] and was only introduced to modern Western yoga in the mid-20th century. Some proponents of newer *yoga-nidrā* approaches are not sure whether *yoga-nidrā* should be a meditation technique, a mindfulness method[597] or a deep relaxation technique, even a 'style of yoga', or all of the above. The commercial demand for 'something new' has led to derivatives and modifications as secondary, tertiary, etc. techniques that often differ widely from the goal of *yoga-nidrā* and have almost created a kind of New Age *yoga-nidrā* jungle.

---

595 See Part III. Chapter 20. *Yoga-nidrā and* Hypnosis.

596 See Part III. Chapter 18. *Effect of Stress and the Importance of Relaxation*.

597 *Mindfulness-Based Stress Reduction* (MBSR) is based on Buddhist *vipāśana* meditation and was developed in the 1980s by Prof. Jon Kabat-Zinn in the USA.

The following is an introduction to the most important secondary *yoga-nidrā* techniques: *iRest Yoga Nidra®* by Dr Richard Miller, USA, then *I AM Yoga Nidra™* by Yogi Amrit Desai, USA, and finally the collaborative work of the *Total Yoga Nidra Network* in the UK. The author has compiled the information about these derivatives or independent developments of *yoga-nidrā* from the official websites and the publications issued by the originators of the techniques. This is only a brief overview and a general comparison that refrains from judging these techniques.

iRest Yoga Nidra® by Richard Miller

Application: Psychotherapy, especially for PTSD[598] patients, practised in social institutions, hospitals, the military and in work with veterans, children and adolescents.

Intended Effect: Coping with everyday stress, dissolving traumas, alleviating depression, anxiety and chronic pain, improving sleep, healing and 'awakening to one's true nature'.

This first Western *yoga-nidrā* method was developed by clinical psychologist, author, researcher, spiritual and yoga teacher Dr Richard Miller (b. 1948), USA. He is one of the pioneers in the integration of the non-dual teachings of Kaśmīri Śaivism, Yoga, Tantra, Advaita, Daoism and Buddhism into Western psychology. He dedicated more than 40 years of his life and work to this goal. His mentors include Jean Klein, T.K.V. Desikachar and Stephen Chang. In the 1970s, he was introduced to the Satyananda Yoga Nidra technique and Svāmī Satyānanda's book *Yoga Nidra* by one of his yoga teachers.[599]

Miller has incorporated the above teachings into his research and into his clinical work with patients in various settings, with a particular emphasis on working with veterans and PTSD-clients. Miller has integrated the above teachings into his research and clinical work with patients in various fields, with a particular focus on work with veterans and PTSD patients. He continued to develop his therapeutic technique until he finally developed

598 PTSD – post-traumatic stress disorder.

599 Miller, Richard. (2015). *Yoga Nidra – A Meditative Practice for Deep Relaxation and Healing*. Colorado: Sounds True Publications. p. 5.

his own method called *iRestYoga Nidra®* — Integrative Restoration Yoga Nidra. By detaching the original technique from its tantric and yogic context, he implemented his therapeutic method in Western society. He referred to the various steps of his method as the '*iRest Yoga Nidra® protocol*', and he researched its effectiveness on health, healing and well-being in various population groups, including active-duty military personnel, veterans, students, children, seniors, homeless people, and people in prison, as well as in people with problems such as sleep disorders, PTSD, drug addiction, chronic pain and similar disorders. The effect of *iRestYoga Nidra®* has been evaluated in several scientific studies since 2007.[600]

Miller's *yoga-nidrā* technique uses strongly suggestive language with affirmations. The focus is on integrating and identifying with sensations and feelings and developing the *draṣṭā* state. Unlike the primary *yoga-nidrā* techniques, Miller says the *iRestYoga Nidra®* protocol can be adapted by any practitioner or trainer to suit their needs. The complete practice consists of ten steps, which can be modularised depending on the length of the session. However, the first three steps of the protocol should be included in every *iRestYoga Nidra®* session. For beginners, the first five steps are recommended as sufficient. As time goes on, the remaining steps are then added. In contrast to the original technique of Svāmī Satyānanda, practitioners decide for themselves which pairs of contrasting sensations and which visualisations to use during the practice.

The Ten Steps of *iRest Yoga Nidra®* by Dr Richard Miller[601]

Step 1: Connect to Your Heartfelt Desire

This step bears similarities to the *saṃkalpa* in Svāmī Satyānanda's technique, although *saṃkalpa* in this sense is not a desire.[602] In this Step of *iRestYoga Nidra®*, the practitioner should become aware of their deepest heartfelt

600 The ten steps of *iRest Yoga Nidra®* are listed on the *iRest* website: https://www.irest.org/irest-research (accessed on 10 April 2020).

601 The ten steps of *iRest Yoga Nidra®* are listed on the *iRest* website, https://www.irest.org/irest-10-step-protocol (accessed on 10.04.2020).

602 See Part II. Chapter 14. *The saṃkalpa – the Essence of yoga-nidrā.*

desire — something they want more than anything in life and their intention should emerge from within. They should feel this heartfelt desire with their whole body and experience it as if it had come true.

Step 2: Set an Intention

Practitioners are free to choose the intention for each individual session. They should reflect on their intention for the day's practice and set a goal for it, such as to relax and rest, to explore a particular sensation, emotion or belief, or to reflect on ways to live their heart's desire in their daily lives. The intention should be welcomed and affirmed with the whole body and mind.

Step 3: Find Your Inner Resource

Attention is drawn to the inner resource, which is a personal safe haven in one's own body, where one experiences a sense of security, serenity, calm and well-being. This inner resource can be accessed at any time during the exercise or in daily life, especially when one feels overwhelmed by an emotion, thought or life situation and wants to feel safe and better.

Step 4: Feel Your Body

This step is similar to Stage 3 — Rotation of Awareness Throughout the Body — of Svāmī Satyānanda's method, and to Step 1 or Step 3 — *śava-yatra* — of Swāmī Rāma's method. Similarly, awareness is moved throughout the body while welcoming the various sensations that arise.

Step 5: Become Aware of Your Breath

This step is similar to Stage 4 — Breath Awareness — by Svāmī Satyānanda. Here, awareness is directed to the natural flow of the breath: the spontaneous flow of air in the nostrils, throat and chest, as well as the rise and fall of the abdomen, and you feel the breath as a flowing energy that permeates the entire body.

STEP 6: Welcome Your Emotions

This step is similar to Stage 5 — Pairs of Opposites — by Svāmī Satyānanda. The momentary sensations or emotions in the body and mind are welcomed. At the same time, the opposite feelings and emotions are also perceived, and all sensations are accepted as they are.

STEP 7: Witness Your Thoughts

In this step, thoughts and memories, as well as inner images that are present in the mind, are welcomed and observed, along with the corresponding sensations in the body. The flow of thoughts is spontaneous; no images are provided. This step resembles both the tantric technique of *antar-mauna* — inner silence, in which the spontaneous flow of thoughts, inner images and emotions is observed, and the Buddhist *vipāśana* meditation.

STEP 8: Experience Joy

The sensations of joy, well-being or bliss are soothing, emanating from the heart or abdomen and radiating throughout the body and into the surrounding space.

STEP 9: Find Lasting Peace

Thought is set aside and dissolved into pure awareness. One is awake and aware. This practice should lead into the *yoga-nidrā* state. This step is similar to Svāmī Rāma's Step 3 (or Step 5) — Sleep with Awareness.

STEP 10: Reflect on Your Practice

After finishing the practice, take a few moments to reflect on the journey you have just taken, to recognise the feeling of peace that is always present, and to integrate it into your daily life, in both pleasant and difficult moments.

I AM Yoga Nidra™ by Yogi Amrit Desai

This method is also called 'Integrative Method of Yoga Nidra for Health and Healing'.

Intended Effects: it is said to alleviate stress and burnout, improve sleep quality, relieve anxiety and depression, alleviate trauma, PTSD and addiction, combat inflammation and type 2 diabetes, and be effective in treating stress-related health issues and self-destructive behaviour.[603]

Yogi Amrit Desai (born 1932) is an academic artist, yoga master and disciple of Svāmī Kṛpālvānanda (1913–1981). He is considered one of the pioneers of yoga in the West and has been teaching yoga in the United States since the early 1960s. The yoga school he founded became so successful that he gave up his career as an artist to devote himself entirely to teaching. In 1969, he received *śaktipāta*[604] from his guru, and in the early 1970s, he became a *guru* himself. He is the initiator of three registered yoga trademarks — Kripalu Yoga (1970) and *I AM Yoga* and *I AM Yoga Nidra* (1996) — and the founder of five yoga and health centres in the United States. In 2005, Jennifer Reis, a Canadian yoga instructor at the Kripalu Yoga School, registered *Divine Sleep® Yoga Nidra* as a trademark.[605]

Yogi Amrit Desai's successor is his daughter Kamini Desai. She is an anthropologist, psychologist, writer, yoga therapist and yoga instructor and has written a book about her father's *yoga-nidrā* method. Desai lists six tools of *yoga-nidrā*: insight, integration, disidentification, intention, relaxation and regeneration. On her website, *yoga-nidrā* is described as 'an ancient sleep-based meditation technique that has the power to take you to the innermost, deepest levels of relaxation where your whole body and being is permeated by peace of mind and profound stillness'.[606]

This technique uses suggestions as well as affirmations. The instructor gives their instructions in the first person. The language used is similar to

603 Desai, Kamini. (2017). *Yoga Nidra – The Art of Transformational Sleep*. Twin Lakes: Lotus Press.

604 *śaktipāta* is a rite of initiation in which a master transmits energy to the disciple.

605 Information about Jennifer Reis, https://jenniferreisyoga.com/events/divine-sleep-yoga-nidra-teacher-training-live-online-7/ (accessed on 25.01.2022).

606 Website of Kamini Desai: https://www.kaminidesai.com/yoga-nidra (accessed on 24.01.2022).

elements of hypnosis. Steps 2, 5, 6 and 9 are related to Svāmī Rāma's method and Stages 7 and 8 to Svāmī Satyānanda's method.

The following is a brief overview of the individual steps. Some instructions are quoted verbatim to make the technical specification clearer.

The *I AM Yoga Nidra*™ Method[607]

STEP 1: Closing the Eyes and Being Present

Still the mind, release thoughts and tension. To give oneself fully to a 'higher power' and relax. 'Feel a deep sense of contentment and peace in your heart'.

STEP 2: Deliberate Tension and Relaxation

Attention is moved around the body to release blocked energy and to achieve a deeper state of total relaxation. The upper body, the lower body and finally the whole body are tensed while inhaling and relaxed while exhaling.

STEP 3: Bumblebee Breath

'Use your thumbs to gently close your ears, [… (the bumblebee breath is practiced for seven rounds)] Feel the stimulating impact of the vibrations extending throughout your whole body.' Then attention is directed to the eyebrow centre. 'And empty your mind into the flood of energy.'

STEP 4: Universal Instructions

'[…] returning to stillness as soon as you are able. Resolve to remain awake staying in touch with the sound of my voice. Allow your entire body to respond directly and non-mentally to my words. […] Drop into the deepest state of tranquillity, stillness and peace in the third eye. […]'

---

607 Desai, Kamini. (2017). *Yoga Nidra – The Art of Transformational Sleep*. Twin Lakes: Lotus Press. pp. 353–363.

Step 5: Complete Yogic Breath

'Now follow my guidance as we begin the relaxation breath.' In this stage, yogi breathing is practised and the body is relaxed even further. 'With each breath in, fill every nerve and cell with pulsating healing energy. […] Empty your body and mind and enter deeper levels of stillness and silence.'

Step 6: Integrate

'Do absolutely nothing from now on. Settle into the silent Source of your being.'

Step 7: Heavy and Light

'As I name the body part bring your total attention accompanied by a feeling of heaviness … sinking … like a stone in water …' etc. This creates a feeling of lightness in the body.

Step 8: Energy Body (optional)

'Be free of all inhibitions and boundaries of your body and mind, past and future.' Furthermore, you should feel freedom and lightness, release the energy body from the physical body; enjoy the spirit freed from all limitations, from the fear of pain, injury and suffering; experience the innate wisdom of the body that heals, frees and functions optimally. 'Now relax back into your physical experience as you remain deeply established in your connection with the Spirit in faith and trust.'

Step 9: Integration — Resting in Awareness/Third Eye

'Bring your attention to the center between your eyebrows and drop into the deepest level of relaxation. (pause…) Hier, there remains nothing to do or achieve, you have entered the domain of grace… Allow yourself to merge into that space and be empty… (pause…) In this domain of integration, you are witness of all that is happening but doing nothing to make it happen … […] Feel completely safe and comfortable as you hand yourself over to the power and protection of the Presence… […]'

STEP 10: Intention

'[...] Repeat your Intentions now silently three times [...] Know that your higher Self recognises, honours and accepts your intention. Have faith and trust that it has been heard and is being acted upon by a higher power of the Source within. [...].'

STEP 11: Affirmations

'Allow your entire Self to respond spontaneously and effortlessly to what I say [...].' The teacher then says up to three affirmations of his choice, which may be general affirmations such as: 'I hold no one responsible for all that has happened in the past. I am free and clear of all that has happened in the past.', 'I go to the Source within that heals all conflict and restores my health and peace of mind.' etc. or health and healing affirmations such as: 'I relax so completely and let go so fully that the inner healing blueprint of my body functions freely and optimally.' etc.

STEP 12: Higher Self and Spiritual Guide

'Establish yourself firmly in faith and trust to receive the grace, protection and guidance of the higher Self within you. [...] Feel the presence of your own spiritual guides, family members or mentors surrounding you and blessing you. [...] You are the emissary of light and love. [...].'

STEP 13: Externalise

The practice is completed by returning to the physical body and sensing how one feels after the practice.

Total Yoga Nidra Network, United Kingdom

The approach of the *Total Yoga Nidra Network* is best described in the words of its two founders, Dr Uma Dinsmore-Tuli and Nirlipta Tuli: 'We resist all attempts to limit, own or otherwise contain and reduce the potential of Yoga Nidra as a force for global healing and evolution.'[608] Furthermore: 'We have not chosen to trademark, own or otherwise commercialise the specific methods of Yoga Nidrā practice that we call *Total Yoga Nidrā*, [...] The term 'Total' Yoga Nidrā indicates that we experience the totality of Yoga Nidrā, Yoganidra and Yoga Nidrā Shakti as essentially interconnected and interdependent. [...] The term 'Total' Yoga Nidrā indicates that we consider the totality of the experience of Yoga Nidrā, Yoganidrā and Yoga Nidrā Shakti as essentially interconnected and interdependent components. Total Yoga Nidrā is not a trademark, but an accurate description of our integrative, diverse and intuitive approach to practice. [...] it is a practice approach that offers a spectrum of different borderline experiences and honours the rich and ancient hybrid history of Yoga Nidrā.'[609]

The Total Yoga Nidra Network invites *yoga-nidrā* teachers from all backgrounds, 'styles' and schools to become part of their network. It offers them a platform for exchange and a place to list their *yoga-nidrā* audio recordings for free download, including in specific national languages. The recordings are made available in the network's audio library.[610]

Uma Dinsmore-Tuli founded the network in the UK in 2010 with her husband Nirlipta Tuli.[611] She has a PhD in communication studies and also works as a writer and yoga therapist. Uma describes herself as a writer, visionary, 'radical yogini', Total Yoga Nidra advocate and eco-feminist activist.[612] Her mother introduced her to yoga in childhood, and she later studied Structural Yoga Therapy, Satyananda Yoga, and Iyengar Yoga. Uma and her husband,

---

608 Total Yoga Nidra Network. *About*. https://www.yoganidranetwork.org/about/ (accessed on 20.12.2021).

609 Total Yoga Nidra Network. *In Defence of the Practice of Yoga Nidrā*. https://www.yoganidranetwork.org/blog/defence-practice-yoga-nidra (accessed on 20.12.2021).

610 Total Yoga Nidra Network. *Free yoga nidras*. https://www.yoganidranetwork.org/downloads (accessed on 20.12.2021).

611 Total Yoga Nidra Network. *Yoga Nidra Network Operating Ethics*. https://www.yoganidranetwork.org/yoga-nidra-network-operating-ethics (accessed on 20.12.2021).

612 Uma Dinsmore-Tuli. https://umadinsmoretuli.com (accessed on 21.12.2021).

Nirlipta, visited the Rikhiapeeth *āśrama* several times, where she personally met Svāmī Satyānanda, who spent the last 20 years of his life there. Her family had a close connection with Svāmī Satyānanda, and in 1997, Uma Dinsmore-Tuli and Nirlipta Tuli were married in the *āśrama* under his guidance, as he had been their family *guru* for several years.[613] Uma specialises in women's health, prenatal yoga, yoga for childbirth and postnatal recovery, and family yoga. In recent years, she has also addressed the ethical issues of abuse and exploitation in the world of yoga, as well as the history, development and therapeutic applications of *yoga-nidrā*.[614] She has developed *Total Yoga Nidra, Wild Nidra* and *Nidra Shakti* as 'radically creative and intuitive approaches to teaching yoga nidra'.[615]

Nirlipta Tuli, a co-founder of the network, is a registered clinical hypnotherapist specialising in perinatal hypnotherapy, including the resolution of birth trauma and birth-related anxiety. He is a trained Satyananda Yoga teacher and has completed further training at the British Wheel of Yoga and the Sivananda Yoga Vedanta Centres in the UK. He became acquainted with Satyananda Yoga through his mother, who had been a *svāmī* at the Rikhiapeeth *āśrama* in the time of Svāmī Satyānanda for over eight years. Nirlipta began practising Satyananda Yoga and *yoga-nidrā* in 1989.[616] He has been teaching yoga since 1990, specialising in pregnancy yoga, yoga therapy and yoga practices for mental health, stress relief and relaxation. He is particularly interested in the therapeutic applications of *yoga-nidrā*, especially for insomnia and sleep-related issues such as lucid dreaming, for stress management, increasing individual and group productivity, and for pain-related issues.[617]

An important concern of the Tuli family is to foster intuitive and creative skills in teachers and practitioners. *Yoga-nidrā* facilitators should be encouraged to develop their own personal intuitive and creative relationship with

---

613 Total Yoga Nidra Network. *Yoga Nidra Network Operating Ethics*. https://www.yoganidranetwork.org/article/total-yoga-nidra-and-swami-satyananda-where-we-stand-now-2014 (accessed on 30.01.2022).

614 Total Yoga Nidra Network. *Uma*. https://www.yoganidranetwork.org/users/uma (accessed on 20.12.2021).

615 Uma Dinsmore-Tuli. https://umadinsmoretuli.com (accessed on 21.12.2021).

616 Total Yoga Nidra Network. *Yoga Nidra Network Operating Ethics*. https://www.yoganidranetwork.org/article/total-yoga-nidra-and-swami-satyananda-where-we-stand-now-2014 (accessed on 30.01.2022).

617 Total Yoga Nidra Network. *Nirlipta*. https://www.yoganidranetwork.org/users/nirlipta (accessed on 20.12.2021).

yoga-nidrā. Both draw on all *yoga-nidrā* 'styles' as well as their own experiences with the various techniques in their teaching. Her thesis is that *yoga-nidrā*-like states have been sought and achieved by all indigenous peoples of the world and that these connections, the shared history and the influence of autogenic and hypnotic methods on the development of modern *yoga-nidrā* have not been sufficiently explained, acknowledged or even concealed by the larger *yoga-nidrā* schools.

With their training, publications and network, they want to counteract the 'rigidity in the methods of facilitating yoga nidrā' [618] and, while honouring the roots of *yoga-nidrā*, promote diversity.

The 'yoga-nidra Recipe' with Nine Ingredients from the *Yoga Nidra Network*[619]

In 2022, the Tuli family published their *yoga-nidrā* method in the form of a recipe book. They present there their nine 'ingredients' for their '*yoga-nidrā recipe*'.

The language of the instructions is based on hypnotic and trauma-therapeutic language—you are 'invited' to do something and questions are asked that should help you to feel better. The aim is 'radical relaxation', which should be achieved through self-determination during the practice.

Ingredient 1: 'Preparing for the start of your process of *yoga-nidrā*—claiming this moment for the radical act of rest.' This phase of the practice is concerned with preparing for the exercise and includes first creating time and space for the exercise in everyday life. Methods for entering and exiting the exercise are discussed here.[620]

---

618 Total Yoga Nidra Network. *In Defence of the Practice of Yoga Nidrā*. https://www.yoganidranetwork.org/blog/defence-practice-yoga-nidra (accessed on 20.12.2021).

619 Tuli, Nirlipta & Dinsmore-Tuli, Uma. (2022). *Yoga Nidra Made Easy*. London: Hay House Publishing, p. 64–263.

620 Ibid. pp. 65–87.

INGREDIENT 2: 'Settling into your process of *yoga-nidrā* — resourcing the body of rest.' During this phase of the practice, the body is settled into a cosy '*nidrā nest*' (sleeping nest) and one tunes in mentally to the exercise. The phase concludes with sensory perception.[621]

INGREDIENT 3: 'Inner listening and/or an invitation for intuitive intention — choosing your flavor of *yoga-nidrā* for now.' This is the third ingredient and the same as 'ingredient' number seven. 'They define the flavour of each individual practice of *yoga-nidrā*. The first time you meet this ingredient, you simply taste it, whereas the second time it shows up — after you have completed the cycle of practice — you are ready to savor its flavor because it has been imbued or marinated with your natural process of *yoga-nidrā*.' You can formulate an intention for the practice or decide whether it is more appropriate for you to simply 'rest in a receptive space of simply being.'

INGREDIENT 4: 'Welcoming attention around the body — journeying through places and spaces.' In this phase, the awareness is guided on a 'journey through the body' from head to toe. Various routes through the body are offered.[622]

INGREDIENT 5: 'Playing with paradox and integration — inviting pairs of opposites.' According to the authors, this is the heart of the '*yoga-nidrā labyrinth*' and can take from five to ten minutes. Two gentle recipes of contrasting sensations are presented in the form of questions. You can use the audio files to choose which version you would like to practice with.[623]

INGREDIENT 6 (optional): 'Connecting to imaginative capacity — feeling into sensory and extrasensory knowing.' This phase can be left out in this method. One should not visualise with the intention of 'visualising', as in the traditional *yoga-nidrā* method, because, according to the authors, most people in this phase are no longer listening and are in a very introverted state. Furthermore, the terms are said to be imposed by the practitioner's imagination. Instead, the images from one's own recipe will not be 'impositions from an external

621 Ibid. pp. 88–130.
622 Ibid. pp. 145–179.
623 Ibid, pp. 180–196.

voice, but instead will arise from within yourself'. This is meant to be a good incentive to learn 'to cook your own *yoga-nidrā* recipes so that you can use this ingredient for inspiration, healing, and nurture'. Another suggestion is to use this time to find creative solutions to problems.[624]

INGREDIENT 7: 'Inner listening and/or an invitation for intuitive intention — savoring your flavor of *yoga-nidrā* now.' This 'ingredient' is the same as 'ingredient' 3. 'It's as if the first intention (ingredient 3) is planting a seed, and the revisiting of this intention is gently checking to see how it has grown'.[625]

INGREDIENT 8: 'Externalising awareness — preparing to complete your process of *yoga-nidrā*.' Here, various 'recipes' for getting out are presented, from which you can choose how to get out.[626]

INGREDIENT 9: 'Completing the cycle of your process — returning to everyday attention.' After a brief reflection on your practice, you begin to make small movements as you return from *yoga-nidrā* to everyday life.[627]

Important Note

THE AUTHOR has deliberately not discussed any further methods of *yoga-nidrā* here. The modern derivatives of the method — with all the ramifications of these techniques developed in the West with influences from Western psychotherapy, hypnosis, autogenic training and also esotericism — are moving further and further away from methods that can still be seen as 'traditional' *yoga-nidrā* of Indian origin. Of course, every tradition and practice is subject to periodic changes, at the personal discretion of some practitioners. Historically, however, aside from the influence of socio-economic factors, changes with lasting effects on a method or a tradition and its teaching usually came from practitioners with sufficient experience, erudition and deep understanding of the material and its principles.

624 Ibid. pp. 197–222.
625 Ibid. pp. 223–235.
626 Ibid. pp. 236–250.
627 Ibid. pp. 251–262.

Ultimately, the theory behind the practice and the effectiveness of modern *yoga-nidrā* methods are at risk of being lost if it is extracted from its integral yoga context[628]. The techniques developed in the time after Svāmī Satyānanda and Svāmī Rāma use the same or very similar stages or steps as the two primary methods, which are then often mixed with each other or supplemented with techniques from mental training, for example. In this sense, Uma Dinsmore-Tuli's assertion that contemporary *yoga-nidrā* methods are 'hybrid' is justified.[629]

The reference to the thesis that the *yoga-nidrā* method of Svāmī Satyānanda draws heavily on the relaxation and hypnosis techniques of the 20th century[630] should not be omitted here. As presented in Part IV. Chapter 17. *Yoga-nidrā and Western Psychology*, sub-chapter *Yoga-nidrā and Hypnosis* a clear distinction can be drawn between the aim and purpose of *yoga-nidrā* or Satyananda Yoga Nidra and hypnosis or all relaxation techniques. The same applies to its sources, as there are clear predecessors to Svāmī Satyānanda's method in yogic and tantric literature of preceding centuries. Svāmī Satyānanda should be seen as a master in the context of his time, who was well-aware of the contemporary findings in neuroscience, psychology, psychotherapy and autogenic training, as well as newer methods in yoga. He was also interested in examining and confirming the effects of yoga using the new scientific methods, as well as in translating the Yoga and Tantra teachings into a contemporary language and making them accessible to Westerners. This is evident from the numerous publications on these topics, in which he re-examined and systematised many historical techniques. The intersection of Western and Eastern approaches was a major topic of interest in Svāmī Satyānanda's time.[631] In his book *Yoga Nidra*, he also makes clear reference to these trends, but also shows where his own insights into his method come from and in what yogic context they stand.

---

628 See Part I. Chapter 2. *Introduction to the Integral Yoga Approach*.

629 This note comes from Nirlipta Tuli and Uma Dinsmore-Tuli, Total Yoga Nidra Network. https://www.yoganidranetwork.org/blog/defence-practice-yoga-nidra (accessed on 20.12.2021).

630 Ibid.

631 See the book of Boyes, Denis. (1973). *Le yoga du sommeil éveillé. Méthode de relaxation – Yoga Nidra*. Paris: FeniXX réédition numérique (Épi), which will be presented in more detail below.

Even if we follow the thesis that Svāmī Satyānanda was influenced by currents from the West, this would not make his method any less effective. It is all the more interesting to see how he was able to integrate new insights into his authentic yogic and tantric knowledge and experience and translate them into a systematic, valuable and easily-accessible teaching. Although Svāmī Satyānanda based his method on the principles and techniques of Tantra and *rājā-yoga*, he never claimed that these were the only way and his only sources. On the contrary, he followed the research of his contemporary Svāmī Rāma and included his findings in his book. We must not forget that before the time of these two masters, no type of *yoga-nidrā* technique had been known or accessible to the general public.

The great contribution of Svāmī Satyānanda is and remains the fact that he separated *yoga-nidrā* from its ritual and religious background in order to make it accessible to all people, regardless of origin, walk of life, sex, gender and religious affiliation. At the same time, while setting aside the theistic components of the practices he uses as a basis, Svāmī Satyānanda did not extract *yoga-nidrā* as a standalone practice, separate from an integral system or yoga, but instead emphasised its synergistic effect when done together with other complementary practices, which aim to address the entirety of human existence as a whole — something supported by recent scientific studies. This approach was very well received in the West at the time. In contrast, over the last decade, Uma Dinsmore-Tuli's *yoga-nidrā* approach has returned to a '[...] worship of the goddess Nidrā Shakti as a powerful manifestation of the deep feminine'[632]. The question arises as to how practitioners from different cultural, religious and spiritual communities deal with this kind of return to ritual and mysticism. The development of *yoga-nidrā* must therefore always be viewed in the temporal, cultural and social context of the teachers and practitioners.

Particularly in the yoga context, as already described in Part I. Chapter 1. *The Schools of Thought of India*, the paths of yoga are open and variegated, yet at the same time rooted in robust oral and textual traditions handed down over time. The serious seeker should really understand well which path can be practised with which goal and which effect in which context. Ultimately,

632 Total Yoga Nidra Network. https://www.yoganidranetwork.org/blog/defence-practice-yoga-nidra (accessed on 20.12.2021).

each practitioner chooses their path for themselves. At this point, it should be remembered that the effect of *yoga-nidrā* is potentiated when combined with the corresponding practices from the integral yoga approach. Ultimately, the aim is to deepen one's own *sādhanā,* be it for spiritual realisation and personal growth.

CHAPTER 20

Yoga-nidrā in Contemporary Literature

THIS CHAPTER ATTEMPTS TO PRESENT a selection of the most important works on the various *yoga-nidrā* approaches, as described in the previous chapter, that have been published up to the year 2023. It contains an up-to-date list of the most important *yoga-nidrā* publications by contemporary yoga schools, masters, practitioners and psychologists, in the order in which they were created. In addition, there are many other publications on the subject, and their number is growing rapidly. However, these publications are largely based on the work of these predecessors, with a focus on emphasising the aspect of relaxation through *yoga-nidrā*, often combined with self-help advice and mental training exercises. Publications of this kind are not included here.

The 1970s

Boyes, Dennis. *Le yoga du sommeil éveillé. Méthode de relaxation — Yoga Nidra*

In 1973, after his stay in various *āśramas* in India between 1967 and 1969, the English Waldorf[633] and yoga teacher Dennis Boyes published his book: *Le yoga du sommeil éveillé. Méthode de relaxation — Yoga Nidra*[634] in French. In 1986, the book was published in German under the title *Autogenes Yoga — Tiefenentspannung im Liegen*[635]. Boyes does not give information on the *āśramas* and institutes he visited during his stay in India, apart from the Yoga-Institute Lonavla, where he was introduced to various scientific studies on the effects of relaxation on the physical body. In his book, he draws a comparison between modern autogenic techniques and the *yoga-nidrā* approach. He mentions 'the *yoga-nidrā* method' which he encountered during his stay in India, without referring to a specific technique or citing any sources. He does, however, refer to the *Yoga-sūtras* of Patañjali (despite the fact that they do not mention *yoga-nidrā*), emphasises the importance of the *draṣṭā* state during the practice and points out the three states of consciousness and the *turyīa* state (the fourth). Furthermore, references are made in the book to the Western master Jean Klein[636], as well as to Jacobson's progressive muscle relaxation and Schultz's autogenic training[637]. Boyes does not present a self-contained *yoga-nidrā* technique, but rather compiles techniques for self-improvement (not *yoga-nidrā* techniques) rooted in 'the *yoga-nidrā* method'. In his techniques he has adapted autogenic

633 A Waldorf teacher is an educator who implements Rudolf Steiner's holistic educational philosophy. Steiner was the founder of Anthroposophy – a new religious movement which was founded in the early 20th century.

634 Boyes, Dennis. (1973). *Le yoga du sommeil éveillé. Méthode de relaxation – Yoga Nidra*. Paris: FeniXX réédition numérique (Épi). 144 pages.

635 Boyes, Dennis. (1986). *Autogenes Yoga – Tiefenentspannung im Liegen*. Düsseldorf: ECON Taschenbuch Verlag. 174 pages.

636 Jean Klein (1912–1998) was a doctor, musician and Advaita Vedānta master. His teachings were influenced by Kaśmīri Śaivaism.

637 Autogenic training was developed in 1926 by the German psychiatrist Johannes Schultz. The method uses repeated visualisations alongside verbal suggestions to induce a state of deep relaxation. It is based on passive concentration on bodily sensations – such as feelings of heaviness or warmth in the limbs – which are brought about through self-suggestion.

training with principles from yoga[638]. The book includes comments from participants in his classes in France. It is an important contribution to clarifying the differences between the Western concept of relaxation, as it was already used, for example, in the autogenic methods of the 1960s and 1970s, and the basic principles of yoga related to the state of *yoga-nidrā*.

Satyananda, Swami. *Yoga Nidra*

Svāmī Satyānanda Sarasvatī (1923–2009) — Indian yoga master and teacher, disciple of Svāmī Śivānanda Sarasvatī, *tāntrika*, lecturer and author of numerous books — published his book *Yoga Nidra*[639] in English for the first time in 1976. This book is the ultimate *yoga-nidrā* classic and bestseller. Since then, new editions have been published annually and the book has been translated into several languages. In his book, Svāmī Satyānanda provides the first systematic introduction to the *yoga-nidrā* technique he developed, freeing it from religious and ritual content. However, the context of holistic yoga, Tantra, Sāṃkhya and Advaita Vedānta is retained. The book focuses on the *pratyāhāra* form of the method. Svāmī Satyānanda translates the technique and the concepts on which it is based into a 'simpler' and more contemporary language, making the technique accessible and useful for people of all cultures and walks of life. The stages of the method described in the book are those that are essential and must be mastered by all practitioners. The aim is to attenuate the externally stimulated impressionability of the mind in order to enable a different, deeper immersion. An important part of the book is the scientific knowledge gained from laboratory research and the implementation of the technique in healthcare. The many effects of the practice are presented, starting with deep relaxation, stress management, improving learning ability, awakening dormant potential by harmonising consciousness, and immersive practice. The practical part includes transcripts of the technique from Svāmī Satyānanda's teaching. However, these require some basic understanding and should be used and studied according to one's own level of progress. A mere one-to-one implementation is discouraged without

638 Boyes, Dennis. (1986). *Autogenes Yoga – Tiefenentspannung im Liegen*. Düsseldorf: ECON Taschenbuch Verlag. p. 13.

639 Satyananda, Swami. (1976). *Yoga Nidra*. Munger: Yoga Publication Trust. 1st edition. 261 pages.

having studied with a qualified teacher. A solid prior knowledge as well as knowledge of Indian philosophy and its concepts are beneficial for understanding the contents of the book. To learn advanced levels of the technique, it is always recommended to seek the guidance of a master.

The 1980s

Rama, Swami. *Enlightenment Without God (Mandukya Upanishad)*

Svāmī Rāma Bhāratī (1925–1996), an Indian yoga master from the Himalayan tradition, lecturer and author, and one of the pioneers who made himself available to Western scientists in the 1970s to study his ability to consciously control bodily processes and brain activity, including the state of *yoga-nidrā*. In 1982, he mentioned the *yoga-nidrā* state and the technique he used to achieve it in his commentary on the *Māṇḍūkya-upaniṣad*.[640] He also explained *yoga-nidrā* and the Steps of the technique he practised in his book *Path of Fire and Light*, Vol. 2[641] in 1988. *Yoga-nidrā* is described here in the integral yoga context and as a way of maintaining awareness in the three states of consciousness and of entering the fourth state (*turīya*).[642]

Ramm-Bonwitt, Ingrid. *Yoga Nidra — Der Schlaf der Yogis*

Ingrid Ramm-Bonwitt is a disciple of Śrī Maheśa (1959–2007), a psychologist and yoga teacher. Her book on *yoga-nidrā*, first published in 1984 and completely revised in 2010, provides a comprehensive introduction to the technique and a thorough overview of the context and background of

640 Rama, Swami. (1982). *Enlightment without God – Mandukya Upanishad*. Honesdale: Himalayan Institute Press. 103 pages. For *yoga-nidrā* go to p. 47–58.

641 Rama, Swami. (2018). *Path of Fire and Light*. Vol. 2. Honesdale: Himalayan Institute Press. 200 pages. For *yoga-nidrā* go to p. 165–182.

642 See Part I. Chapter 9. *The states of consciousness and yoga-nidrā*.

yoga-nidrā based on the technique of Svāmī Satyānanda and Yoga and Tantra philosophy. The book is currently only available in German in antiquarian bookshops.[643]

Flak, Micheline & de Coulon, Jacques. *Des enfants qui réussissent. Le yoga dans l'éducation*

Micheline Flak (Svāmī Yogabhakti, 1934*), a French middle school teacher and student of Svāmī Satyānanda's, began to implement yoga, including *yoga-nidrā*, in a holistic and integral way in her school lessons in the 1970s. She founded the international movement RYE — Research on Yoga in Education — in 1987. In her book *Des enfants qui réussissent. Le yoga dans l'éducation*[644], she published her experiences and insights from her work in the school context using practical examples. The educator Jacques de Coulon is a co-author of the book. This book is a pioneering work in terms of introducing yoga and *yoga-nidrā* into the education system and has been translated into English and Spanish. Yoga is now highly valued in the French education system and has been integrated into the national school programme, largely thanks to the efforts of Micheline Flak.

The 2000s until 2025

Miller, Richard. *Yoga Nidra — A Meditative Practice for Deep Relaxation and Healing*

Dr. Richard Miller (1948*) is one of the leading clinical psychologists in the USA and also one of the pioneers in the integration of yoga techniques

643 Ramm-Bonwitt, Ingrid. (2010). *Yoga Nidra – Der Schlaf der Yogis*. Darmstadt: Schirner Verlag. (überarbeitete Auflage), 379 pages.

644 Flak, Micheline & de Coulon, Jacques. (1985). *Des enfants qui réussissent. Le yoga dans l'éducation*. Paris: Editions Desclée de Brouwer. pp. 119–124.

into the clinical context. He originally came to yoga through the teachings of Svāmī Satyānanda and learned about his technique of *yoga-nidrā* in the 1970s.[645] From there, he continued his spiritual search by training with various teachers and subsequently became a disciple of Jean Klein (1912–1989). Miller developed a *yoga-nidrā* technique based on his experiences in clinical psychology, particularly his work with patients diagnosed with PTSD, and the non-dual teachings of Kaśmīri Śaivism. Miller presents the different stages of his method and suggests ways to combine them for personal application. His book on *yoga-nidrā* was first published in 2005.[646]

Miller, Richard. *The iRest Program for Healing PTSD*[647]

In this book, Miller explains how he uses his *iRest*® programme — *Integrative Restoration Yoga Nidra* — to treat PTSD patients, particularly war veterans. He describes techniques based on the principles of *yoga-nidrā* as well as on approaches from Jacobson's progressive muscle relaxation and Schultz and Luthe's autogenic training. Breathing and breathing patterns are emphasised as an important aspect in the treatment of PTSD symptoms, and exercises are presented that relax and deepen breathing. In addition, elements from mental training for self-acceptance, stabilisation and strengthening are combined with stages of *yoga-nidrā*.

Prakashananda, Swami. *Yoga Nidra — Neue Erkenntnisse*

Svāmī Prakashānanda (1938–2020) from Germany, a disciple of Svāmī Satyānanda Sarasvatī, published her book *Yoga Nidra — Neue Erkenntnisse* (Yoga Nidra — New Insights) in 2003. This publication contains a compilation of articles by several authors on new research findings in the Satyananda

645 Miller, Richard. (2016). Developing Interoception – The Power of Body Sensing. [*YogaUOnline*] https://www.youtube.com/watch?v=EqdtKjukF7k&t=484s (Time: 11:16 min.) (accessed on 01.04.2019)

646 Miller, Richard. (2010). *Yoga Nidra – A meditative practice for deep relaxation and healing*. Colorado: Sounds True Publications. 2nd edition. 108 pages.

647 Miller, Richard, (2015). *The iRest Program For Healing PTSD. A Proven-Effective Approach to Using Yoga Nidra Meditation and Deep Relaxation Techniques to Overcome Trauma*. Oakland: New Harbinger Publications. 398 pages.

Yoga Nidra technique and also sheds light on aspects of Swami Satyananda's method. The book can be considered a contemporary addition to Swami Satyananda's book *Yoga Nidra*. It is currently only available in German.[648]

Panda, N. C. *Yoga-Nidrā: Yogic Trance—Theory, Practice and Applications*

Dr. Nursingh Charan Panda (1929–2015) was an Indian scientist, scholar, philosopher, *yogin*, *tāntrika* and author. He obtained his Master of Science and his doctorate in philosophy from the University of Missouri, USA. Panda has made numerous interpretations of Vedic literature based on modern science. In his book, first published in 2003, he presents *yoga-nidrā* as a scientific discipline. He discusses the theory of its psychological foundations, techniques and applications to show its importance as a method for strengthening the body's immune system, preventing and healing diseases and regulating lifestyle habits. The book includes comparative analyses of yogic trance and hypnotic trance and juxtaposes Yoga Vedānta and Freudian psychology.[649]

Online publications on the *iRest®* research results since 2007

A very rich source of scientific research on the topic of *iRest®* and the psychological and mental effects of the method in various social settings is the official *iRest®* website *iRest®*[650]. Miller has scientifically researched his method based on his academic and scientific training, as well as his thematic proximity to the field of healthcare, over several years. Numerous research results from 2007 to the present can be found on this website.

648 Prakashananda, Swami. (2010). *Yoga Nidra – Neue Erkenntnisse*. Köln: Satyananda Yoga Zentrum e.V. (reprint), 86 pages.

649 Panda, Nursingh, Charan. (2011). *Yoga-Nidrā: Yogische Trance – Theorie, Praxis und Anwendungen*. New Delhi: D.K. Printworld (P) Ltd. (2nd edition), 324 pages.

650 See https://www.irest.org/irest-research (accessed on 17.02.2022).

Kumar, Kamakhya. *A Handbook of Yoga-Nidra*

Dr Kamakhya Kumar is a scholar, author and recognised researcher in the field of yoga science. He studied applied yoga sciences at the Bihar School of Yoga and the T.M.B. University in Bhagalpur and completed his doctorate in 2006 with a research paper on the topic *Psychophysiological Changes in Connection with Yoga Nidrā*, based on Satyananda Yoga Nidra. Kumar is the author of several renowned books and over fifty research articles in national and international journals, a leading member of the Indian Association of Yoga and editor-in-chief of the International Journal of Yoga and Allied Sciences. He works as an associate professor in the Department of Yoga and Health at Dev Sanskriti University, Haridwar, India. In his book *Handbook of Yoga-Nidrā*[651], he provides a comprehensive overview of Svāmī Satyānanda's *yoga-nidrā* method, its history, written sources, the views of various authors, and the research results on *yoga-nidrā*.

Bharati, Veda, Swami. *My Experiments with Yoga Nidra*

Svāmī Rāma's disciple Svāmī Veda Bhāratī (1933–2015) was a well-known scholar and lecturer. In his words he was considered a child prodigy, lecturing on a wide range of topics from an early age and translating a large number of ancient texts that he learned to read through a state of intuitive guidance from the 'Himalayan Masters'. When he met his *guru* Svāmī Rāma at the age of 36, he learned about his *guru*'s *yoga-nidrā* technique and realised that he had already experienced the *yoga-nidrā* state spontaneously in his early childhood. In this state, he had learned several languages. He shared his personal experiences with *yoga-nidrā* in a publication available as an e-book from 2014[652].

---

651 Kumar, Kamakhya. (2013). *A Handbook of Yoga-Nidra*. New Delhi: D.K. Printworld (P) Ltd. 146 pages.
652 Bharati, Veda, Swami. (2014). *My Experiments with Yoga Nidra*. [Kindle]. Himalayan Yoga Publications Trust. 28 pages.

Desai, Kamini. *Yoga Nidra — The Art of Transformational Sleep*

Dr Kamini Desai was trained at the Kripalu Yoga Center for Yoga and Health and is currently the director of training at the Amrit Yoga Institute. She developed the *I AM Yoga Nidra*™ method in the late 1990s together with her father Amrit Desai (born 1932), a disciple of Svāmī Kṛpālvānanda (also Svāmī Kṛpālu, 1913–1981). Amrit Desai came to the West in the 1960s and founded Kripalu-based yoga system and the Kripalu Yoga Center for Yoga and Health in Massachusetts, USA. After retiring from the Kripalu Yoga Center in 1994, he founded the Amrit Yoga Institute in Florida, where he has taught together with his daughter Kamini Desai since 2002.

In her book[653], Kamini Desai presents the I AM Yoga Nidra™ method as a relaxation and mindfulness-oriented meditation technique. She discusses the connection between traditional yogic concepts and *yoga-nidrā* and draws on insights from modern scientific research that focuses on the physiological, psychological and mental effects of meditation, in particular mindfulness meditation. The author presents a considerable number of results from mindfulness meditation research and equates them with the effects of *yoga-nidrā*. However, Desai hardly refers to research that explicitly addresses *yoga-nidrā*, or the *I AM Yoga Nidra*™ method. The various stages of the *I AM Yoga Nidra*™ method are practised flexibly, at the discretion of the practitioner. In the book's epilogue, she presents a transcript of the *I AM Yoga Nidra*™ technique.

Janakananda, Swami. *A Deeper Yoga and Yoga Nidra*

Svāmī Janakānanda (born 1939) is one of the first students of Svāmī Satyānanda, a *yogin*, *tāntrika* and internationally renowned yoga and meditation teacher. After completing his apprenticeship with his *guru*, he returned to his native Denmark and founded the renowned Scandinavian Yoga and Meditation School.

Svāmī Janakānanda was instructed in tantric *kriyā-yoga* by his guru and always kept his teachings close to the authentic teachings of Svāmī

653 Desai, Kamini. (2017). *Yoga Nidra – The Art of Transformational Sleep*. Twin Lakes: Lotus Press. 388 pages.

Satyānanda. Over more than four decades, he trained many yoga teachers and taught countless students in *kriyā-yoga* and other higher practices. At the same time, he was involved in several scientific research projects in Europe on yoga and meditation, including *yoga-nidrā*. He currently lives at Håå International Retreat Center in southern Sweden.

His e-book *A Deeper Yoga and Yoga Nidra*[654] is practice-oriented and based on the direct personal teachings of Svāmī Satyānanda and the living Tantric tradition. It summarises the background concepts, ideas and theories of yoga and Tantra succinctly and in a simple way to put *yoga-nidrā* in its integral context and make it accessible. The symbolic language of Tantra and *yoga nidrā* has a special place in these explanations. Svāmī Janakānanda establishes connections to other ancient traditions and compares them with Yoga, Tantra and *yoga-nidrā*. In addition, he explains the effects of *yoga-nidrā* on body and mind, health and sleep, as well as the results of the research projects in which he participated. For personal practice, the e-book includes several audio instructions spoken by Svāmī Janakānanda. His *yoga-nidrā* instructions are accompanied by meditative music composed by Roop Verma. This may come as a surprise, since it is not advisable to practice 'classical' *yoga-nidrā* with background music or sound, and Svāmī Satyānanda never taught with music. This e-book and audio files have also been translated into German, Swedish and Danish.

Tuli, Nirlipta & Dinsmore-Tuli, Uma. *Yoga Nidra Made Easy*[655]

Uma Dinsmore-Tuli and Nirlipta Tuli, the founders of the Yoga Nidra Network in Great Britain, present their intuitive approach in the spirit of their network in their book *Yoga Nidra Made Easy*. They present various '*yoga-nidrā recipes*' of their own creation and offer practitioners a variety of options for designing their own practice. You learn how to 'prepare' a *yoga-nidrā* 'tailor-made' for yourself and your current state of mind. This *yoga-nidrā cookbook* also includes a number of little songs and poems to help the reader remember

654 Janakananda, Swami. (2022). *A Deeper Yoga and Yoga Nidra*. [eBook edition]. Hamneda: Bindu Publishers, 197 pages.

655 Tuli, Nirlipta & Dinsmore-Tuli, Uma. (2022). *Yoga Nidra Made Easy*. London: Hay House Publishing, 272 pages.

the sequence of the process. The book purports to provide a brief overview of *yoga-nidrā* history and explains that the methods presented there are rooted in ancient practices and draw on the best of all four major modern schools[656], each of which has presented its own *yoga-nidrā* technique. The authors utilise their own interpretations of technical terms used in Sanskrit sources, e.g. '*nidrā*' or '*nidrā-śakti*' are, for example, mentioned as an important component for drawing strength. This is surprising, because in Indian literature the state of *nidrā* alone is more often described as a state of unconsciousness or torpor (*tamas*). In Pātañjala yoga it is defined as one of the patterns of mind (*vṛtti*) which should be overcome in order to reach the *turīya* state — analogous with *yoga-nidrā*. In this book, the nine phases of this method are explained, as well as general effects and practical instructions given. Throughout the book, there are short testimonials from the author's students. The book is accompanied by audio 'recipes'.

Dinsmore-Tuli, Uma. *Nidrā Shakti: The Power of Rest — An Illustrated Encyclopaedia of Yoga Nidrā*[657]

Nidrā Shakti: The Power of Rest is a visionary (bri)collage, which reflects Uma Dinsmore-Tuli's inner mythology and social and political convictions. For some readers, it can serve as a political and spiritual affirmation. However, for those seeking an accurate, source-based, practical, and lineage-respecting guide to *yoga-nidrā*, this book may not be the best choice. It puts forward concepts largely developed within Dinsmore-Tuli's own teaching system, such as *Total Yoga Nidra*, *Wild Nidra*, *Yoni Nidra*, and *Nidra Shakti*. The volume spans around 700 pages, with full-colour illustrations, poetic entries, a glossary, and practice scripts — all framed within a strong ideological undercurrent.

At first glance, *Nidrā Shakti* presents itself as a generous, encyclopaedic work. However, despite its aesthetic design and spiritual branding, the book does not deliver a coherent, historically accurate account of *yoga-nidrā* which is pedagogically useful outside Dinsmore-Tuli's own system. Readers should keep in mind that it offers a personal, ideologically-charged, and

656 This refers to Satyananda Yoga Nidra™, Svāmī Rāma's *yoga-nidrā* technique, *iRest Yoga Nidra*® by Dr Richard Miller and *I AM Yoga Nidra*™ by Amrit Desai, which have already been presented in this volume.
657 Dinsmore-Tuli, Uma. (2024). *Yogā Nidra – The Power of Rest*. Stroud: Sitaram and Sons Ltd., 705 pages.

highly-syncretic reinterpretation of what was originally a structured and lineage-based yogic method.

One of the book's central perspectives is its 'de-colonialising' and feminist framing. In this context, *yoga-nidrā* is no longer presented as 'merely' an immersive technique but rather as 'a tool of resistance' against capitalism and patriarchy, as well as for promoting unity in diversity. 'Rest' becomes a political rebellion, 'sleep'—a form of social activism. While these metaphors may be emotionally evocative, they introduce ideological distortion into a practice originally oriented toward neutrality and self-inquiry, aiming instead at ascent through constructed identity. The author explicitly blends her personal spiritual interpretation and political agendas, resulting in a synthesis of yoga and contemporary activist discourse.

In the book, the figure of 'Yoganidrā Śakti Devī' is invoked as a central deity embodying both dreams and deep sleep. While this contributes to the book's own poetic and devotional tone, it gives rise to a form of romantic syncretism in which yoga becomes a vessel for neo-goddess-worship, shamanic ritual, 'storytelling' and 'intuitive creativity'. While this blending of neo-goddess-mysticism, 'indigenous' references, and New Age therapeutic discourse may be meaningful to the author and her community, it generates more ambiguity than coherence.[658] The title—*Nidrā Shakti*—itself illustrates this tension in both its choice of orthography and its intended meaning. In Sanskrit, the compound *nidrā-śakti* would denote a *tāmasic* force of consciousnesslessness[659]—a meaning far-removed from the author's translation—'the power of rest'. Furthermore, the author equates the deity Yoga-Nidrā[660] with the Śaiva-Śākta goddess Kālī[661] and proceeds to use the two names interchangeably. The Sanskrit term *yoga-nidrā*, on the other hand, specifically highlights the aspect of awareness necessary for reaching higher states of consciousness and ultimately the superconscious state of *turīya*. Removing *yoga-* removes the awareness aspect of the term.[662] There are also other creative combinations in the book using the term *nidrā* such as *bhakti-nidrā* etc., which are equally problematic. This highlights the agenda of

658 See Part IV. Chapter 17. *Yoga-nidrā and Western Psychology; Interpretatio occidentis vs. interpretatio orientis?*
659 See the book review of *Yogā Nidra Made Easy* above.
660 Ibid., p. 34.
661 Dinsmore-Tuli, Uma. (2024). *Yogā Nidra – The Power of Rest.* Stroud: Sitaram and Sons Ltd, p. 37.
662 See Part I, Chapter 4. *History and Origins of yoga-nidrā; Yoga-nidrā vs. nidrā-śakti.*

the author aiming to redefine existing terms rather than engage with their established meanings.

The book's broader attempt to politicise *yoga-nidrā*—casting 'rest as resistance', 'sleep as social justice', and 'dreaming as anti-capitalist subversion'—is conceptually novel but ultimately projects modern ideologies onto pieces of ancient Indic frameworks. This issue is further compounded by the author's one-to-one comparison of myths and practices from disparate cultures, which are often removed from their complex original contexts and reassembled to support her interpretative agenda.

Despite its claim to objectivity, the book's treatment of Satyananda Yoga Nidra, the Bihar School of Yoga, and Svāmī Satyānanda Sarasvatī is also problematic. Much of the related material is both inaccurate and presented in a misleading way (for example, stating that the Satyananda Yoga Nidra method has ten Stages), which compromises the reliability of the book's broader claims. This is particularly puzzling given the author's former close association with the Bihar School of Yoga and Svāmī Satyānanda himself, with whom she and her family are well-known to have had a personal and longstanding connection[663]. The descriptions and interpretations of other *yoga-nidrā* techniques included in Dinsmore-Tuli's book are not the subject of this review, though the reader is advised to compare them with their original sources or consult with their authorised representatives in light of these facts.

In summary, *Nidrā Śakti: The Power of Rest* is a richly imaginative but interpretatively unstable text. It is best approached not as a historical or pedagogical resource, but as a creative and ideologically expressive artefact which reflects current cultural, political, and spiritual preoccupations within some Western yoga movements.

663 Total Yoga Nidra Network. *Yoga Nidra Network Operating Ethics*. https://www.yoganidranetwork.org/article/total-yoga-nidra-and-swami-satyananda-where-we-stand-now-2014 (accessed on 30.01.2022).

CHAPTER 21

From Descent to Ascent
Final Reflections

THIS VOLUME IS THE OUTCOME of five years of intensive research and collaboration with specialists across various scientific disciplines and presents *yoga-nidrā* from multiple perspectives. It is also grounded in the practical experience I have accumulated through my own practice, teaching and conducting one-year-long *yoga-nidrā* training courses in Vienna with participants from a wide range of yogic backgrounds. Throughout these training courses, it became increasingly evident that there was a pressing need for terminological clarity across yogic communities—to establish a common language and conceptual foundation. Only through this mutual understanding could meaningful dialogue and deeper exploration of *yoga-nidrā* truly unfold. This book therefore seeks to clarify some of the traditional yoga terminology found in Sanskrit and align contemporary interpretations with its original meanings in context, establishing a shared framework for accurate communication and further study.

The intention behind this book has been to reconnect *yoga-nidrā* to its sources—to emphasise its rootedness in the Indic philosophical and spiritual traditions, and thereby allow contemporary practitioners to appreciate its true potential as a means of transformation and self-realisation. The aim has been to establish a sound basis for the correct use of the term '*yoga-nidrā*', to clarify its historical context, and to situate it properly within the theoretical and practical frameworks of Yoga, Vedānta, Sāṃkhya and Tantra. In doing so, I have sought to illuminate its profound depth and multifaceted potential.

Yoga-nidrā, in its oldest sense, refers to a specific state of consciousness and, in modern times, also to the systematic process through which awareness is developed across progressively subtler levels of mind. Although the concept has been known in Indian thought for millennia, it was not formulated as a structured method until the 20th century.

The modern method of *yoga-nidrā* which later became widely known, was developed by Svāmī Satyānanda Sarasvatī in the 1960s. Drawing upon more than two thousand years of Indian philosophy, debate and practice, as well as upon his own extensive yogic and tantric experience, Svāmī Satyānanda created a systematised and universally accessible method. By removing religious and ritualistic components, he made the practice available to individuals of all walks of life, cultural backgrounds, gender, and faith, without the need for prior yogic preparation.

This publication seeks to clarify, contextualise, and restore the original intent and scope of *yoga-nidrā* as taught by Svāmī Satyānanda Sarasvatī within the integral yoga system of his Bihar School of Yoga, with which I have been engaged since 2001. I was blessed and honoured to have met Svāmī Satyānanda in the later years of his life; his radiant presence and vision moved me deeply and have remained a lasting source of inspiration. His direct successor and my *guru*, Svāmī Nirañjanānanda Sarasvatī, continues to embody the essence of discipleship and unwavering dedication on the spiritual path.

The present work offers a detailed, stage-by-stage exposition of Svāmī Satyānanda's *yoga-nidrā* method, examining its structure, components, sequence, and rationale. Each stage is analysed in relation to both its practical function and its philosophical underpinnings. A particular focus has been to trace the interconnections between Satyananda Yoga Nidra and other components of integral yoga. This aspect has assumed special importance given its near absence in much of the Western understanding of yoga today.

After its introduction to the West, Svāmī Satyānanda's method underwent significant decontextualisation in many settings. In a number of Western therapeutic and popular adaptations, the method has been simplified, combined with techniques from hypnotherapy, cognitive approaches, and mindfulness, or reduced to a stress-management tool. Such assimilations have often obscured the method's integrative place within an overarching system of yoga and its traditional aims. The present volume therefore documents these tendencies and argues for a careful, contextualised reinterpretation which recognises both the method's therapeutic benefits and its broader soteriological aspirations. Similarly, the relationship between Satyananda Yoga Nidra, meditation, and Western psychological currents has been explored in order to dispel prevalent misconceptions.

From a philosophical standpoint, this book also seeks to highlight the fundamental differences between *interpretatio occidentis* and *interpretatio orientis*, or between Western and Indic conceptions of consciousness. In Western christianised thought, descent is often associated with inferiority or moral decline — epitomised by the fall of Lucifer or of Adam — whereby the subconscious and unconscious are regarded as primitive or darker strata of the mind. By contrast, within the Indic paradigm, the descent into subtler layers of consciousness is a process of 'ascent' — an inward movement leading towards self-realisation. This approach resonates with C.G. Jung's notion of integrating the 'shadow', yet goes further by focusing on the revelation of the Self or Ultimate Reality rather than the confrontation of a psychological adversary.

In essence, while Western traditions have often viewed the unconscious as a realm to be subdued or corrected, in the yogic framework this descent is not a fall into darkness but a disciplined illumination of the hidden recesses of the mind. It involves integrating the sub- and unconscious contents through awareness and understanding rather than suppression or control.

Furthermore, whereas Western Enlightenment thought — outside select streams of certain esoteric traditions — has lacked a systematic framework for mapping states of consciousness, the Indic sciences have developed such frameworks over millennia. In the East, these systems were not merely speculative but grounded in direct experiential methods, enabling precise inquiry into the structure and functioning of the human mind. It is precisely this scientific and experiential spirit that Satyananda Yoga Nidra preserves and brings to the contemporary world.

A major objective of this book has been the compilation and analysis of existing scientific data specifically on the Satyananda Yoga Nidra method.

Until now, no comprehensive collection of such studies has been available. The present volume therefore aims to provide an important foundation for future research, summarising and comparing empirical findings on the psychophysiological, psychological, and therapeutic effects of the practice.

While the list of studies presented is not exhaustive, it establishes a framework for systematic comparison and critical discussion, contributing to the growing dialogue between the spiritual traditions and modern science.

Certain advanced topics, such as the use of Satyananda Yoga Nidra in conjunction with *cakra* practices or higher forms such as *prāṇa-yoga-nidrā*, have been intentionally omitted from this work. These require adequate framework, preparation, guidance, and maturity of practice. Similarly, applications of Satyananda Yoga Nidra in specialised contexts — such as pregnancy, clinical treatment of patients, education, or military and correctional environments — have only been briefly mentioned and should be addressed further in future publications.

This work aspires to bridge Indian traditions of spiritual exploration and modern empirical enquiry — to restore *yoga-nidrā* to its contextual roots while offering a transparent, reproducible account amenable to scientific scrutiny and responsible practice. My hope is that it will serve both as a practical guide for dedicated practitioners and as a scholarly resource for yoga teachers, researchers, and clinicians, enabling further, disciplined engagement with a unique method that is at once based on ancient knowledge and strikingly relevant to contemporary concerns about consciousness, health, and human development.

Part Five

Appendix

APPENDIX 1

Introduction to Bihar Yoga

Origin and Tradition

THE YOGA SYSTEM AND TEACHING method known as Bihar Yoga, also Satyananda Yoga is inspired by the teachings of Ādi Śankarācārya (ca. 788–820 CE), the founder of the Daśanāmi-saṃnyāsa tradition from ancient times. The system was developed by the tantra and yoga master Paramahaṃsa Satyānanda Sarasvatī (1923–2009) and sometimes named after him by his disciples. In 1964, he founded the renowned Bihar School of Yoga in the city of Munger in the district of Bihar, North India, where the ancient knowledge is preserved, recaptured, passed on and disseminated. The Bihar Yoga Bharati training facility was founded in 2000 and officially declared a university. It is considered to be the first yoga university in the world. Today it is an institution officially recognised by the Indian government as a research and training institute.

Paramahaṃsa Satyānanda Sarasvatī was assigned by his *guru* Svāmī Śivānanda Sarasvatī (1887–1963) with the mission of popularising and spreading yoga throughout the world. He dedicated his life to this mission and handed it over to his successors Paramahaṃsa Nirañjanānanda Sarasvatī (*1960) and Paramahaṃsa Satyasaṅgānananda Sarasvatī (*1953). Both continue to enrich and carry on the Bihar Yoga tradition to this day.

Paramahaṃsa Nirañjanānanda Sarasvatī currently lives and teaches at Ganga Darshan, Munger, Bihar in India, where the Bihar School of Yoga is based. As a yoga master and teacher, he combines tradition and modernity and is an inexhaustible source of wisdom in all areas of yoga philosophy and practice as well as the yogic lifestyle. In Munger, he teaches according to his *guru*'s mission of preserving the ancient traditions of Indian Vedānta, Sāṃkhya, Tantra and Yoga while at the same time opening up the teachings to modern culture.

Paramahaṃsa Satyasaṅgānananda Sarasvatī is a yoga master, inspired teacher, speaker and gifted writer. She is the author of several important contemporary texts on Yoga and Tantra. She has been living and teaching in Rikhiapeeth (Svāmī Satyānanda's last *sādhanā* place) since 1989 and works tirelessly for her *guru*'s vision — because, like him, she supports the impoverished villagers in the surrounding rural areas. By expanding the Sivananda Math, a non-profit organisation, she has succeeded in significantly improving the living conditions of the people in this region. In Rikhiapeeth, she created a vibrant, dynamic centre of spirituality and education.

As the traditional teachings are constantly being developed in line with the needs of the present day, we can speak of a 'living tradition'.

What is Bihar Yoga?

Bihar Yoga provides us with a system with a rich variety of practical techniques to harmonise mind, emotion and action ('head, heart and hands') in our daily lives. It combines the wisdom of three ancient traditions — Vedānta, Tantra, Sāṃkhya and Yoga proper. It is therefore referred to as an integral yoga system and as such addresses the entire personality. This is achieved through the synthesis of selected techniques from the traditional branches of Yoga (*haṭha*, *rāja*, *jñāna*, *karma*, *bhakti* and *kriyā-yoga*), whereby the individual combination of techniques is orientated towards the individual personality and thus adapts perfectly to people in the modern world. A central message of Bihar Yoga is that everyday life and yoga are one. Ideally, everyday life becomes a yoga practice as we become closer to ourselves through awareness and conscious exploration.

Bihar Yoga is a complete system that addresses all levels of being and supports us in expanding the awareness of our gross and subtle layers.

Bihar Yoga Can Be Practised By Anyone

Bihar Yoga is suitable for people at all stages and walks of life. It is a gentle, awareness-oriented system of yoga that can be adapted to a wide range of physical conditions. It is understood as a form of lived awareness rather than a practice driven by athletic ambition, while still incorporating appropriate *āsanas* (postures) as an integral component. These contribute to physical, energetic, and overall well-being.

The progression of a Bihar Yoga session

A Bihar Yoga session usually lasts ninety minutes and is structured in such a way that perception is gradually guided from the gross material level — the body — through the energetic layer to the more subtle aspects of our being (mental, emotional, intuitive). Through the observer stance — *draṣṭā-bhāva* — the mind is trained in witnessing awareness at each stage of the practice, with the aim of deepening and expanding the *draṣṭā* and integrating this perspective into everyday life.

Typically, following a brief centring phase at the beginning, the session proceeds through *āsana*, then *prāṇāyāma* (techniques for breath control), followed by *pratyāhāra* practices (Satyananda Yoga Nidra and/or various immersive techniques), each of which is practised with full awareness and presence.

Systematic and Progression

The aim of Bihar Yoga is to provide practitioners with the tools to harmonise their daily lives over time and to enable them to become aware and cultivate this awareness. Awareness and breathing are the key factors here. The practices are developed systematically and progressively, focussing on the specific benefit to the individual. Each component of the practice is seen as an integral part of the whole. Between each practice, practitioners are given time to contemplate its effects so that participants maintain focus on the practice throughout the session.

The main goal of the practice is to build a personal *sādhanā* at home in order to integrate yoga into everyday life and gradually cultivate yoga as a lifestyle.

Experience-orientated

The teacher enables the participants to gain experience by guiding their awareness throughout the practice, using neutral language and tone of voice. Apart from the shared experience of being in the same yoga class and engaging in the same techniques, each individual perceives the effects of the practices in their own way and can learn at their own pace. The experience of each practitioner is valued, and the development of an intuitive approach is supported. They learn what suits their body and mind—and what does not.

Participant-orientated

The focus is on the participants, not the teachers. Classes are non-competitive and comparisons with other practitioners or teachers are discouraged. This approach empowers participants to develop their own practice through self-awareness and promotes confidence in practice through self-responsibility. It also promotes introversion and the ability to prepare for more extensive states of immersion.

It is usually practised with eyes closed, without music and under neutral verbal guidance. The teacher never touches the participants. Assistance is only given verbally and by demonstration. The teacher does not practise together with the participants during the session. New techniques are first demonstrated and explained, and then practised by the group.

Code of Ethics

Bihar Yoga qualified teachers follow an agreed code of ethics as a condition of their accreditation. The code is based on the *niyamas* of Patañjali and underpins the qualities and professional responsibilities of a yoga teacher in this tradition.

Professional Standard

Teachers are trained, assessed and accredited by the international Satyananda Yoga Academies and the Bihar School of Yoga to ensure high quality and professionalism in teaching. Through a system of lifelong learning, teachers regularly update their skills and knowledge by keeping abreast of new developments from India and other countries. The accreditation system also upholds the standards, ethics and tradition of Bihar Yoga.

Bihar Yoga Today

Bihar Yoga is practised all over the world and offers profound training opportunities to those interested at the Bihar School of Yoga in India and through its yoga academy abroad — Satyananda Yoga Academy Europe (SYAE). The numerous publications of the Bihar School of Yoga spread profound knowledge about yoga throughout the world and have been regarded as yoga classics for decades.

Further links

- Bihar School of Yoga: https://www.biharyoga.net
- Satyam Yoga Prasad — is a free digital library of all the collected publications of the Bihar Yoga Tradition: https://www.satyamyogaprasad.net
- Rikhiapeeth Ashram: https://rikhiapeeth.in
- Yoga Magazine: http://www.yogamag.net
- Satyananda Yoga Akademie Europe (SYAE): https://syae.eu
- European Satyananda Yoga Family: https://www.esyf.eu
- Ananda Verlag — Publications in German: https://www.yoga-anandaverlag.de

APPENDIX 2

Summary of Clinical Studies and Scientific Findings on Satyananda Yoga Nidra

Yoga-nidrā as Reducer of Physical and Mental Tension, Stress and Anxiety

In his book *Yoga Nidra*[664], Svāmī Satyānanda refers to the four stages of stress disorder pathogenesis which Kodethur Udupa (1979)[665] defined based on his research on stress and stress management through yoga. In the first phase, mental symptoms such as anxiety and irritability occur due to overactivation of the sympathetic nervous system. The second stage is characterised by corresponding physical symptoms such as high blood pressure and increased heart rate. In the third phase, the deviations manifest clinically in the organ systems. In the fourth stage, severe symptoms occur in certain organs that require long-term medical treatment. The parameters measured by Udupa included blood pressure and the concentration of stress hormones (catecholamines) in the blood and urine.

The study showed that regular yoga practice is significantly more effective than state of the art pharmacologic antihypertensive treatment of the time when the study was conducted. The studies also showed that conventional physical training, such as gymnastics and fitness exercises, increase catecholamine levels. However, yoga *āsanas* can also have the same undesirable effect – if they are practised as a sporting performance or in some strenuous

664 Satyananda, Swami. (2006). *Yoga Nidra*. (12th reprint). Munger: Yoga Publications Trust, p. 187.

665 Kodethur Narasimha Udupa (1920–1992) was an Indian surgeon, pioneer of integrative medicine, and founding member and director of the Institute of Medical Sciences at Banaras Hindu University.

way, the stress-reducing effect is not only lost, but reversed. Udupa in fact recommends *śavāsana* as prophylaxis against stress.[666]

Bahrke (1979)[667] concluded that yogic relaxation (understanding *yoga-nidrā*) is effective in reducing psychological tension and significantly improves psychological well-being in individuals suffering from anxiety.

Carrington et al. (1980)[668] showed in their research, that *yoga-nidrā* has a wide range of applications as a preventive measure that should be practised by healthy, active people to reduce built-up psychological tension, increase stress resistance and alleviate psychosomatic illnesses.

In another study, **Seth et al. (1981)**[669] compared the relative effectiveness of *śavāsana* ('corpse pose') as one of the most important components of *yoga-nidrā* practice with the then-current medical therapy for reducing the severity of symptoms of tension headaches.

> **INTERVENTION:** 13 subjects (16–45 years of age, otherwise healthy, clinically presenting with muscular contraction headache) suffering from tension headaches were evaluated through a clinical history of their general health and a subsequent examination with detailed cardiovascular, neurological, ENT and ophthalmological findings. They were randomly assigned to either EMG biofeedback or *śavāsana* sessions for a period of four weeks and examined on an ongoing basis.

> **RESULTS:** In a comparative analysis, the results of EMG biofeedback and *śavāsana* were found to be equally effective as medical therapy in treating tension headaches. It was found that in the younger age group (16–25 years), more patients experienced a more significant improvement with both treatment methods than in patients in

666 Janakānanda, Swami. (2022). *A deeper yoga and Yoga Nidra*. [eBook edition]. Hamneda: Bindu, p. 99–104.

667 Bahrke, M., S. (1979). Exercise, meditation and anxiety reduction: A review. American Corrective Therapy Journal, 33(2). In Kamakhya Kumar. (2013). *A Handbook of Yoga-Nidrā*. New Delhi: D. K. Printworld (P) Ltd., p. 105.

668 Carrington, Patricia et al. (1980). The Use of Meditation–Relaxation Techniques for the Management of Stress in a Working Population. Journal of Occupational Medicine, 22(4). In Swami Satyananda Saraswati. (2006). *Yoga Nidra*. Bihar: Yoga Publications Trust. p.195

669 Sethi, B. B., Trivedi, J. K. & Anand, R. (1981). A comparative study of relative effectiveness of biofeedback and Shavasana (Yoga) in tension headache. *Indian Journal of Psychiatry*, 23(2), 109–14. https://www.ncbi.nlm.nih.gov/pmc/articles/PMC3013159/pdf/IJPsy-23-109.pdf (accessed on 12.09.2023)

the older groups (26–35 years and 36–45 years). A further study by Chesney and Shelton (1976) found that both *śavāsana* alone and EMG biofeedback after *śavāsana* to be superior to feedback alone, which Masur (1976) and White and Alaxender (1976) found to be no different from placebo. Furthermore, only 13 sessions of *śavāsana* were needed to achieve the same result as 16 sessions of EMG Biofeedback.

Kumar (2004)[670] conducted a six-month study at the Yoga Clinic of the Dev Sanskriti Vishwavidyalaya University in Haridwar, India, on the effects of *yoga-nidrā* on stress, anxiety and general well-being. Eighty students were selected as subjects, along with 30 people between the ages of 20 and 30 for the control group.

INTERVENTION: Both the experimental and control groups completed postgraduate yoga courses, so they could all demonstrate regular *āsana*, *prāṇāyāma* and *ṣaṭkarman* practice. The only difference for the subjects in the experimental group was that they additionally practised *yoga-nidrā* for half an hour every day.

RESULTS: The result showed a significant reduction in the stress level of the subjects in the *yoga-nidrā* group, whereas no significant change in the anxiety level was observed. The general well-being of the subjects was also positively influenced by *yoga-nidrā*.

In a follow-up study **(2008)**[671] **Kumar** observed a significant change in the stress and anxiety levels, however, anxiety decreased significantly in male subjects only.

Kumari und Tripathi (2020)[672] examined the short-term effect of *yoga-nidrā* on 20 patients with stress syndrome at Sir Sundar Lal Hospital, BHU, Varanasi.

670 Kumar, Kamakhya. (2004). A Study on the Impact on Stress and Anxiety Through Yoga Nidra. In Yoga Mimamsa. *Indian Journal of Traditional Knowledge*, 36(3), 136–160. https://de.scribd.com/document/364474553/A-Study-on-Stress-Anxiety-Yoga-Nidra-Yoga-Mimansa (accessed on 12.09.2023).

671 Kumar, Kamakhya. (2008). A study on the impact on stress and anxiety through Yoga Nidra. In *Indian Journal of Traditional Knowledge*, 7(3), 401–404. https://nopr.niscpr.res.in/bitstream/123456789/1700/1/IJTK%207%283%29%20401–404.pdf (accessed on 12.09.2023).

672 Kumari, Priyanka & Tripathi, J. S. (2020). A Pilot Study on Effect of Yoga Nidra in the Management of Stress. *International Journal of Science and Research* (IJSR), 9(1), 1101–1103.https://www.ijsr.net/archive/v9i1/ART20204197.pdf (accessed on 12.09.2023).

INTERVENTION: The ten patients in the experimental group were treated with *yoga-nidrā*, while the ten patients in the control group took herbal medication. Each patient in the experimental group practised *yoga-nidrā* for 30 minutes a day for a total of seven days.

RESULTS: Results were measured using the DASS (Depression-Anxiety-Stress-Scale)[673] and showed a significant reduction in stress and anxiety levels in both groups. However, the reduction in stress levels in the experimental group was greater in relation to the control group. It can therefore be assumed that the *yoga-nidrā* practice promises better results in managing stress than taking herbal medication. A follow-up study by the same authors from 2023 add further credulity to these findings.

Jayshree and Choudhury (2022)[674] conducted a pilot study on the effect of a *yoga-nidrā* programme on depression, anxiety and stress in patients with chronic kidney disease treated with haemodialysis.

INTERVENTION: The subjects for the study were randomly selected and divided into an experimental and a control group. A pre- and post-test was used for both groups to assess stress, anxiety and depression.

RESULT: No significant reduction in stress, anxiety or depression was observed in the control group (without intervention), while the test group showed a significant improvement. The results of the study show that *yoga-nidrā* is a very effective relaxation technique for reducing stress, anxiety and depression in haemodialysis patients.

---

673 DASS is a test with 21 questions that is used to measure psychological stress.

674 Jayshree, Kalita & Choudhury, Purujit. (2021) A pilot study on effect of yoga-nidra programme on depression, anxiety, and stress among patients with chronic kidney disease receiving haemodialysis. *International Journal of Applied Research*, 2022; 8(6), 346–349. https://doi.org/10.22271/allresearch.2022.v8.i6e.9893 (accessed on 12.09.2023).

Yoga-nidrā in the education system — anxiety and stress reduction, improvement of emotional intelligence, increased learning ability and memory, well-being and creativity, reduction of cortisol levels

Another study by **Kumar (2004)**[675] looked at anxiety levels in young people in the education system. It showed that *yoga-nidrā* could reduce stress in students at university level and significantly increase their well-being. Kumar then recommended the introduction of *yoga-nidrā* for students at universities.

Bhushan und Sinha (2001)[676] conducted a study on the effects of *yoga-nidrā* on reducing stress levels, increasing concentration, changing behavioural patterns and increasing feelings of happiness in school students.

INTERVENTION: The selected students, aged 17 to 18, attended the 11th and 12th grades and participated continuously in *yoga-nidrā* courses at their school for a year and a half.

RESULTS: *Yoga-nidrā* proved to be a significantly helpful technique in a school environment for reducing stress levels, increasing concentration, changing behavioural patterns and enhancing feelings of happiness. The researchers also suggested that *yoga-nidrā* practice could awaken students' innate creativity and enhance their learning and memory skills.

Verma (2004)[677] — a lecturer at the Department of Applied Yogic Sciences, Bihar Yoga Bharati — conducted a study to examine the memory performance of 30 students aged 13 to 15 years, who were divided into an experimental and a control group of 15 students each.

INTERVENTION: At the beginning and end of a 15-day period, a test was conducted with both groups that included verbal and non-verbal

---

675 Kumar, Kamakhya. (2004). Yoga Nidra and its Impact on Students' Well-Being. In *Yoga Mimamsa, Indian Journal of Traditional Knowledge*, 36(1), 31–35.

676 Bhushan, S. & Sinha, P. (2001). Yoganidra and management of anxiety and hostility. *Journal of Indian Psychology*, 19(1–2), 44–49.

677 Verma, Veena (Sannyasi Soumyashakti). (2004). Possibilities of Revolutionizing the Education System Through Yoga Nidra. *Yoga Magazine*. 5. Bihar: Bihar School of Yoga. http://www.yogamag.net/archives/2000s/2004/0405/0405pred.html (accessed on 15.09.2023).

material to measure the performance of long-term and immediate memory, short-term, very short-term, medium-term and long-term memory. During the study period, the *yoga-nidrā* practice was only carried out in the experimental group, for 30 to 35 minutes daily.

RESULTS: The memory performance of the experimental group had improved significantly. The different *yoga-nidrā* levels may help to strengthen willpower, and the positive affirmations in the visualisation phase have a strong effect on the subconscious, which is where memory draws its strength from. The results showed that *yoga-nidrā* had a positive effect on the memory of the students.

CONCLUSIONS: The researchers concluded that it would be highly beneficial if the school authorities were to include a 15- to 20-minute *yoga-nidrā* phase in the daily schedule. If just 15 days of practice can produce such a notable improvement in memory performance as shown in the above study, regular *yoga-nidrā* practice could not only improve memory and academic performance, but also have a positive impact on overall personal development. According to the study, *yoga-nidrā* can help enhance academic performance, by helping students to develop their creative potential.

Gupta (2004)[678] conducted a comparative study of *yoga-nidrā* with sports and games lessons over a period of one month to examine the effect of *yoga-nidrā* on the creativity of school children aged between 10 and 12.

INTERVENTION: The subjects were divided into two groups — 30 students who participated in a 25-minute *yoga-nidrā* session every weekday and 30 students who attended their usual sports and games lessons. A creativity test with ten parameters, compiled by the researcher himself, was used as the evaluation method: 1) ability to associate objects and ideas, 2) creativity in dealing with geometric forms, 3) ability to think about consequences/imagine consequences,

678 Gupta, K. S. S. (2004). Effect of Yoga Nidra on creativity in School Children. In Yoga Research Foundation: Volume three. (2018). *Promotion of Health 1988–2007*. Bihar: Yoga Publication Trust. pp. 242–249.

4) ability to foresee/recognise a problem, 5) ability to think/talk about alternatives, 6) sequential thinking, 7) ability to solve a mechanical problem (play-making test), 8) ability to solve a mechanical problem (tool-making test), 9) ability to convert abstract thought into a phrase/shape, and 10) ability to express curiosity.

RESULTS: The creativity test showed significant improvement in all the creativity dimensions for the *yoga-nidrā* group except for dimensions 1 and 6. These results suggest a global activation of creative potential and not only in particular aspects.

Bhushan (2006a)[679] found in his study that *yoga-nidrā* can address an individual's entire personality and that *yoga-nidrā* practice can be considered an effective means of qualitatively affecting the personality.

In a follow-up study, **Bhushan (2006b)**[680] concluded that the practice of *yoga-nidrā* promotes self-confidence in teenagers.

Jensen et al. (2012)[681] examined the effects of a *yoga-nidrā* session on chest and abdominal breathing patterns in boys with disruptive behaviour disorders using respiratory inductive plethysmography[682]. The seven participants were aged 10 to 15 years and attended special schools for children with disruptive behaviour (DB). The results were compared with the values of three students aged 15 without DB.

INTERVENTION: The seven boys with DB had previously participated in a 13-week yoga programme. During this programme, the participants were gradually introduced to the *yoga-nidrā* method. The comparison group did not participate in this yoga programme, but underwent the same data collection procedure as the yoga group.

679 Bhushan, S. (n.d.). Qualitative Transformation in Personality: A Function of Yoga Nidra, Journal of Indian Psychology, 24(1/2). In Kamakhya Kumar. (2013). *A Handbook of Yoga-Nidrā*. New Delhi: D. K. Printworld (P) Ltd. p. 64.

680 Bhushan, S. (n.d.). Yoga-Nidra as Intervenor to Promote Self-Confidence among Teenagers, Indian Journal of Psychometry and Education, 37(1). In Kamakhya Kumar. (2013). *A Handbook of Yoga-Nidrā*. New Delhi: D. K. Printworld (P) Ltd., p. 64.

681 Jensen, P. S., et al. (2012). Respiratory patterns in students enrolled in schools for disruptive behaviour before, during, and after yoga nidra relaxation. In *Journal of Child and Family Studies*, 21(4), 667–681. https://doi.org/10.1007/s10826-011-9519-3 (accessed on 12.09.2023)

682 A non-invasive method of monitoring breathing.

RESULTS: The study showed that the boys with DB generally had unstable breathing patterns throughout the entire recording period and that they showed more stable breathing during *yoga-nidrā* compared to the periods before or after the recording. There were also examples of a reduction in the predominance of thoracic breath during *yoga-nidrā*. The breathing patterns of the comparison group without DB were stable during the three phases of the process — before, during and after the practice.

Rani et al. (2013)[683] conducted a pre-experimental study with 50 subjects which aimed to evaluate and compare the stress levels of first-year B.Sc nursing students before and after regular practice of *yoga-nidrā*. The data was collected using a modified stress rating scale, originally prepared by M. Singh, Senior Psychologist in Dev Sanskriti Vishwavidyalaya, Haridwar, which was altered for the purpose of the study. The tool consisted of forty statements on a three point scale of Always, Sometime and Never scored as 3, 2 and 1 respectively. The maximum and minimum scores of the modified stress assessment tool were 80 and 0 respectively. The stress level was assessed according to five categories: severe (57–80), high (47–56), moderate (37–46), low (27–36) and very low (0–26).

RESULTS: The study showed that the mean stress value after *yoga-nidrā* (17.8) was lower than the mean stress value before *yoga-nidrā* (28.82). This indicates that the nursing students' stress levels had decreased as a result of *yoga-nidrā*.

In a study by **Singh et al. (2015)**[684], the influence of *yoga-nidrā* on the general state of health of 30 healthy medical students aged 18 and 20 was examined who served as their own controls.

---

683 Rani, K., Kumar, A., Sharma, P. (2013). Effect of Yoga Nidra on Stress Level among B.Sc. Nursing first year students. *Nursing and Midwifery Research Journal*, (9), pp. 47–55. http://doi.org/10.33698/NRF0156 (accessed on 12.09.2023).

684 Singh, I., Beena & Singh, H. (2016). To Study the Effect of Yoga Nidra on Anxiety and Stress in Medical Students. *European Journal of Biomedical and Pharmaceutical Sciences*, 3(2), 178–180. https://storage.googleapis.com/journal-uploads/ejbps/article_issue/volume_3_february_issue_2/1454068178.pdf/ (accessed on 12.09.2023).

INTERVENTION: The students practised *yoga-nidrā* for 45 minutes a day at a fixed time for three months. The answers to a questionnaire on their general state of health were evaluated before and after the practice.

RESULTS: After three months of *yoga-nidrā* practice, a significant decrease in stress and anxiety levels was observed. *Yoga-nidrā* proved to be an effective means of balancing the sympathetic and parasympathetic nervous systems and of better managing anxiety and stress.

CONCLUSION: This study was on medical students and the researchers concluded that as curriculum and teaching modalities change, it would be beneficial to introduce students to techniques such as *yoga-nidrā* that could help them improve their academic performance and adopt healthy lifestyles.

Sachdeva (2016) conducted a study[685] with 21 students in grades 11 and 12 to examine the effectiveness of a once-weekly *yoga-nidrā* practice at school to reduce stress levels, increase concentration, change behavioural patterns and increase happiness in students.

RESULTS: The study showed changes in those students who participated continuously in *yoga-nidrā* classes at school for a year and a half, despite them rarely practicing at home. *Yoga-nidrā* proved to be a helpful technique for stress management, increasing concentration, changing behaviour patterns and increasing happiness levels among students. This study was repeated and the results confirmed by Graham (2021–2022)[686].

685 Sachdeva, Sachi. (2018). To Study the Effects of Yoga Nidra on Reduction of Stress, Increase in Concentration, Changes in Behaviour and Increase in Happiness among School Going Students. In *International Journal of Science and Research* (IJSR), 7(12), 5–11. https://www.ijsr.net/archive/v7i12/ART20193216.pdf, (accessed on 12.09.2023).

686 Graham, M. (2022). Effect of Yoga Nidra on Reducing Stress, Increasing Attention, Changing Behaviour and Increasing Happiness of School Students. *Journal of Inovation and Social Science Research*, 9(4), 239–245.

Vaishnav et al. (2018)[687] conducted a study with different methods to examine the effect of *yoga-nidrā* on the well-being of students aged 13 to 15.

INTERVENTION: 36 students participated in 30-minute *yoga-nidrā* sessions three days a week for one month. The primary outcome measures were subjective feelings of happiness, decrease of perceived stress, general quality of life and general psychological well-being. Dimensions of experience such as enthusiasm, alertness, calmness, clarity of thought, control over anger, self-confidence and self-awareness were assessed before and after the intervention. Qualitative observations were recorded from the participants, their teachers and parents.

RESULTS: The *yoga-nidrā* intervention led to significant improvements in all primary outcome measures. Participants reported significant increases in feelings of happiness, enthusiasm, calmness, inspiration, alertness, activity, clarity of thought, control over anger, and self-confidence at the end of the study period.

CONCLUSION: *Yoga-nidrā* has a positive effect on several dimensions of well-being in adolescents.

Lakshmipathy and Easvaradoss (2018)[688] conducted a study to examine the *yoga-nidrā* method as an effective strategy for coping with perceived stress and for self-regulation in 70 teacher trainees. The subjects were divided into an experimental group and a control group, each with 35 participants. The age range was between 21 and 23 years.

INTERVENTION: The *yoga-nidrā* intervention used in the experimental group consisted of 20 sessions. There were three sessions per week, with each session lasting 1 hour and 30 minutes. Psychological tests

---

687 Vaishnav, S. B., Vaishnav, V. S. & Varma, J. R. (2018). Effect of Yoga-nidra on Adolescents Well-being: A Mixed Method Study. *International journal of yoga*, 11(3), 245–248. https://doi.org/10.4103/ijoy.IJOY_39_17 (accessed on 12.09.2023).

688 Lakshmipathy, Shalini & Easvaradoss, Veena. (2018). Impact of Yoga Nidra Meditation on Perceived Stress and Self Regulation in Teacher Trainees. *International Journal of Indian Psychology*, 6(3), 89–93. https://ijip.in/wp-content/uploads/2020/06/18.01.049.20180603.pdf (accessed on 12.09.2023).

were used to measure stress levels and self-regulation ability. These tests were carried out in both groups before and after the intervention.

RESULTS: The study showed that the *yoga-nidrā* method significantly reduced the stress levels of the participating teacher trainees compared to the control group.

Bhalendu et al. (2019)[689] also examined the qualitative effects of *yoga-nidrā* on the physical, emotional, cognitive and spiritual dimensions of well-being in prospective teachers.

INTERVENTION: 77 college students participated in *yoga-nidrā* sessions over a three-month period. Approximately 86% of the participants submitted their diaries, which contained their observations and experiences during the *yoga-nidrā* sessions and were thematically analysed.

RESULTS: The main observations recorded in the total of 475 notes taken by the subjects were the experience of calmness, freshness or disappearance of tiredness, clarity of thought, improved concentration, improved memory and a reduction in anxiety, depression and worry. Over the weeks, the transformative effects of *yoga-nidrā* were seen in the form of an improved ability for self-reflection and self-awareness and for behavioural modification.

CONCLUSION: *Yoga-nidrā* can be used to reduce stress and anxiety and increase emotions such as happiness, enthusiasm and alertness. *Yoga-nidrā* can lead to experiences of cognitive, emotional and behavioural stability and clarity and can be considered a useful tool for increasing well-being.

---

689 Bhalendu, Suriakant, Vaishnav et al. (2019). Transformative effects of yoga nidra on hedonic and eudemonic dimensions of well-being: A qualitative study in trainee teachers. *International Journal of Yoga – Philosophy, Psychology and Parapsychology*, 7(1), p 17–23.

Chowdhary (2019)[690] conducted a study to determine the effect of *yoga-nidrā* and *prāṇāyāma* on selected physiological variables in adolescents. 90 students aged 17 to 22 were randomly selected as subjects. All subjects were randomly assigned to three groups (A, B and C), with A and B serving as the experimental group and C as the control group, each with 30 subjects.

> **INTERVENTION:** Two experimental groups participated in a training programme for 12 weeks. Group A received *prāṇāyāma* training (*bhastrikā-*, *ujjāyī-* and *anuloma-viloma prāṇāyāma*), while group B practised *yoga-nidra*. The control group (group C) did not participate in any yoga programme. The quantitative measurements of the subjects' values were taken using standard equipment before and after the twelve-week training.

> **RESULTS:** The study showed that *yoga-nidrā* and *prāṇāyāma* were able to significantly improve the adolescents' physiological values (resting heart rate, breathing rate and vital capacity).

Pandey and Dalal (2020)[691] examined the effects of the yoga techniques *nāḍi-śodhana prāṇāyāma* and *yoga-nidrā* on the mental health and emotional maturity of 30 young adults.

> **INTERVENTION:** A yoga-specific practice programme that included *nāḍi-śodhana*, *prāṇāyāma* and *yoga-nidrā* was completed by the participants daily from 6 to 7.15 am for one month. The subjects were asked to complete the Emotional Maturity Scale (a five-point self-assessment scale) before and after the training, and their mental state was assessed using the Mental Health Scale before and after the test.

---

690 Chowdhary, Binod. (2019). Effect of yoga nidra and pranayama on selected physiological variables of tribal youths. *International Journal of Physiology, Nutrition and Physical Education*, 4(1), 2011–2015. https://www.journalofsports.com/pdf/2019/vol4issue1/PartAQ/4-2-105-195.pdf (accessed on 12.09.2023).

691 Parasar Pandey A. O. & Dalal S. (2020). Effects of nadi-shodhan pranayama and yoga-nidra on emotional maturity and mental health of young adults. *International Journal of Indian Psychology*, 8(4), 1657–1668. doi:10.25215/0804.180 (accessed on 12.09.2023).

RESULTS: The yoga practices *nāḍi-śodhana*, *prāṇāyāma* and *yoga-nidrā* were both shown to significantly increase the level of mental health and emotional maturity.

Ganpat (2020)[692] tested the influence of *yoga-nidrā* on the emotional intelligence values of university students. Emotional intelligence can be measured with a test which includes essential psychological dimensions such as emotional sensitivity, emotional maturity and emotional competence. These parameters represent the motivation to truly recognise the dynamics of behavioural patterns, to interpret them honestly and to deal with them tactfully.

INTERVENTION: 60 students with an average age of 25 years participated in this research study. They were randomly assigned to two groups: 30 students in the yoga group and the other 30 in the control group. The subjects in the yoga group practised *yoga-nidrā* for three weeks, while the participants in the control group followed their usual daily routine. Emotional intelligence data was collected before and after a three-week period in both groups using a test.

RESULTS: The tests showed a significant increase in all psychological dimensions for the yoga group, while no significant change was observed in the control group.

CONCLUSION: The test results of the students show that *yoga-nidrā* leads to an improvement in emotional intelligence, which could have a positive effect on academic performance.

Tiwary et al. (2020)[693] conducted a stress-reduction study for medical students with two experimental groups and assigned the subjects to a yoga group and a control group with 26 and 27 participants, respectively.

---

692 Ganpat, Tikhe, Sham. (2020). Yoga Nidra Practice Enhances Emotional Intelligence in University Students. In *Alternative and Complementary Therapies*, 26(5), 214–218. https://doi.org/10.1089/act.2020.29294.tsg (accessed on 12.09.2023).

693 Tiwari, V. K., Pandey, S., & Mishra, R. (2020). Yoga is an effective technique of stress reduction within the medical population: a biochemical study in MBBS students of BRD Medical College,

INTERVENTION: The yoga group practised selected *āsanas*, *prāṇāyāma* and *yoga-nidrā* for three months. Contact was maintained with the control group, who went about their usual activities. The morning serum cortisol level measured between 8 am and 9 am was used as a stress marker for both groups before and after the experimental period.

RESULTS: The yoga group showed a significant reduction in morning serum cortisol levels (a marker of stress levels), while the cortisol levels of the control group participants showed no significant changes.

CONCLUSIONS: Yoga is an effective technique for stress reduction. Introducing yoga classes in the first year of medical school could result in our future healthcare providers adopting a healthy lifestyle. In the long term, the practice of yoga by healthcare providers could have a positive impact on the healthcare system.

D'souza et al. (2021)[694] examined the effectiveness of *yoga-nidrā* in alleviating the psychosocial stress of school-age adolescents.

INTERVENTION: The study was conducted with tenth-grade students (14 to 16 years old) and included two groups — a control group and an experimental group that practised *yoga-nidrā* for 21 consecutive days. The Modified Youth Stress Questionnaire was used to assess students' stress before and after the intervention.

RESULTS: The results indicated that practising *yoga-nidrā* significantly reduced overall stress, including important areas such as stress in the home, stress concerning school performance, interaction with teachers, uncertainty about the future, and conflicts at school and during leisure time.

Gorakhpur, Uttar Pradesh, India. *International Journal of Research in Medical Sciences*, 8(4), 1326–1330. https://doi.org/10.18203/2320-6012.ijrms20201318 (accessed on 12.09.2023).

694 D'souza, O. L., Jose, A. E., Suresh, S., & Baliga, M. S. (2021). Effectiveness of Yoga Nidra in reducing stress in school going adolescents: An experimental study. *Complementary therapies in clinical practice*, 45, 101462. https://doi.org/10.1016/j.ctcp.2021.101462 (accessed on 12.09.2023).

CONCLUSIONS: This study shows that *yoga-nidrā* is effective in reducing psychosocial stress in adolescents and can be useful in a school setting.

Kanchibhotla et al. (2021)[695] addressed the issue that the academic performance of visually impaired children is affected by the loss of vision. A pilot study was conducted to determine whether the verbal memory of children with visual impairment can be improved by practising a yoga module.

INTERVENTION: 113 children from a School For The Blind in Surat took part in a seven-hour workshop based on yoga and *prāṇāyāma*. The intervention included three *prāṇāyāmas* (breathing techniques), 'Super-Brain-Yoga' and *yoga-nidrā*. The subjects were tested for their verbal memory before and after the intervention.

RESULTS: The results after the intervention indicated a significant improvement in the memory performance of the participants.

CONCLUSION: Holistic techniques can have a positive effect on the academic performance of visually impaired children.

Jaiganesh et al. (2022)[696] conducted a study to determine the effects of *sūrya-namaskāra* exercises with and without *yoga-nidrā* on the stress levels of high school students. The hypothesis was that the *sūrya-namaskāra* exercise with and without *yoga-nidrā* would lead to significant differences in the stress levels of high school students. For this purpose, 45 secondary school students aged 12 to 15 were selected and divided into two experimental groups and one control group, each with 15 students.

INTERVENTION: For a period of six weeks, the experimental group I. practised the *sūrya-namaskāra* exercise with *yoga-nidrā* for one hour

695 Kanchibhotla, Divya et al. (2021). Enhancement of the Cognitive Abilities in Visually Impaired Children Following a Yoga Based Intervention. *Annals of Yoga and Physical Therapy*, 5(1), 1046. https://doi.org/10.26420/ANNYOGAPHYSTHER.2021.1046 (accessed on 08.02.2023).

696 Jaiganesh, D. K., Parthasarathy, D. S., & Mr. Duraisamy. (2022). Effect of Suryanamaskar Practices with and Without Yoga Nidra On Stress Among High School Students – A Randomized Controlled Trial: Life Sciences-Health. *International Journal of Life Science and Pharma Research*, 12(SP25), L28–L33. https://doi.org/10.22376/ijpbs/lpr.2022.12.6.SP25.L28–33 (accessed on 12.09.2023).

every morning, while the experimental group II. practised *sūrya-namaskāra* without *yoga-nidrā*. The control group did not receive any specific training but took part in regular school activities. All three groups were tested before and after the training period.

RESULTS: The study showed that *sūrya-namaskāra* with and without *yoga-nidrā* significantly reduced students' stress levels. However, *sūrya-namaskāra* in combination with *yoga-nidrā* proved to be even more effective than *sūrya-namaskāra* alone.

Gupta and Singh (2022) conducted a study[697] to examine the role of yoga practices in improving the psychological well-being of 60 adolescent girls aged 13 to 15.

INTERVENTION: The subjects were randomly assigned to an experimental or a control group, each with 30 participants. The experimental group completed a structured yoga programme in 24 sessions, using techniques such as *sūrya-namaskāra*, *prāṇāyāma* and *yoga-nidrā*. A checklist was used to assess the psychological well-being of the adolescents, which was evaluated at the beginning and after three months.

RESULTS: The results of the participants in the experimental group showed significant changes in various areas of psychological well-being compared to the participants in the control group.

CONCLUSION: Yoga practices can significantly improve the psychological well-being of female students during puberty. As an intervention, yoga techniques have the potential to promote mental health, self-awareness and mental relaxation.

---

697 Madhu K. Gupta & Amool R. Singh. (2022). Exploring the Therapeutic Effect of Yoga to Enhance Psychological Well-Being Among Adolescent Girl Students. *Journal of Education, Society and Behavioural Science*, 35 (2), 13–19. https://doi.org/10.9734/jesbs/2022/v35i230402. (accessed on 12.09.2023).

Yoga-nidrā as a reducer of symptoms of fatigue and its beneficial effects on mental and psychosomatic disorders

Gersten (1978)[698] concluded in his study that *yoga-nidrā* can increase the practitioner's sense of self-efficacy in such a way that he can recognise and systematically work through his personal problems as well as interpersonal conflicts.

Mathew (1981)[699] found that *yoga-nidrā* is a successful therapy for both acute and chronic mental disorders of all kinds, especially for excessive anxiety and neurotic behavioural patterns.

Kumar (2006)[700] conducted a study on the effects of *yoga-nidrā* on regressive responsiveness, guilt, arousal and fatigue symptoms with 55 male and 55 female students aged 20 to 30 years, who were each assigned to a test and a control group. The subjects attended postgraduate yoga courses at the Indian University Dev Sanskriti Vishwavidyalaya in Shantikunj, Haridwar.

> RESULTS: In the course of the study, the yoga group showed a significant change in regressive responsiveness and a reduction in guilt, arousal and fatigue. These results were confirmed in a further study on regressive responsiveness and feelings of guilt by **Kumar (2010)**[701].

Köksoy et al. (2017) conducted[702] a study to examine the efficacy of yoga in 12 patients with diagnosed chronic subjective tinnitus. Their mean age was 52.5 years, and the mean duration of their tinnitus was 5.4 years.

---

698 Gersten, D. J. (1978). Meditation as an Adjunct to Medical and Psychiatric Treatment, American Journal of Psychiatry, 135, 5. In Swami Satyananda Sataswati. (2026). *Yoga Nidra*. Bihar: Yoga Publication Trust. p. 196.

699 Mathew, R. J., Ho, B. T., Kralik, P., Weinman, M., & Claghorn, J. L. (1981). Anxiety and platelet MAO levels after relaxation training. *The American Journal of Psychiatry*, 138(3), 371–373. https://doi.org/10.1176/ajp.138.3.371 (accessed on 13.09.2023)

700 Kumar, Kamakhya. (2013). *A Handbook of Yoga-Nidrā*. New Delhi: D. K. Printworld (P) Ltd, p. 107–116

701 Kumar, Kamakhya (2010). Psychological changes as related to Yoga Nidra. In *International Journal of Psychology: A Biopsychosocial Approach*. 6, 129–137. https://www.researchgate.net/publication/213341724_Psychological_changes_as_related_to_Yoga_Nidra (accessed on 12.09.2023).

702 Köksoy, S., Eti, C. M., Karataş, M., & Vayisoglu, Y. (2018). The Effects of Yoga in Patients Suffering from Subjective Tinnitus. *International Archives of Otorhinolaryngology*, 22(1), 9–13. https://doi.org/10.1055/s-0037-1601415 (accessed on 12.09.2023).

INTERVENTION: Patients participated in a weekly yoga session and also practised yoga at home with the help of a worksheet for three months. Each yoga session consisted of physical postures (*āsanas*), breathing practices (*prāṇāyāma*) and meditation (*śavāsana* and *yoga-nidrā*). Tinnitus scores before and after the yoga sessions were compared.

RESULTS: There were statistically significant differences in the questionnaire scores for stress, restrictions due to tinnitus and its severity.

CONCLUSION: This study suggests that yoga practices can reduce everyday stress caused by tinnitus, as well as the subjectively perceived tinnitus symptoms.

Yoga-nidrā as an effective aid for sleep disorders, chronic insomnia, and improved sleep quality

Datta et al. (2012–16)[703] conducted a comparative study between conventional treatment of insomnia with cognitive behavioural therapy and treatment with guided *yoga-nidrā* in 41 patients with chronic insomnia, who were divided into two groups.

INTERVENTION: The results were measured both subjectively, using a sleep diary, and objectively using polysomnography. In addition, the cortisol level in saliva was measured. The measurement was carried out on all patients before the intervention and only repeated on those who had volunteered for it.

RESULTS: The results showed an improvement in subjective total sleep time, sleep efficiency, frequency of waking after falling asleep, a reduction in total daily waking time and an improvement in subjective sleep

703 Datta, Karuna et al. (2021). Yoga nidra practice shows improvement in sleep in patients with chronic insomnia: A randomized controlled trial. In *National Medical Journal India*, 34(3), 143–50. https://nmji.in/yoga-nidra-practice-shows-improvement-in-sleep-in-patients-with-chronic-insomnia-a-randomized-controlled-trial/ (accessed on 12.09.2023).

quality. Objectively, both interventions improved total sleep time and total waking time. Furthermore, it was additionally observed that salivary cortisol levels decreased significantly only after *yoga-nidrā*.

CONCLUSION: *Yoga-nidrā* with guided practice can be used to treat chronic insomnia.

Datta et al. (2017)[704] demonstrated the effect of *yoga-nidrā* on insomnia in two patients in a case study. Patient 01, a 60-year-old widower, had been suffering from sleep disorders for twenty years. He was already worried about falling asleep during the day, which worsened before bedtime. He had a history of benign prostatic hypertrophy and was not taking any medication for sleep or other medical conditions. Patient 02 was a 78-year-old company owner who had suffered from sleep disorders for 15 years. During the day, he felt quite energetic due to work demands, but in the evening he was increasingly worried about his sleep problems, and at bedtime his anxiety about insomnia increased. He had been taking sleeping pills repeatedly for a year.

INTERVENTION: After a thorough medical examination, a *yoga-nidrā* intervention was initiated, followed by five supervised sessions, after which the patients were instructed to practice *yoga-nidrā* independently every day with the help of an audio recording. Regular follow-up visits were conducted every second week until four weeks after the start of the *yoga-nidrā* sessions. Repeated polysomnographic tests and assessments of various organ functions were offered if patients were willing to undergo them. The parameters of the sleep diaries kept by the subjects were also analysed.

RESULTS: After practising *yoga-nidrā*, both patients experienced improvements in sleep quality, insomnia severity, depression, anxiety and stress levels. These improvements were still present three months after the start of the intervention.

---

704 Datta, Karuna, Tripathi, M. & Mallick, H.N. (2017). Yoga Nidra: An innovative approach for management of chronic insomnia – A case report. *Sleep Science Practice*, 1(7). https://doi.org/10.1186/s41606-017-0009-4 (accessed on 12.09.2023).

Kohler et al. (2017)[705] examined the effect of *yoga-nidrā* meditation on reducing sleepiness and improving sustained attention after acute sleep deprivation.

INTERVENTION: Before and after a 21-day training programme with a concentrative form of *yoga-nidrā*, the participants in the experimental group completed tests measuring sustained attention and attention interference control. While attention interference control was maintained, sustained attention and alertness were impaired after a single night of sleep deprivation before the start of the study.

RESULTS: After only one *yoga-nidrā* session, sustained attention improved and drowsiness decreased. Rest alone did not have the same effect. These results demonstrate that *yoga-nidrā* can improve attention deficits after a lack of sleep. The effects of *yoga-nidrā* on attention could be explained by a lower mobilisation of mental processes, as this improvement was accompanied by less sleepiness.

CONCLUSION: Short-term implementation of *yoga-nidrā* appears to be sufficient to improve attention adversely affected by sleep deprivation.[706]

Sharpe et al. (2021)[707] examined how *yoga-nidrā* affects perceived relaxation and the extent to which the effect of *yoga-nidrā* compare with contemporary non-pharmaceutical interventions that could improve sleep quality.

INTERVENTION: The experiences of participants after a single 30-minute *yoga-nidrā* session (conducted in a total of 6 groups) were analysed using qualitative and quantitative methods.

---

705 Kohler, M., Rawlings, M., Kaeding, A.et al. (2017). Meditation is Effective in Reducing Sleepiness and Improving Sustained Attention Following Acute Sleep Restriction. *Journal of Cognitive Enhancement*, 1, 210–218. https://doi.org/10.1007/s41465–017-0032–5 (accessed on 12.09.2023).

706 The duration of the improvement after *yoga-nidrā* meditation training is not apparent from the study.

707 Sharpe, E., Tibbitts, D., Wolfe, B., Senders, A., & Bradley, R. (2021). Qualitative Impressions of a Yoga Nidra Practice for Insomnia: An Exploratory Mixed-Methods Design. *Journal of Alternative and Complementary Medicine* (New York, N.Y.), 27(10), 884–892. https://doi.org/10.1089/acm.2021.0125 (accessed on 12.09.2023).

RESULTS: The results of this analysis showed that *yoga-nidrā* was well received in the sample group, and the participants' descriptions suggested that *yoga-nidrā* could be useful for deeper relaxation, for falling asleep more easily, for alleviating anxiety and for pain relief.

Verma et al. (2021)[708] conducted a randomised study to examine the effects of yoga practice on coping with insomnia and on the associated complications such as cognitive failure, stress and impairment of the quality of life in individuals with acute insomnia.

INTERVENTION: Subjects were divided into a yoga group and a control group, each with 12 participants. The yoga group participated in yoga exercises for 60 minutes every day for 30 days, and for 30 days they practised *jala-netī* three times a week and *yoga-nidrā* once a week. The control group received conventional treatment.

RESULTS: After the intervention, the reduction in stress and improvement in sleep quality were significantly better in the yoga group than in the control group. Significant improvements were also seen in three aspects of quality of life — physical, mental and social — in the yoga group.

Datta et al. (2021)[709] studied 41 patients with chronic insomnia who participated in a study conducted between 2012 and 2016. 20 patients were assigned to cognitive behavioural therapy for insomnia and 21 to *yoga-nidrā*. The *yoga-nidrā* technique was conducted using the copyrighted audio CD of the Bihar School of Yoga after prior approval. The supervised sessions were conducted in a laboratory, and the *yoga-nidrā* intervention model was standardised for *yoga-nidrā* practice by developing guidelines for the observer.

---

708 Verma, K., Srivastava, A. & Singh, D. (2022). Effects of Yoga on Psychological Health and Sleep Quality of Patients With Acute Insomnia: A Preliminary Study. *Advances in Mind-Body Medicine*, 36(4), 4–11. https://pubmed.ncbi.nlm.nih.gov/36351185/ (accessed on 15.09.2023).

709 Datta, Karuna et al. (2021). Yoga nidra practice shows improvement in sleep in patients with chronic insomnia: A randomized controlled trial. In *National Medical Journal India*, 34(3), 143–50. https://nmji.in/yoga-nidra-practice-shows-improvement-in-sleep-in-patients-with-chronic-insomnia-a-randomized-controlled-trial/ (accessed on 12.09.2023).

RESULTS: The results were evaluated both subjectively and objectively using a sleep diary and polysomnography (PSG), respectively. Salivary cortisol levels were also examined. The PSG was performed on all patients before the intervention and repeated on a voluntary basis afterwards. The results showed that both behavioural therapy and *yoga-nidrā* improved overall wake time and subjective sleep quality. After a *yoga-nidrā* intervention, salivary cortisol levels decreased significantly.

CONCLUSION: According to the researchers, the *yoga-nidrā* method can be used to treat chronic insomnia after supervised exercise sessions.

Sharpe et al. (2023)[710] chose 22 adults who reported suffering from insomnia as test subjects to investigate the physiological and psychological effects of *yoga-nidrā*. Brain waves were measured using electroencephalography, heart rate variability and respiratory rate were recorded, and the mood reported by the participants themselves was evaluated.

INTERVENTION: During the first visit to the research centre, participants were asked to lie quietly for 90 minutes in a supine position. The primary outcome measured was changes in brain waves as detected by electroencephalography. During the second visit, the same protocol was followed, except that half of the participants were randomly selected to practice *yoga-nidrā* for the first 30 of the total 90 minutes.

RESULTS: In response to *yoga-nidrā*, the breathing rate was significantly reduced. This preliminary clinical study provided initial evidence that *yoga-nidrā* is a well-tolerated and easy-to-use intervention for adults suffering from insomnia.

---

710 Sharpe, E., Butler, M. P., Clark-Stone, J., Soltanzadeh, R., Jindal, R., Hanes, D. & Bradley, R. (2023). A closer look at yoga nidra- early randomized sleep lab investigations. *Journal of psychosomatic research*, 166, 111169. https://doi.org/10.1016/j.jpsychores.2023.111169 (accessed on 12.09.2023).

Datta et al. (2023)[711] used objective parameters to investigate the effects of *yoga-nidrā* practice on cognitive performance and nighttime sleep.

INTERVENTION: 41 healthy volunteers were included in the study, and a sleep diary was kept at the beginning of the study. The subjects underwent overnight polysomnography and cognitive tests which consisted of a motor practice test, an emotion recognition task, a task for replacing digital symbols, a task for learning visual objects, an abstract matching task, a task for orientation along a line, a task for logical thinking in a matrix, a fractal-2-back test, a task for psychomotor vigilance and an analogue balloon risk task[712]. *Yoga-nidrā* was practised for two weeks after the cognitive training. The tests were repeated for comparison one week and two weeks after *yoga-nidrā* was started. Polysomnography was performed before and after to evaluate the effects of the *yoga-nidrā* intervention.

RESULTS: Shorter (faster) reaction times were observed for all ten cognitive tasks. Polysomnography revealed a significant difference after the intervention compared to the baseline. The change data showed an improvement in sleep efficiency, waking up after sleep onset, and delta wave activity in deep sleep. Cognitive performance was significantly increased after two weeks of *yoga-nidrā* practice. After two weeks of *yoga-nidrā* practice, there were increased levels of recognition of emotions such as happiness, fear and anger.

CONCLUSION: The *yoga-nidrā* method improves cognitive performance and leads to higher sleep quality, even in yoga beginners.

---

711 Datta, Karuna., Bhutambare, A., V L, M., Narawa, Y., Srinath, R., & Kanitkar, M. (2023). Improved sleep, cognitive processing and enhanced learning and memory task accuracy with Yoga nidra practice in novices. *PloS one*, 18(12), e0294678. https://doi.org/10.1371/journal.pone.0294678 (accessed on 12.09.2023).

712 The Balloon Analogue Risk Test (BART) is a decision-making task that tests behavioural risk-taking, which is associated with greed.

Yoga-nidrā alleviating migraines

Kisan et al. (2014)[713] investigated the effectiveness of yoga techniques as a supportive therapy for migraine patients by analysing clinical outcomes and tests of autonomic function.

> **INTERVENTION:** 60 migraine patients were randomly assigned to either conventional treatment or yoga with conventional treatment. The yoga group performed a yoga programme consisting of *āsanas*, *śavāsana*, and *yoga-nidra* five days a week for six weeks in addition to conventional treatment. Clinical assessment (frequency, intensity, and impact of headaches) and autonomic function testing were performed at baseline and at the end of the intervention.

> **RESULTS:** Significant improvements in clinical variables were observed in both the yoga therapy and conventional therapy groups, but the improvements were more pronounced in the yoga therapy group. In migraine patients who received yoga as an adjunct therapy, headache frequency and intensity were reduced more than in the group with conventional treatment alone. Furthermore, yoga therapy increased vagal tone and decreased sympathetic drive, thereby improving cardiac autonomic balance. It can be concluded that yoga therapy can be effectively used as an adjunctive therapy for individuals with migraine.

Shashikiran et al. (2022)[714] conducted a study in which 60 participants examined the effect of *yoga-nidrā* on brain activity in migraine patients.

> **INTERVENTION:** The 30 subjects in the intervention group completed *yoga-nidrā*, while the 30 subjects in the control group lay in a supine position (resting position without guided practice). The electroencephalographic data of the participants in both groups were recorded and evaluated both at the beginning and after the intervention.

---

713 Ibid.

714 Shashikiran, H. C., Shetty, P., Akshay, R., Venugopal, A. & Shetty, S. (2022). Effect of yoga nidra on the brain activity in individuals with migraine. *Yoga-Mimansa, Indian Journal of Traditional Knowledge*, 54(1), 18–23. DOI: 10.4103/ym.ym_35_22 (accessed on 12.09.2023).

RESULTS: The results showed increased frequency of alpha waves in the intervention group compared to the control group. The control group showed no significant changes in brain activity.

CONCLUSION: The results suggest that *yoga-nidrā* leads to relaxation indicated by increased alpha wave activity. This shows that *yoga-nidrā* contributes to the dominance of the parasympathetic nervous system and thus reduces the activation of the sympathetic nervous system. This study therefore suggests that *yoga-nidrā* could be used as an effective means of treating stress and neuropsychological symptoms in migraine patients.

Yoga-nidrā as a promoter of physical, mental and psychological health, general well-being and self-confidence

Kumar (2006)[715] found in a six-month study that practising *yoga-nidrā* reduced stress and anxiety in practitioners and that, due to the deep relaxation, a significant positive change in the alpha wave frequency in the brain and an improvement in the electrodermal activity of the subjects could be recorded. This indicates an improvement in physical and mental health as a result of practising *yoga-nidrā*.

Tripathi (2018) conducted a study[716] on 100 male participants aged 35 to 45 to investigate the effects of *yoga-nidrā* on physical and mental health. The subjects were examined in advance for their physical and mental health and then introduced to a training programme for *yoga-nidrā*.

715 Kumar, Kamakhya. (2006). A Study on the Improvement of Physical and Mental Health Through Yoga Nidra. In *Dev Sanskriti Inter-disciplinary Research Journal*, 4(4), 39–46. https://www.researchgate.net/publication/215451321_A_study_of_the_improvement_of_Physical_and_Mental_Health_through_Yoga_nidra (accessed on 12.09.2023).

716 Tripathi, R. C. (2018). Effects of yoga nidra on physical and psychological health. In M. Karasawa, M. Yuki, K. Ishii, Y. Uchida, K. Sato, & W. Friedlmeier (Eds.), Venture into cross-cultural psychology: Proceedings from the *23rd Congress of the International Association for Cross-Cultural Psychology*. https://doi.org/10.4087/CVPP9404 (accessed on 12.09.2023).

INTERVENTION: Participants were assigned to an experimental or a control group. The training programme for the experimental group was scheduled for 12 weeks, five days a week. Participants completed the training programme in the morning for about 60 minutes. The *yoga-nidrā* technique was facilitated by a yoga expert. Both groups underwent testing before and after.

RESULTS: The results indicated positive effects of *yoga-nidrā* on the overall physical and psychological health of middle-aged participants.

Ozdemir and Saritas (2019)[717] conducted a study with 110 patients to examine the effect of *yoga-nidrā* on self-esteem and body image in patients with burns.

INTERVENTION: This study was conducted with a quasi-experimental model. The participants were patients at the adult burn unit of a university hospital. The subjects were given tests before and after the intervention and a control group was tested as well. Data were collected using the Self-Description Form, the Rosenberg Self-Esteem Scale, and the Body Image Scale.

RESULTS: After practising *yoga-nidrā* there was a statistically significant increase in self-esteem and an improvement in body image in the experimental group. In the patients in the control group, a statistically significant decline was observed in body image perception in both testings.

CONCLUSION: Practising *yoga-nidrā* can increase the self-esteem of burn patients and significantly improve their body image.

Dwivedi (2020)[718] examined the effectiveness of *yoga-nidrā* for improving well-being in an experimental study. The 200 participants were divided

---

717 Ozdemir, Ahmdet & Saritas, Serdar. (2019). Effect of yoga nidra on the self-esteem and body image of burn patients. In *Complementary Therapy in Clinical Practice*, 35(5), 86–91. https://doi.org/10.1016/j.ctcp.2019.02.002 (accessed on 12.09.2023).

718 Dwivedi, Manish Kumar. (2022). Effectiveness of Yoga Nidra Intervention (Meditation) in Improving well-being of an Individual. *Indian Journal of Social Psychiatry*, 38(1):p 73–85, DOI: 10.4103/ijsp.ijsp_32_20 (accessed on 14.09.2023).

into two groups of 100 subjects, with Group 1 serving as a control group in which no interventions were implemented and Group 2 serving as the main experimental group.

INTERVENTION: The participants in Group 2 did *yoga-nidrā* once a week for a month and were also asked to practice at home. The data were collected before and after the application of *yoga-nidrā*. Then a follow-up examination was carried out to determine the degree of well-being according to four fundamental aspects on a comprehensive scale: 1) sense of meaning in life; 2) psychological needs for autonomy, competence and relatedness according to the self-determination theory; 3) domain-specific and general life satisfaction and 4) happiness at different levels — physical, mental, emotional.

RESULTS: The results showed that practising *yoga-nidrā* could significantly improve an individual's general well-being at different levels — physical, mental, and emotional.

Yoga-nidrā for excessive weight/obesity

Selvam and Elangovan (2018)[719] studied the effect of brisk walking combined with *yoga-nidrā* on selected psychological variables in obese college students.

INTERVENTION: 30 overweight college students aged between 19 and 24 were randomly assigned to an experimental group or a control group, each with 15 participants. The experimental group practised brisk walking for a maximum of one hour, followed by *yoga-nidrā*, 5 days a week in the morning for 12 weeks. The control group spent the exercise time in a resting position without any further intervention. Psychological tests were conducted in both groups before and after the experiment.

---

719 Selvam, A.S. & Elangovan, R. (2018). Effect of Brisk Walking with Yoga Nidra on Selected Psychological Variables among Obese College Boy. *Journal of Yoga, Physical Therapy and Rehabilitation*, 1(01), 1–4. http://doi.org/10.29011/YPTR-143.%20000043 (accessed on 13.09.2023).

RESULTS: Compared to the control group, the experimental group showed significantly improved emotional maturity and reduced anxiety compared to before as a result of the brisk walking combined with *yoga-nidrā*.

Yoga-nidra supporting and strengthening the immune system and affecting Complete Blood Count (CBC)

Pandya und Kumar (2007)[720] studied the effect of *yoga-nidrā* on a range of physiological variables in 80 college students and a control group of 30 students in a 6-month study. The subjects were selected from postgraduate yoga courses. The study was conducted at the Yoga Arogya Polyclinic of the Dev Sanskriti Vishwavidyalaya University in Haridwar, India.

INTERVENTION: The practice time of *yoga-nidrā* was 30 minutes.

RESULTS: The results showed an increase in alpha brain waves and electrodermal activity and a decrease in resting pulse and respiratory rates, as well as a drop in blood pressure. Consequently, it can be assumed that *yoga-nidrā* also has a beneficial effect on the immune system.

Kumar (2007)[721] observed in a further study that *yoga-nidrā* has a positive effect on blood cell formation, in particular on haemoglobin levels and the total leukocyte count.

Kumar und Joshi (2009)[722] observed a significant increase in alpha brain wave activity and galvanic skin response levels in 40 students aged 18 to 25

720 Pandya, Pranav & Kumar, Kamakhya. (2007). Yoga-Nidra and its Impact on Human Physiology- In *Yoga Vijñāna – The Science of Yoga Journal*. New Delhi, India, 1(1), pp. 1–18 https://www.researchgate.net/publication/260268130_Yoga_Nidra_Its_impact_on_Human_Physiology (accessed on 13.09.2023).

721 Kumar, Kamakhya. (2007). The Healing Sleep, Yoga Magazine Mind Body Spirit. 3(50), 42–44. In Kumakhya, Kumar. (2013). *A Handbook of Yoga Nidra*. New Delhi: D. K. Printworld (P) Ltd., p. 64.

722 Kumar, K.& Joshi, Bhanu (2009). Study on the Effect of Pranakarshan Pranayama & Yoga Nidra on Alpha EEG & GSR, Indian Journal of Traditional Knowledge, 8(3), 453–454. In Kumakhya, Kumar. (2013). *A Handbook of Yoga Nidra*. New Delhi: D. K. Printworld (P) Ltd., p. 65.

years after 40 days of *prāṇākarṣaṇa-prāṇāyāma* and *yoga-nidrā* practice.[723] From the measured values, it can be concluded that yoga practice aids in improving the students' immunity.

Kumar und Pandya (2012)[724] conducted a six-month study on the effect of *yoga-nidrā* in particular on the erythrocyte sedimentation rate (ESR)[725] in healthy subjects. The study was conducted at the Yoga Arogya Polyclinic of the Dev Sanskriti Vishwavidyalaya in collaboration with the Brahmavarchas Research Institute, Haridwar.

INTERVENTION: For the experimental group, 80 students with regular yoga practice who additionally practised *yoga-nidrā* for 30 minutes a day were selected. The control group consisted of another 30 students.

RESULTS: As a result of *yoga-nidrā* practice, there was a significant change in the ESR value in the subjects. The study found that *yoga-nidrā* lowered the ESR value in both male and female subjects, thus promoting immune health.

CONCLUSION: The researchers recommend conducting further studies to examine the effect of *yoga-nidrā* on patients with high ESR levels, i.e. with weak immunity.

723 The galvanic skin response is a measure of the individual physiological response to external and internal stimuli.

724 Kumar, Kamakhya & Pandya, Pranav. (2012). A study on the impact on ESR level through Yogic Relaxation Technique Yoga Nidra, Indian Journal of Traditional Knowledge. 11(2), 358–361. In Kumakhya, Kumar. (2013). *A Handbook of Yoga Nidra*. New Delhi: D. K. Printworld (P) Ltd., p. 67.

725 The erythrocyte sedimentation rate, or abbreviated ESR, is based on how quickly red blood cells settle in a test tube. This indirectly determines whether there is a disease causing inflammation in the body.

Yoga-nidrā regulating high blood pressure and helping with heart disease

Datey und Bhagat (1977)[726] showed that extended *śavāsana* practice, which is a part of *yoga-nidrā*, also contributes toward lower blood pressure in hypertensive patients.

Bali (1979)[727] conducted a study at the Langley Porter Neuropsychiatric Institute at the University of California to examine the long-term effect of relaxation through *yoga-nidrā* for lowering blood pressure and anxiety. Eighteen male patients with significantly elevated blood pressure were examined.

> RESULTS: Relaxation was able to significantly reduce both blood pressure and anxiety levels. The effect lasted for twelve months after the *yoga-nidrā* training.

Agras (1980)[728] conducted a study at Stanford University School of Medicine (USA) which showed that regular *yoga-nidrā* practice lowers blood pressure and has a lasting effect that lasts throughout the day and is not just a temporary effect limited to the hour of practice.

Nirmalānanda and Choudhary (2006–2007)[729] conducted a controlled study on the efficacy of techniques of the Bihar Yoga system, with integrated *yoga-nidrā* practice as a complementary treatment for hypertension. Thirty-four subjects were assigned to the yoga group and 12 subjects to the control group, and were examined over a period of 12 months using symptoms, objective clinical observations and medication use as parameters.

---

726 Datey, K. K. & Bhagat, S. J. (1977). Stress and Heart Desease and How to Control It with Biofeedback and Shavasana, Quart. Journal for Surgical Science, Banaras Hindu University, 13. In Kamakhya Kumar. (2013). *A Handbook of Yoga-Nidrā*. New Delhi: D. K. Printworld (P) Ltd., p. 55.

727 Bali, Lekh Raj. (1979). Long-Term Effect of Relaxation on Blood Pressure and Anxiety Levels of Essential Hypertensive Males: A Controlled Study, Psychosomatic Medicine, 41(8), p. 637–646. In Kamakhya, Kumar. (2013). *A Handbook of Yoga-Nidrā*. New Delhi: D. K. Printworld (P) Ltd., p. 118

728 Agras W. S., Taylor C. B., Kraemer H. C., Allen R. A. & Schneider J. A. (1980). Relaxation Training: Twenty-four-Hour Blood Pressure Reductions. *Archives of General Psychiatry*, 37(8), 859–863. doi:10.1001/archpsyc.1980.01780210017001 (accessed on 13.09.2023).

729 Nirmalananda, Swami. (n.d.). Research III: Effect of Satyananda Yoga on Hypertension. In Yoga Research Foundation: Volume two. (2017). *Promotion of Health 1988–2007*. Bihar: Yoga Publication Trust., p. 48–82.

RESULTS: The results show highly significant relief in four out of six symptoms — reduction in systolic and diastolic blood pressure, reduction in medication use, improvement in symptoms such as shortness of breath, dizziness, discomfort and heaviness in the chest, clinically significant improvement in headaches and sleep disorders, and a significant change in BMI[730]. No significant change in waist/hip circumference and no effect on hypertensive retinopathy were observed.[731]

CONCLUSION: Bihar Yoga and *yoga-nidrā* are effective complementary therapies for the treatment of hypertension.

Kumar (2005)[732] conducted a study that aimed to determine the effect of *yoga-nidrā* on high blood pressure and its psychological side effects.

INTERVENTION: The practice time was 30 minutes for 15 days. 40 subjects between the ages of 30 and 60 were selected for the study: 30 businessmen and 10 housewives, all with mild hypertension.

RESULTS: The result showed a significant change in the values. It can be concluded that *yoga-nidrā* has a positive effect on blood pressure (both systolic and diastolic) as well as pulse rate, respiratory rate, stress, anger and anxiety.

Pandya and Kumar (2007)[733] observed significant changes in pulse rate, respiratory rate, blood pressure and electrodermal activity in the subjects of their study. They also found that *yoga-nidrā* practice increased practitioners' immunity.

---

730 High blood pressure is associated with an increased waist circumference in many people.

731 Hypertensive retinopathy is a disease of the retina caused by high blood pressure.

732 Kumar, Kamakhya. (2005). Effect of Yoga Nidra on Hypertension and other Psychological Co-relates. In *Yoga the Science Journal*, Yoga Publiations, Hubli, Karnataka, 3(7), 29–36. https://www.researchgate.net/publication/215451330_Effect_of_Yoga_nidra_on_hypertension_other_psychological_co-relates (accessed on 13.09.2023).

733 Kumar, Kamakhya & Pandya, Pranav. (2007). Yoga-Nidra and its Impact on Human Physiology. In *Yoga Vijñāna – The Science of Yoga Journal*, New Delhi, India, 1(1), pp. 1–18, https://www.researchgate.net/publication/260268130_Yoga_Nidra_Its_impact_on_Human_Physiology (accessed on 13.09.2023)

On the basis of his studies, **Kumar (2009)**[734] suggested that *yoga-nidrā* should also be used as a preventive measure against coronary heart disease.

Markil et al. (2012)[735] conducted a comparative study in a university laboratory for movement physiology to examine whether the effect of *yoga-nidrā*, practiced on its own, differs from *yoga-nidrā* practiced in combination with physical-mental practices (*haṭha-yoga*). The acute heart rate variability (HRV) reactions were used for the measurement. HRV data are often used as an index of the balance of the autonomic nervous system and thus of the stability of the heart muscle. Previous studies suggested that relaxation or physical-mental exercises can positively influence the balance of the autonomic nervous system measured by HRV, but may work through different mechanisms.

INTERVENTION: 20 adult male and female subjects with a mean age of 29 years were studied, who completed a yoga plus *yoga-nidrā* session and a pure *yoga-nidrā* session.

RESULTS: The intervention led to significant changes in heart rate and HRV indices in both cases. The *yoga-nidrā*-only group also showed significant changes in heart rate compared to the baseline. These changes showed a favourable shift in the autonomic balance towards the parasympathetic branch of the autonomic nervous system for both interventions.

CONCLUSION: Whether practised alone or preceded by *haṭha-yoga*, *yoga-nidrā* as a method for relaxation can produce positive changes in HRV measurements.

---

734 Kumar, Kamakhya & Joshi, Bhanu. (2009). Reversing the Ischemic Heart Disease through Yoga Nidra. *Nature and Wealth*, 8(1), 453–454. https://www.researchgate.net/publication/215585754_Reversing_the_Ischemic_Heart_Disease_through_Yoga_Nidra (accessed on 13.09.2023).

735 Markil, N., Whitehurst, M., Jacobs, P. L., & Zoeller, R. F. (2012). Yoga Nidra relaxation increases heart rate variability and is unaffected by a prior bout of Hatha yoga. *Journal of alternative and complementary medicine* (New York, N.Y.), 18(10), 953–958. https://doi.org/10.1089/acm.2011.0331 (accessed on 13.09.2023).

Devi and Kala (2015)[736] conducted a study on the effect of *yoga-nidrā* and *śiro-dhāra* (an Āyurvedic treatment where therapeutic oil is allowed to pour or drip over the forehead) on patients with high blood pressure.

INTERVENTION: 32 hypertensive patients aged between 30 and 60 years participated in the study. A pre-post single-group design was used.

RESULTS: The hypertensive patients who practised *yoga-nidrā* and *śiro-dhārā* showed a significant reduction in systolic and diastolic blood pressure.

Bajpai (2015)[737] conducted a study to determine whether regular practice of *bhrāmarī prāṇāyāma* and *yoga-nidrā* over a period of three months can reduce cardiovascular hyperreactivity to a blood pressure test in 94 young, healthy medical students.

INTERVENTION: Before and after the yoga practice, each participant's blood pressure was tested.

RESULTS: Hyperreactivity to the blood pressure test decreased by 79%—the number of people with hyperreactivity decreased from 32 before the start of the study to seven after three months of the yoga practice. Among the hyperreactive individuals, the systolic and diastolic blood pressure increases decreased significantly. The mean systolic blood pressure decreased in all 94 subjects, and the mean diastolic blood pressure also decreased significantly.

CONCLUSION: *Bhrāmarī-prāṇāyāma* and *yoga-nidrā* in combination can significantly mitigate stress-related changes in cardiovascular parameters.

---

736 Devi, Saraswati & Kala, Saraswati. (2015). Role of Yoga-nidra and Shirodhara on Hypertensive Patients. *International Journal of Yoga and Allied Sciences*, 4 (1), 22–27. http://indianyoga.org/wp-content/uploads/2015/05/v4-issue1-article4.pdf (accessed on 13.09.2023.)

737 Bajpai, R., Rajak, C., & Rampalliwar, S. (2015). Effect of Bhramari Pranayama and Yoga Nidra on cardiovascular hyper-reactivity to cold pressor test. *International Journal of Medical Science Research and Practice*, 2(1), 24–26. https://www.ijmsrp.com/wp-content/uploads/2015/04/07_Ritu_Bajpai.pdf (accessed on 08.02.2023).

Manik and Gartia (2016)[738] conducted a comparative study to find out the effect of *yoga-nidrā* and *nāḍī-śodhana-prāṇāyāma* on essential hypertension. A sample of 120 people was randomly selected from the Sambalpur district in Odisha, India. The subjects' ages ranged from 21 to 65 years.

> **INTERVENTIONS:** The subjects were divided into two groups of 60 each: a *yoga-nidrā* group and a *nāḍī-śodhana* group. Objective parameters such as systolic blood pressure, diastolic blood pressure, pulse rate, respiratory rate, body mass index (BMI) and the Hamilton Anxiety Rating Scale were used as a basis for measurement.[739] The *yoga-nidrā* group participated in *yoga-nidrā* for one hour in the morning over a period of four weeks. The *nāḍī-śodhana* group practised *nāḍī-śodhana-prāṇāyāma* for 30 minutes every day over a period of four weeks. The subjective and objective parameters were recorded for both groups before and after the programme.

> **RESULTS:** The *yoga-nidrā* group showed a significant reduction in blood pressure (systolic and diastolic), pulse rate, respiratory rate, BMI and anxiety scale scores. In the *nāḍī-śodhana*-only group, there was a particularly noticeable significant reduction in respiratory rate.

Thangam und Bharati (2019)[740] conducted a study to evaluate the effect of *yoga-nidrā* on older people with hypertension. With the help of a random sample, 35 older people were selected from a nursing home. 20 of the subjects were assigned to the experimental group and 15 to the control group.

> **INTERVENTION:** The *yoga-nidrā* practice was performed once a day in the morning between 6 and 8 am for 15 days. On the first and the 15th day, blood pressure was measured and the values were documented.

---

738 Manik, Ricardo & Gartia, Rajendra. (2016). A Comparative Study of Yoga Nidra and Nadisodhana Pranayam on Essential Hypertension. In *Advanced Science Letters*, 22(2), pp. 437–441(5), https://www.researchgate.net/publication/303808615_A_Comparative_Study_of_Yoga_Nidra_and_Nadisodhana_Pranayam_on_Essential_Hypertension (accessed on 13.09.2023).

739 The Hamilton Anxiety Scale contains fourteen questions on different symptom groups to determine the severity of an anxiety disorder through external assessment.

740 Thangam, F. E. & Bharathi, A.D. (2019). Effect of Yoga-nidra on Blood Pressure among Elderly with Hypertension Residing at Selected Old Age Homes, Coimbatore. *International Journal of Nursing Education and Research*, 7(1), pp. 30–32. http://dx.doi.org/10.5958/2454-2660.2019.00006.1(accessed on 13.09.2023).

RESULTS: The study showed a significant reduction in both the mean systolic and diastolic blood pressure of the subjects in the *yoga-nidrā* group. It can therefore be concluded that *yoga-nidrā* is an effective measure for lowering blood pressure in older people with hypertension.

Chhetri at al. (2020) conducted a study[741] to examine the immediate effects of *yoga-nidrā* on heart rate variability (HRV) parameters in young healthy volunteers.

INTERVENTION: 52 male medical students were divided into two groups of 26 subjects each. The participants in one group were to lie on their backs for a certain period of time, while the other group practised *yoga-nidrā*. The HRV indices were recorded before and after lying on one's back and practising *yoga-nidrā* respectively and compared within and between groups.

RESULTS: Compared to mere supine position, *yoga-nidrā* led to a significant change in HRV values, indicating that the parasympathetic modulating response with *yoga-nidrā* was more effective than that of supine lying. *Yoga-nidrā* produced a better relaxation response than supine lying alone, as indicated by the significantly improved HRV indices.

Rajagopalan et al. (2022)[742] recruited 80 patients with diagnosed hypertension for a study, randomly assigning them to either an experimental or control group.

INTERVENTION: The experimental group participated in a combination of *oṃ*-repetition/chanting and *yoga-nidrā* five days a week for a period of two months. The control group continued to take their regular

---

741 Chhetri, Praghosh et al. (2020). Immediate Effects of Yoga Based Relaxation Technique on Heart Rate Variability in Young and Healthy Volunteers. *Journal of Karnali Academy of Health Sciences*, 3(2), 65–72. https://doi.org/10.3126/jkahs.v3i2.30807 (accessed on 13.09.2023).

742 Rajagopalan, A., Krishna, A. & Mukkadan, J. K. (2022). Effect of Om chanting and Yoga Nidra on depression anxiety stress, sleep quality and autonomic functions of hypertensive subjects - a randomized controlled trial. *Journal of Basic and Clinical Physiology and Pharmacology*, 34(1), 69–75. https://doi.org/10.1515/jbcpp-2022–0122 (accessed on 13.09.2023).

medication. Depression Anxiety Stress Scale, Pittsburgh Sleep Quality Index[743] and heart rate variability (HRV) scores were determined for both groups at baseline and then at 30 and 60 days respectively.

RESULTS: The study confirms the efficacy of *oṃ*-repetition/chanting and *yoga-nidrā* in reducing depression, anxiety and stress, and in improving sleep quality and autonomic function in hypertensive patients.

CONCLUSION: The interventions used in this study can be considered a safer form of complementary therapy for managing stress and hypertension.

Anjana et al. (2022)[744] conducted a randomised controlled trial to examine the effect of *ōṃ*-recitation and *yoga-nidrā* (as a relaxation technique) on blood pressure and lipid profiles in individuals with hypertension.

INTERVENTION: Eighty patients with diagnosed hypertension were randomly assigned to either an experimental or a control group. Patients in the experimental group performed a combination of *ōṃ*-recitation and *yoga-nidrā* for two months, five days a week, while patients in the control group continued to take their regular medication. Blood pressure and lipid profile parameters were measured in both groups at baseline, on day 30 and on day 60.

RESULTS: After two months, a significant reduction in blood pressure and lipid profile was observed in the experimental group compared to the control group. In addition, a significant increase in HDL-cholesterol[745]-levels was observed in the experimental group. During the study, no adverse effects were reported by the subjects in the experimental group who were not taking medication.

---

743 The Pittsburgh Sleep Quality Index is a standardised self-assessment questionnaire used to assess sleep quality over a period of one month.

744 Anjana, K., Archana, R., & Mukkadan, J. K., (2022). Effect of om chanting and yoga nidra on blood pressure and lipid profile in hypertension – A randomized controlled trial. In *Journal of Ayurveda Integrative Medicine*, 13(4). https://doi.org/10.1016/j.jaim.2022.100657. (accessed on 13.09.2023).

745 The so-called 'good' cholesterol.

Yoga-nidrā and asthma

Nirmalānanda and Tiwari (2006–2007)[746] studied the effectiveness of the integral system of Bihar Yoga (*ṣaṭkarman-*, *āsana-*, *prāṇāyāma-*, *yoga-nidrā* and other *pratyāhāra*-techniques) as an additional treatment for people in the older age group (mean 55.8 years) with long-standing asthma and chronic obstructive pulmonary disease (COPD) (mean duration of illness 12.4 years).

INTERVENTION: The health status of the 20 subjects in the yoga group and the 21 participants in the control group was assessed on the basis of symptoms, objective clinical observations, spirometry and medication over a period of one year. The results showed a relief of symptoms, an improvement in breath holding time and a reduction in the use of medication in the yoga group.

RESULTS: Spirometry tests showed improvement in forced expiratory volume in the first second and forced vital capacity.

CONCLUSION: The study concludes that Bihar Yoga (including *yoga-nidrā*) is effective in the treatment of long-standing asthma and COPD.

Yoga-nidrā alleviating physical and psychological menstrual disorders and having a positive effect on the endocrine system and hormonal status

Rani et al. (2011)[747] conducted a study on the effectiveness of *yoga-nidrā* for mental health issues such as emotional insecurity, stress, and symptoms of depression and/or anxiety of varying severity in patients with menstrual disorders. The 150 subjects were selected at the Department of

746 Ibid., p. 85–134.

747 Rani, K., Tiwari, S., Singh, U., Agrawal, G., Ghildiyal, A., & Srivastava, N. (2011). Impact of Yoga Nidra on psychological general wellbeing in patients with menstrual irregularities: A randomized controlled trial. *International Journal of Yoga*, 4(1), 20–25. https://doi.org/10.4103/0973-6131.78176 (accessed on 13.09.2023).

Obstetrics and Gynaecology at Chhatrapati Sahuji Maharaj Medical University, Lucknow, India.

INTERVENTION: The subjects were randomly divided into two groups: one group of 75 women did *yoga-nidrā*, while the control group of 75 subjects did not take part in any yoga programme. In both groups, psychological well-being was assessed at the beginning of the study and then after six months.

RESULTS: The results showed that after six months of regular yoga therapy with *yoga-nidrā*, there was a significant reduction in anxiety and depression and a significant improvement in the psychological well-being, general health and vitality of the subjects compared to the control group.

In a follow-up study using the same format, **Rani et al. (2011)** investigated[748] the effects of complementary *yoga-nidrā* treatment in patients with menstrual disorders and somatoform symptoms[749], who had previously been treated with medication.

RESULTS: The results showed a significant improvement in pain symptoms as well as gastrointestinal, cardiovascular and urogenital symptoms after six months of *yoga-nidrā* therapy in the intervention group compared to the control group.

In yet another study, **Rani et al. (2012)**[750] were able to show that *yoga-nidrā* is a promising complementary therapy for both acute and long-standing hormonal mental disorders of all kinds, in particular for depression, anxiety disorders and neurotic patterns. In patients with mild to moderate anxiety

748 Rani, K., Tiwari, S. C., Singh, U., Agrawal, G. G., & Srivastava, N. (2011). Six-month trial of Yoga Nidra in menstrual disorder patients: Effects on somatoform symptoms. *Industrial Psychiatry Journal*, 20(2), 97–102. https://doi.org/10.4103/0972–6748.102489 (accessed on 13.09.2023).

749 Somatoform symptoms are a relatively common form of physical discomfort that can be clearly described by the person affected, but for which no organic cause can be found on medical examination.

750 Rani, K., Tiwari, S., Singh, U., Singh, I., & Srivastava, N. (2012). Yoga Nidra as a complementary treatment of anxiety and depressive symptoms in patients with menstrual disorder. *International Journal of Yoga*, 5(1), 52–56. https://doi.org/10.4103/0973–6131.91715 (accessed on 13.09.2023).

and depressive symptoms, mental well-being improved significantly after six months of yoga therapy with *yoga-nidrā* compared to the control group.

Monika et al. (2012)[751] studied the effect of *yoga-nidrā* on the physiological variables for establishing balance between the sympathetic and parasympathetic nervous systems in patients with menstrual cramps, in particular, the effect on the functions of the autonomic nervous system.

> RESULTS: After six months of *yoga-nidrā* practice, lasting 35 to 40 minutes five times a week, a significant improvement in blood pressure, postural hypotension, and sustained isometric handgrip[752] was observed in the *yoga-nidrā* group compared to the control group, as well as in the regulation of heartbeat and breathing rhythm.

Rani et al. (2013)[753] studied the effect of *yoga-nidrā* on menstrual abnormalities, particularly on the hormonal profile of patients with menstrual irregularities.

> RESULTS: A six-month *yoga-nidrā* practice with 35 to 40 minutes of daily practice, five days a week, proved helpful for patients with hormonal menstrual disorders such as dysmenorrhea, oligomenorrhea, menorrhagia, metrorrhagia, and hypomenorrhea. Thyroid-stimulating, follicle-stimulating and luteinising hormones, as well as prolactin, were significantly reduced in the intervention group compared to the control group.

Gawali et al. (2015)[754] tested the effectiveness of *sūrya-namaskāra* (salutation to the sun) and *yoga-nidrā* on the physical and mental problems of 180 adolescent girls (average age 13 years) during their menstruation.

---

751 Monika, Singh, U., Ghildiyal, A., Kala, S., & Srivastava, N. (2012). Effect of Yoga Nidra on physiological variables in patients of menstrual disturbances of reproductive age group. *Indian Journal of Physiology and Pharmacology*, 56(2), 161–167. https://ijpp.com/IJPP%20archives/2012_56_2_%20Apr%20-%20Jun/161-167.pdf (accessed on 13.09.2023).

752 The isometric handgrip is routinely used to measure the response to a pressure stimulus. This test involves a complex set of multiple factors, including sympathetic and parasympathetic output.

753 Rani, Monika., Singh, U., Agrawal, G. G., Natu, S. M., Kala, S., Ghildiyal, A., & Srivastava, N. (2013). Impact of Yoga Nidra on menstrual abnormalities in females of reproductive age. *Journal of Alternative and Complementary Medicine* (New York, N.Y.), 19(12), 925–929. https://doi.org/10.1089/acm.2010.0676 (accessed on 13.09.2023).

754 Gawali, Minakshi Haribhau. (2015). Effect of suryanamaskar and yoga nidra on menstruation problems of adolescent girls. *Semantic Scholar*. https://www.semanticscholar.org/paper/Effect-of-suryanamaskar-and-

INTERVENTION: The subjects were divided into three groups of 60 girls each, who either practised sūrya-namaskāra or *yoga-nidrā* or formed the control group. A 24-week *sūrya-namaskāra* or *yoga-nidrā* programme was conducted in the respective yoga groups, while the control group did not participate in any yoga practice. The self-concept scale of Saraswat (1981) and Sinha's Comprehensive Anxiety Test (1973) were used to collect data.

RESULTS: Both *sūrya-namaskāra* and the *yoga-nidrā* programme appeared to reduce the girls' physical problems during menstruation and lower their anxiety levels, as well as improve their self-concept from an average to a high level within 24 weeks.

Rani et al. (2016)[755] confirmed in a study conducted in the same format that the mean values for anxiety, depression, subjective well-being, general state of health and vitality, as well as the hormone levels of female subjects with menstrual disorders in the intervention group, differed significantly and in a positive way from the values of the control group.

Vanitha et al. (2018)[756] examined the effect of a 12-week *yoga-nidrā* intervention on resting cardiovascular parameters in 40 women aged between 18 and 35 years who suffered from polycystic ovary syndrome.

INTERVENTION: The daily 40-minute *yoga-nidrā* intervention in a lying position was led by a yoga teacher and doctor of yoga and naturopathy. The cardiovascular parameters such as systolic blood pressure, diastolic blood pressure and heart rate were recorded as standard before and after the intervention.

---

yoga-nidra-on-problems-Gawali/739d6d988b7018a65484d96915458c9ef81c0715 (accessed on 08.02.2023.)

755 Rani, Khushbu., Tiwari, S. C., Kumar, S., Singh, U., Prakash, J., & Srivastava, N. (2016). Psycho-Biological Changes with Add on Yoga Nidra in Patients with Menstrual Disorders: a Randomized Clinical Trial. *Journal of Caring Sciences*, 5(1), 1–9. https://doi.org/10.15171/jcs.2016.001 (accessed on 13.09.2023).

756 Vanitha, A., Pandiaraja, M., Maheshkumar, K. & Venkateswaran S. T. (2018) Effect of yoga nidra on resting cardiovascular parameters in polycystic ovarian syndrome women. *National Journal of Physiology, Pharmacy and Pharmacology*, 8 (11), 1505–1508. http://dx.doi.org/10.5455/njppp.2018.8.0411112082018 (accessed on 13.09.2023)

RESULTS: There was a significant reduction in resting cardiovascular parameters such as heart rate, systolic and diastolic blood pressure.

Yoga-nidrā and pain management

Li et al. (2018)[757] conducted a study in which the effects of *yoga-nidrā* and relaxation music for pain management in patients undergoing a colonoscopy were compared.

INTERVENTION: A quasi-experimental design was used. The 144 patients scheduled to undergo a colonoscopy were assigned to three different treatment groups. Group 1 was an untreated control group, Group 2 listened to relaxation music, and Group 3 listened to a recording of *yoga-nidrā* instructions. Pain level was determined as the primary outcome measure. Secondary outcome measures of the effectiveness of the intervention were overall patient satisfaction, willingness to repeat the procedure, and difficulty in inserting the colonoscope. Secondary objective measurements of treatment effects included systolic and diastolic blood pressure and total procedure duration.

RESULTS: Results showed significant reductions in perceived pain and practitioner-rated difficulty of colonoscope insertion in Groups 2 and 3. Overall patient satisfaction was significantly improved in groups 2 and 3. Patients' willingness to repeat the procedure and the total duration of the procedure were significantly improved and shortened, respectively, in the *yoga-nidrā* group, although there were no significant differences compared to the music group. No statistically significant differences were found between the three groups in terms of blood pressure. The results showed that both the *yoga-nidrā* recording and relaxation music helped to reduce the pain felt by participants during

757 Li, L., Shu, W., Li, Z., Liu, Q., Wang, H., Feng, B. & Ouyang, Y. Q. (2019). Using Yoga Nidra Recordings for Pain Management in Patients Undergoing Colonoscopy. *Pain Management Nursing: Official Journal of the American Society of Pain Management Nurses*, 20(1), 39–46. https://doi.org/10.1016/j.pmn.2018.04.005 (accessed on 13.09.2023)

the colonoscopy. The *yoga-nidrā* instructions proved, however, to be the more successful intervention.

Maniket al. (2017)[758] conducted a study to examine the effect of selected yogic practices on pain conditions in lumbar spondylitis. 172 patients with lumbar spondylitis aged between 21 and 79 years from the outpatient neurosurgery department at AIIMS in Bhubaneswar, India, were randomly assigned to yoga therapy.

INTERVENTION: The module of selected yoga practices consisted of the Bihar Yoga series *pavana-muktāsana* 1 (loosening and strengthening), other *āsana*, *prāṇāyāma*, and *yoga-nidrā*. Within-group and between-group comparative tests were conducted. Correlation and regression analysis was performed to determine the degree of linear relationship between yoga therapy and pain sensation.

RESULTS: Significant differences were found in the yoga therapy group. Immediate relief was observed even with short-term practice. The results showed a significant reduction in pain intensity in that group over the long term. The selected yoga practices achieved good results in the treatment of pain in lumbar spondylitis.

Yoga-nidrā and its effect on diabetes patients

Nirmalānanda (1998) conducted research[759] at the Yoga Research Foundation in Ganga Darshan (*āśrama*) in Munger, India, on the effect of the Bihar Yoga integral yoga system on the blood sugar levels of people with type 2 diabetes mellitus who are not insulin-dependent.

---

758 Manik, Rajesh Kumar., Mahapatra, Ashok Kumar., Gartia, Rajendra., Bansal, Sumit., Patnaik, Ashis. (2017). Effect of Selected Yogic Practices on Pain and Disability in Patients with Lumbar Spondylitis. *International Journal of Yoga*, 10(2), 81–87. https://doi.org/10.4103/0973-6131.205516 (accessed on 13.09.2023).

759 Nirmalananda, Swami. (n.d.). Research 1: Effect of Yoga on Blood Sugar in Diabetics. In *Yoga Research Foundation: Volume Two*. (2017). Promotion of Health 1988–2007. Bihar: Yoga Publication Trust, p. 22–25.

INTERVENTION: The 66 participants were to spend 18 days on site, completing a special daily routine and yoga programme, as well as following an adapted diet as part of a course in diabetes health management. The yoga programme included a 90-minute *āsana* session, a one-hour *prāṇāyāma* session and a mantra session in the morning, with the *āsana* session being replaced by a *ṣaṭkarman* practice once a week. This was followed in the afternoon by an hour of *yoga-nidrā* and meditation, as well as an hour to repeat the exercises and *satsaṅga*[760] and, in the evening—an hour of *bhakti-yoga*. In addition, the subjects took part in the morning cleaning of the premises for an hour and in *sevā* (selfless service) in the *āśrama* for an hour. Overall, the subjects completed a 15-day integral yoga programme.

RESULTS: The results of this study showed significant improvement in blood sugar levels.

Nirmalānanda (2002 and 2003) conducted a study[761] with 15 type 2 diabetes patients in the summer of 2002, followed by five further studies in the summer of 2003. The subjects completed six weeks of intensive yoga practice based on the integral system of Bihar Yoga with *ṣaṭkarman*, *āsana*, *prāṇāyāma*, *yoga-nidrā* and other *pratyāhāra* techniques. In addition, the participants followed the daily *āśrama* routine. A continuation over five years was planned.

RESULTS: The preliminary results showed significant improvement in fasting and mid-morning blood sugar levels, as well as diabetes risk factors such as body mass index (BMI), waist-hip ratio and lipid profile. Some subjects were able to reduce their medication dosage.

Amita et al. (2009)[762] examined the effect of *yoga-nidrā* as a complementary treatment for stabilising blood sugar levels in 41 type 2 diabetics taking oral hypoglycemic agents.

---

760 *Satsaṅga* – the company of a master and listening to his lectures.

761 Nirmalananda, Swami. (n.d.). Research II: Effect of Yoga on Blood Sugar and Cardiac Risk Factors in Diabetics. In Yoga Research Foundation: Volume two. (2017). *Promotion of Health 1988–2007*. Bihar: Yoga Publication Trust, p. 29–43.

762 Amita, S., Prabhakar, S., Manoj, I., Harminder, S., & Pavan, T. (2009). Effect of yoga-nidra on blood glucose level in diabetic patients. *Indian Journal of Physiology and Pharmacology*, 53(1), 97–101. https://

INTERVENTION: Patients were divided into two groups: 20 patients who were treated with oral hypoglycaemic agents (blood-sugar-lowering medication) and additionally practised *yoga-nidrā* and 21 patients who took medication only. The *yoga-nidrā* practice extended over 90 days and was performed daily for 30 minutes. Blood sugar levels were recorded at 30-day intervals.

RESULTS: The results showed that there was significant improvement in most symptoms and that the mean blood sugar level had significantly decreased after only three months of *yoga-nidrā* practice. The results of this study clearly showed that subjects taking blood sugar lowering medication who regularly practised *yoga-nidrā* were able to better control their fluctuating blood sugar levels and the symptoms associated with diabetes than those who were treated only with hypoglycaemic medication.

Yoga-nidrā promoting the mental health of people who have suffered physical or emotional abuse

Lata and Singh (2014)[763] conducted a study to assess the effect of *yoga-nidrā* on 20 male and 20 female adolescents aged between 13 and 19 who had been victims of emotional and physical abuse. The subjects came from various schools and tutoring centres in the Chandausi district of Uttar Pradesh in India.

INTERVENTION: The subjects were assessed using the Emotional Abuse Test and the Mental Health Battery[764]. They were offered a *yoga-nidrā* course under supervised conditions that lasted for two months.

---

pubmed.ncbi.nlm.nih.gov/19810584/ (accessed on 13.09.2023)

763 Rajpoot, Lata, Pushp & Sanwat, Singh. (2014). A study of the effect of Yoga Nidra on mental health of emotionally abused adolescents. In Academia: *An International Multidisciplinary Research Journal*, 4(12), 6–14. https://www.academia.edu/76315471/A_study_of_the_effect_of_Yoga_Nidra_on_mental_health_of_emotionally_abused_adolescents (accessed on 14.09.2023).

764 The Mental Health Battery measures the level of mental health in adolescents based on psychological, physical, emotional and social aspects.

The results of the Mental Health Battery were used to evaluate the effectiveness of the experimental intervention.

RESULTS: In a before-and-after comparison, there was a significant reduction in the scores on the Mental Health Battery. The subjects felt that they had learned skills with *yoga-nidrā* that they could use in stressful situations to relax and better cope with stress and anxiety. They found that the yoga programme helped to reduce nervousness, tension, depression, dejection, hopelessness, illness and physical discomfort. They felt happier, contented, cheerful and carefree, and gained a new perspective on life.

CONCLUSION: According to this study, *yoga-nidrā* appears to have the potential to have a positive effect on the mental and physical well-being of emotionally and physically abused adolescents.

Yoga-nidrā strengthening the immune system of HIV/AIDS patients

Mishra (2013)[765] conducted a study on 30 HIV-positive patients from the Ayurvedic Panchkarma Hospital, East Champaran, Motihari, Bihar, India. Of this group, 20 patients were male and 10 were female. The age range was between 18 and 50 years.

INTERVENTION: The HIV-positive patients were divided into two groups. The 20 patients in Group A performed a *yoga-nidrā* technique in which they were asked to become aware of the movement of *prāṇa*. The *yoga-nidrā* practice lasted 40 minutes each day for three months. The ten patients in Group B practiced *pavana-muktāsana*-1 for the same period.

765 Mishra, Brajeshwar. (2013). Immunological Effect of Yoga Nidra on HIV/AIDS. In Collection Volume. (2013). *Experience of Yoga*. Bihar School of Yoga – Golden Jubilee 2013. Bihar: Yoga Publication Trust, p. 183–186.

RESULTS: The results of the study showed an increase in the CD4 figure[766] in Group A after three months of *yoga-nidrā* practice. At the beginning of the study, the CD4 figure in Group A was 155/mm3 on average, and after three months of *yoga-nidrā* practice it rose to around 228/mm3. In Group B, which practised *pavana-muktāsana*-1, the CD4 figure remained unchanged. Furthermore, *yoga-nidrā* led to an improvement in symptoms such as weight loss, fatigue, memory loss, depression, recurrent fever and skin problems. Cough, breathing difficulties and diarrhoea improved moderately, and cases of pulmonary tuberculosis improved slightly. Overall, based on observation, 50% of the patients in the *yoga-nidrā* group showed a significant improvement, 25% a moderate improvement and 15% a slight improvement.

CONCLUSION: *Yoga-nidrā* can be successfully used as a complementary method to alleviate the symptoms of HIV-positive patients.

Yoga-nidrā as a method of promoting self-efficacy and self-care in a professional context

Rani et al. (2013)[767] tested the effect of *yoga-nidrā* on the stress levels of first-year nursing students.

RESULTS: The study's results showed that practising *yoga-nidrā* significantly reduced the students' stress levels. The subjects also reported that practising *yoga-nidrā* made them feel relaxed, peaceful and calm.

CONCLUSION: Nurses play a vital role in helping patients manage stress by interacting with them as a whole person rather than just as medical cases. To meet the physical, emotional and mental needs of patients, a nurse should be mentally relaxed and balanced. Therefore,

766 CD4 cells are white blood cells that activate the immune system and are destroyed by HIV.

767 Rani, Ruchika., Kumar, A., Sharma, P. (2013). Effect of Yoga Nidra on Stress Level among B.Sc. Nursing first year students. *Nursing and Midwifery Research Journal*, (9), pp. 47–55. http://doi.org/10.33698/NRF0156 (accessed on 12.09.2023).

the researchers recommend training programmes for nurses to familiarise themselves with techniques that promote their own physical, psychological and mental health.

Kim (2014)[768] conducted a randomised control study on the effect of yogic practice on life stress and blood sugar levels in 27 nursing students (12 in an exercise group and 15 in a control group).

INTERVENTION: The yoga techniques were performed for 60 minutes one day a week for 12 weeks. The practice consisted of physical exercises (*sūrya-namaskāra*) combined with relaxation-associated practices (*śavāsana* and *yoga-nidrā*). Life stress was measured using the Life Stress Scale for College Students, and postprandial blood glucose levels[769] were measured using a digital blood glucose meter.

RESULTS: Compared to the control group, both life stress and postprandial blood glucose levels were significantly lower in the exercise group.

Anderson et al. (2017) conducted a pilot study[770] to examine the effect of *yoga-nidrā* on the stress levels of psychiatric nurses.

INTERVENTION: Nine nurses participated in six weekly *yoga-nidrā* sessions. Measurements of sleep quality, perceived stress and muscle fatigue were taken to determine whether the method had a positive effect on quality of life and stress reduction.

RESULTS: Although the sample of nurses was small, the results suggested a positive effect on both perceived stress levels and muscle fatigue. This pilot study demonstrated the potential benefits of *yoga-nidrā* for stress relief, muscle relaxation and self-care for nurses.

---

768 Kim, Sang Dol. (2014). Effects of yogic exercises on life stress and blood glucose levels in nursing students. *Journal of Physical Therapy Science*, 26(12), 2003–2006. https://doi.org/10.1589/jpts.26.2003 (accessed on 14.09.2023).

769 The postprandial blood sugar level is usually measured two hours after a meal.

770 Anderson, Roberta et al. (2017). Using yoga nidra to improve stress in psychiatric nurses in a pilot study. *Journal for Alternative and Complementary Medicine*, 23(6). https://doi.org/10.1089/acm.2017.004 (accessed on 14.09.2023).

Christine (2017)[771] conducted a study with nursing students with the following objectives: 1) to compare morning and evening stress levels before and after *yoga-nidrā* in the experimental group, 2) to compare morning and evening stress levels after the same test in the control group, 3) to determine differences in morning and evening stress levels as a function of background factors of the subjects, such as age, birth order, economic status, teaching medium, academic performance, friends, relationship with teachers, chronic illness, painful experience, health practices, availability of parents, conflicts between parents, financial support, living in a dormitory, academic year. 40 nursing students were assigned to an experimental group and 40 to a control group. The main study was conducted at selected colleges in Hyderabad. Data were collected using a scale developed by the researcher.

> **RESULTS:** The results of the study showed a significant difference in the experimental group compared to the control group between the stress level experienced before and after the test. Furthermore, there was a significant difference in the assessment of morning and evening stress levels in the experimental and control groups. With regard to the background factors, there was no significant correlation.

> **CONCLUSION:** The stress levels of nursing students could be reduced by practising *yoga-nidrā*. *Yoga-nidrā* can therefore be recommended as an accompanying measure in the training of nurses.

Reddy at al. (2018)[772] examined the effect of *yoga-nidrā* on the mental state of 60 people seeking to start their own business.

> **INTERVENTION:** The selected individuals were randomly assigned to an experimental or control group and evaluated. The subjects in the experimental group were instructed in the practice of *yoga-nidrā* for

---

771 Christine, Michael (2017). Effect of Yoga Nidra on Stress among Nursing Students in Selected Colleges of Nursing. *Asian Journal of Nursing, Education and Research*, 7(3), 429–440. https://doi.org/10.5958/2349–2996.2017.00085.4 (accessed on 14.09.2023).

772 Reddy, Dhrithi B., et al. (2018). Effect of Yoga Nidra on Mental Status Among Self-Employment Aspirants. *Journal of Emerging Technologies and Innovative Research*, 5(8), 412–419.https://www.jetir.org/papers/JETIR1808961.pdf (accessed on 14.09.2023).

30 minutes once a day for ten days. The subjects in the control group were instructed to rest in a supine position for 30 minutes.

RESULTS: A significant improvement in positive attitude was observed in the *yoga-nidrā* group.

CONCLUSION: *Yoga-nidrā* can therefore be considered a viable and cost-effective method for achieving a positive attitude towards career decisions.

Yoga-nidrā having a positive effect on athletic performance

Deuskar et al. (2006)[773] found a significant improvement in the concentration of archers who practised *yoga-nidrā* in comparison with those who did not. **Sethi and Singh (2016)**[774] studied the effect of *yoga-nidrā* on the reaction and anticipation times of wrestlers. 40 Indian wrestlers aged 18 to 25 took part in the study.

INTERVENTION: The subjects were divided into a group that completed *yoga-nidrā* training and a control group. The measurements quantified the wrestlers' fast and slow reactions, i.e. their reaction and anticipation times.

RESULTS: The archers' concentration and attention improved significantly as a result of practising *yoga-nidrā* (45 minutes a day for 54 days). Compared to the control group, the experimental group's simple visual reaction time and anticipation time were significantly faster.

773 Deuskar, Megha. Poonawala, N. & Bhatewara, Sunit. (2006). Effect of Yoga Nidra and Applied Relaxation Technique on Steadiness and Performance of Archers. *Psychological Studies*. University of Callicut, 51(1), 64–68. https://www.researchgate.net/publication/285875486_Effect_of_Yoga_Nidra_and_Applied_Relaxation_technique_on_steadiness_and_performance_of_archers (accessed on 14.09.2023)

774 Sethi, Pramod, Kumar & Singh, Vikram. (2016). Effect of Yoga Nidra on reaction time and anticipation time of wrestlers. In *International Journal of Physical Education, Sports and Health*, 3(5), 504–507. https://www.kheljournal.com/archives/2016/vol3issue5/PartI/3-5-99-152.pdf (accessed on 14.09.2023).

Mahesh and Sanjit (2016)[775] conducted a comparative study on the effect of *āsanas* and *yoga-nidrā* on the anxiety levels of 100 college football players between the ages of 18 and 24. The aim of this research was twofold: 1) to equip the participants with the best tools to deal with competition anxiety and performance anxiety, and 2) to try and scientifically verify the effect of yoga techniques.

INTERVENTION: Subjects were randomly assigned to one of two groups, one practicing *āsanas* and the other practicing *yoga-nidrā*. They completed all sessions during the two-week training programme and did not seek any other treatment during this time. Anxiety levels were measured in all subjects before and after the two-week training programme.

RESULTS: There was no significant difference in anxiety levels between the āsana and *yoga-nidrā* groups before the start of the exercise sessions. Participants with mild to moderate anxiety symptoms showed a significant reduction in their anxiety levels after two weeks of *yoga-nidrā* training. Those with severe anxiety symptoms showed only a very slight qualitative improvement, while quantitatively there was a greater reduction in anxiety levels.

CONCLUSION: This study shows that *yoga-nidrā* can be an effective tool for treating psychological issues such as fear of failure.

Das and Pandey (2020) conducted[776] a comparative study to examine the immediate effect of audiovisual biofeedback therapy and *yoga-nidrā* on lactate reduction and heart rate during the recovery phase of ten badminton players aged 18 to 23.

---

775 Yadav, Mahesh & Sardar, Sanjit. (2016). Comparative effect of yoga asana and yoga Nidra on the anxiety level of intercollegiate level football players. In *International Journal of Physical Education*, Sports and Health, (2), 148–150. https://www.kheljournal.com/archives/2016/vol3issue2/PartC/3-2-26.pdf (accessed on 14.09.2023)

776 Das, Payel & Pandey, Vivek. (2020). Comparative Effect of Audio-Visual Biofeedback Therapy and Yoga Nidra on Lactate Clearance and Heart Rate during Recovery of Badminton Players. *International Journal of Science and Research* (IJSR), 9(5), pp. 158–164. https://www.ijsr.net/archive/v9i5/SR20501010219.pdf (accessed on 14.09.2023).

INTERVENTION: Each subject underwent repeated treatment with either audiovisual biofeedback therapy or *yoga-nidrā* and completed a control training session lasting 30 minutes. Blood lactate (using a lactic acid analyser) and heart rate (using a heart rate monitor) data were collected before and after the three sessions, which were conducted on different days immediately after a three-set badminton match.

RESULTS: There was a clear interaction effect between the time of lactate breakdown and the interventions. The lactic acid concentration in the blood and the heart rate decreased significantly (depending on the time) with *yoga-nidrā* and biofeedback therapy, respectively. When compared to the biofeedback training and control groups, the lactate values for the *yoga-nidrā* treatment group showed a significant difference. No difference was found between *yoga-nidrā* and biofeedback in terms of heart rate reduction.

CONCLUSION: *Yoga-nidrā* is more effective than the audiovisual biofeedback method for faster recovery from athletic exertion, since *yoga-nidrā* increases alpha wave activity in the brain and activates the parasympathetic nervous system, which leads to an overall reduction in psychophysiological reactions and muscle tension.

Datta et al. (2022)[777] conducted a comparative study to find a strategy that could help improve the sleep of competitive athletes. The effects of *yoga-nidrā* and progressive muscle relaxation on the sleep profile of 57 male athletes from a total of seven sports were investigated.

INTERVENTION: *Yoga-nidrā* was practised in the morning and compared to the effect of progressive muscle relaxation before bedtime. The subjects' baseline data and data after the four-week intervention were collected using a 14-day sleep diary and a sleep recording using a sleep tracker. The data of 45 athletes were evaluated.

---

777 Datta K, Yadav N, Narawade Y, Mahajan U, Joseph T, Kumar A. (2022). Sleep Strategies for Sportsmen; What can they be? A Randomised Controlled Trial, *Sleep Vigilance*, 6(1), 165–171. https://doi.org/10.1007/s41782-021-00188-8 (accessed on 14.09.2023).

RESULTS: Both interventions improved all subjective sleep variables. However, when comparing the groups, time to sleep onset, time spent in bed and sleep efficiency were significantly better in the *yoga-nidrā* group than in the group that practised progressive muscle relaxation.

The effect of *yoga-nidrā* on cancer patients

In a pilot study by **Loudon et al. (2014)**[778] preliminary data were obtained on the effect of yoga on women with Stage I. breast cancer-related lymphedema[779].

INTERVENTION: Subjects were randomly assigned to two groups after a baseline examination. 15 patients participated in an 8-week yoga intervention consisting of weekly 90-minute sessions with an instructor and a daily 40-minute session with instruction via DVD. The yoga sessions included selected breathing exercises, physical postures, meditation and relaxation techniques (*yoga-nidrā*) according to the Bihar Yoga tradition. The 13 patients in the control group received usual care. The respective arm volume of the lymphedema, measured by girth, and extracellular fluid were defined as primary outcome measures. As secondary outcome measures, tissue induration, the extent of paraesthesia, pain, fatigue and their restrictive effects were measured, and quality of life was assessed using the lymphedema quality of life tool. Measurements were taken at baseline, at Week 8 of the intervention and at Week 12 (four weeks after the end of the intervention).

RESULTS: At Week 8, the intervention group had greater reductions in arm tightness and the symptom subscale of quality of life compared with the control group. There was no difference in lymphedema

---

778 Immnik, A. Maarten, Loudon, A., Barnett, T., Piller, N. & Williams, A. D. (2014). Yoga management of breast cancer-related lymphoedema: a randomised controlled pilot-trial. *BMC complementary and alternative medicine*, 14, 214. https://doi.org/10.1186/1472–6882–14–214 (accessed on 14.09.2023)

779 Secondary arm lymphedema continues to affect at least 20% of women after breast cancer treatment and requires lifelong professional treatment and self-management.

volume or extracellular fluid volume between the intervention and control groups at Week 8; however, arm volume increased more in the intervention group than in the control group at Week 12.

CONCLUSION: Holistic yoga practice may offer benefits as a complementary self-management option for early-stage lymphedema.

Govardhan et al. (2018)[780] attempted to develop and validate a structured yoga programme for cervical cancer patients.

INTERVENTION: A detailed search of historical and contemporary yoga literature was conducted to compile a basic yoga programme. Five yoga experts validated the programme. Finally, 27 practices were classified as either non-essential, useful but not essential, or essential.

RESULTS: Eighteen of the 27 practices were found to be beneficial. *Yoga-nidrā* was added as a special practice on days when the patients were very tired.

CONCLUSIONS: The yoga programme designed is suitable for cervical cancer patients. The programme should be applied to other patients in the future to better evaluate acceptance and feasibility.

D'cunha et al. (2021)[781] investigated the effectiveness of *yoga-nidrā* for stress reduction in 48 women undergoing curative radiotherapy for cervical cancer.

INTERVENTION: The subjects were assigned to an experimental or a control group, each with 24 participants. The pre-test data were collected using a stress scale. The experimental group participated in *yoga-nidrā* sessions at the end of each radiotherapy session. The post-test data were then collected using the same instrument.

---

780 Govardhan HB. et al. (2018). Development of Comprehensive Yoga Program for Cervical Carcinoma. In *Journal for Inerative Oncology*, 7(1), 206. doi:10.4172/2329–6771.1000206 (accessed on 14.09.2023).

781 D'cunha, R.; Pappachan, B.; D'souza, O., Loyster; Tonse, R.; Saldanha, E. and Baliga, M. Shrinath (2021). Effectiveness of Yoga Nidra in Mitigating Stress in Women Undergoing Curative Radiotherapy for Cervical Cancer. *Middle East Journal of Cancer*, 12(1), 117–127. https://doi.org/10.30476/mejc.2020.82648.1093 (accessed on 14.09.2023).

RESULTS: At the beginning of the study, the subjects in both groups experienced moderate to severe stress due to the radiation treatment. In the post-test, the stress level in the group that practised *yoga-nidrā* was significantly lower than in the control group.

CONCLUSION: The results of the study clearly indicate that *yoga-nidrā* can effectively reduce the experience of stress in patients undergoing curative radiotherapy.

Sandeep et al. (2016)[782] elected 60 alcohol-dependent individuals in a detoxification camp for their study. The subjects in Group 1 practised *yoga-nidrā* for a period of 10 days, while Group 2 went about their routine activities. Both groups were examined for balance, gait and withdrawal symptoms on the first and tenth day.

RESULTS: When the two groups were compared, the *yoga-nidrā* group was found to have significantly better results in terms of withdrawal symptoms. There were no significant differences in balance and gait.

CONCLUSION: Practising *yoga-nidrā* is effective in reducing withdrawal symptoms in alcohol addicts.

Bhatia et al. (2022)[783] developed a meditation programme for a study to test its feasibility, acceptability and efficacy in combination with yoga training for individuals with schizophrenia.

INTERVENTION: The meditation programme consisted of *ānāpāna* (observation of natural breathing) and *yoga-nidrā* practice (quiet awareness while lying down). In a randomised, controlled, single-blinded study, outpatients with schizophrenia who were receiving medication

---

782 Sandeep, C., Shivaprasad & Shetty, Prashant. (2016). Effects Of Yoga Nidra (Psychic Sleep) On Alcohol Dependent Individuals – A Randomized Control Trial. In *Journal of Dental and Medical Sciences* (IOSR-JDMS), 15(9), 8–13. https://www.iosrjournals.org/iosr-jdms/papers/Vol15-Issue%209/Version-11/C1509110813.pdf (accessed on 14.09.2023).

783 Nimgaonkar, V. L. & Deshpande, S. N. (2022). Feasibility, acceptability and evaluation of meditation to augment yoga practice among persons diagnosed with schizophrenia. *Acta Neuropsychiatrica*, 34(6), 330–343. https://doi.org/10.1017/neu.2022.14 (accessed on 14.09.2023).

and were clinically stable were randomly assigned to receive either the usual treatment supplemented by yoga practice or the newly developed meditation and yoga programme for three weeks. Acceptability, clinical, social and cognitive functioning were assessed at three weeks and three months using within-group and between-group analyses of tests and repeated measurements.

RESULTS: Changes observed were in the desired direction for all six clinical variables assessed, with effects slightly greater in the meditation yoga group than in the other group.

CONCLUSION: The meditation programme developed is feasible and acceptable for patients with schizophrenia and shows modest benefits in quality of life and clinical symptoms compared to yoga practice alone.

Effects of *yoga-nidrā* on brain activity and neuroplasticity

Nilson[784] reports that in the early 1980s, in an extensive research project at the University Hospital in Cologne, Germany, the brain waves of a group of experienced yoga teachers from the Scandinavian Yoga and Meditation School were measured while they were practising Satyananda Yoga Nidra.

INTERVENTION: The subjects had many years of daily practice in *kriyā-yoga*[785], which they each practised with *yoga-nidrā* in the morning before the experimental sessions. The researchers, in turn, were familiar with suggestive relaxation and wanted to find out whether *yoga-nidrā* could have a more profound effect than methods based on suggestion or hypnosis.

784 Nilson, Robert. (n. d.) Der entspannte Zustand und die Wissenschaft. In Swami Prakashananda. (2003). *Yoga Nidra – Neue Erkenntnisse*. Satyananda Yoga Zentrum e. V., Germany, Köln: Ananda Verlag, p. 43.

785 This refers to *kriyā-yoga* as taught by Svāmī Satyānanda in the tantric tradition.

RESULTS: During *yoga-nidrā*, the alpha waves occurred in all brain areas and remained constant throughout the practice, while with other relaxation methods they were only partially and irregularly measurable. Furthermore, it was found that, in contrast to other relaxation techniques, the level of alpha waves remained constant throughout the entire *yoga-nidrā* session. The balance of the electrodermal activity of the two brain hemispheres was also improved by *yoga-nidrā*, which means that there was improved communication between the two brain hemispheres.

These results were confirmed in a study by the neuroscientists **Kjær and Lou (1997)**[786] in which consciousness during *yoga-nidrā* was measured.

INTERVENTION: The brain activity of seven yoga teachers at the Scandinavian Yoga and Meditation School, including Svāmī Janakānanda Sarasvatī, was measured in the PET scanner at the State University Hospital in Copenhagen. All subjects practised *kriyā-yoga* regularly and had also practised *kriyā-yoga* in the morning before going to the hospital for the scan.

RESULTS: From the images of the PET scanner[787], it was clearly visible that clearly defined centres in the brain were activated alternately —corresponding to the Stage of *yoga-nidrā* the subject was at. The results showed that the distinct mental activity during the different Stages of *yoga-nidrā* activated exactly the same brain regions in the different participants, which surprised the researchers at the time. The measurements confirmed for the first time that it is possible to be fully aware in such a deeply relaxed state, i.e. to consciously experience and control the altered brain activity. The PET image, which was taken before and after the exercise, showed that the forebrain, the brainstem and the cerebellum were activated, i.e. the control for processing the signals of the deeper emotional and instinctive brain areas and the readiness to act were present. In the image

786 Satyananda, Swami. (2006). Yoga Nidra. (12th reprint). Munger: Yoga Publications Trust, p. 238–244.
787 Images of brain activity recorded in the PET scanner during this research experiment are shown in Satyananda, Swami. (2006). *Yoga Nidra*. (12th reprint). Munger: Yoga Publications Trust, p. 243–244.

representing the general state during *yoga-nidrā*, the visual and tactile centres were active and in contact with the limbic system, suggesting increased visualisation capacity and better access to emotions. In some subjects, most likely due to their regular practice of *kriyā-yoga*, which affected the depth of their *yoga-nidrā* practice, activity was also observed in the centre of long-term memory. On the scans during Stage 3 — Rotation of Awareness Throughout the Body — and Stage 6 — Visualisation — the vision and feeling centres were particularly active, while in Stage 5 — Opposing sensations — the speech and language centre was particularly active.

The researchers found that not only did the contents of the various Stages of *yoga-nidrā* very precisely influence certain parts of the brain, but the subjects also exhibited a high degree of concentration, and did so completely effortlessly. As the EEG showed, they were in a completely relaxed, sleep-like state from start to finish, while still being conscious. Alpha wave activity decreased insignificantly (2%), while theta wave activity increased significantly by 11%. This alpha/theta activity was observed to be constant and homogeneously distributed throughout the brain during the forty-five minutes of *yoga-nidrā* practice.

CONCLUSION: During *yoga-nidrā*, consciousness is in a very deep and stable state. At the same time, the measurements confirmed that it is possible to be fully conscious in such a state of deep immersion — i.e. the altered brain activity can be consciously experienced and controlled. Furthermore, the practice consistently activated specific regions of the brain in a particular order and across subjects.[788]

Gosh (1998)[789] conducted a series of control studies at Charing Cross Medical School in London and found that *yoga-nidrā* is a method that can be used to change brain activity from beta to alpha and then to delta waves

788 Janakānanda, Swami. (2022). *A deeper yoga and Yoga Nidra*. [eBook edition]. Hamneda: Bindu, p. 64–70.

789 Gosh, A.K. (Mangalteertham, Sannyasi). (1988). Brain Electrical Activity Mapping During Yoda Nidra. In Yoga Research Foundation. (2015). Volume One, *YRF Journals 1989–1990*. Bihar: Yoga Publication Trust, p. 26–31 and Yoga Nidra: Altered State of Consciousness. In Swami Satyananda Saraswati. (2006). *Yoga Nidra*. Bihar: Yoga Publication Trust, p. 245–253.

INTERVENTION: For this study, 34 subjects were divided into three groups: Group 1 consisted of 13 experienced practitioners aged between 35 and 43 years with 4 to 15 years of *yoga-nidrā* experience; Group 2 was randomly selected Charing Cross medical students aged 20 to 25 years with no previous experience of meditation or yoga. Both groups practised *yoga-nidrā* for the study. Group 3, the control group, was made up of medical students from the same pool as group 2. The investigation was carried out using brain electrical activity mapping[790] in a Faraday cage, and were thus shielded from external electromagnetic interference.

RESULTS: The results showed that the subjects in Groups 1 and 2 were able to maintain increased alpha wave activity on average during their *yoga-nidrā* practice, which was significantly more pronounced in the occipital areas of the brain during Stage 1 of the practice. At the beginning of Stage 3 — Rotation of Awareness Throughout the Body — there was heightened alpha wave activity. At the beginning of Stage 6 — Visualisation — a distinctly pronounced asymmetrical distribution of alpha waves was recorded over the occipital region of the brain, as well as an asymmetry indicating more pronounced activity in the right cerebral hemisphere. Delta waves slowly appeared in the right hemisphere and gradually became more prominent in both hemispheres, indicating a very calm state at the end of the visualisation and *yoga-nidrā* session. The occurrence of alpha wave blocking in both groups of subjects during Stage 3 points to increased alertness. At Stage 6, the delta wave activity and the appearance of a characteristic pattern of a slow-rhythmed delta wave indicated that the brain had entered a state similar to deep sleep. However, most of the subjects in Groups 1 and 2 remained fully conscious throughout the entire experiment. At the end of Stage 6 (Visualisation), the brain showed complete, synchronised, very slow and low activity, indicated by the appearance of blue colouration in both hemispheres.

790 Electrical Activity Mapping creates a kind of 'map' of the brain.

CONCLUSION: These results suggest that *yoga-nidrā* is a 'sleepless sleep' state in which the space between sleep and wakefulness can be entered into without loss of consciousness. This supports the assumption that *yoga-nidrā* induces a state of deep relaxation in a short period of time, which is, however, characterised more by awareness than by 'unconsciousness' as in deep sleep proper, and that the different stages of the method bring about concrete, clearly measurable changes in differentiated brain areas. The two hemispheres of the brain rarely work together equally. The potential of *yoga-nidrā* to generate synchronous and symmetrical alpha and delta waves indicates its likely beneficial application to a wide range of psychosomatic problems, among other ailments.

Kjær, Lou et al. (1999)[791] investigated whether the neuronal structures underlying the *yoga-nidrā* method can be reproducibly measured and whether they differ from those that support the resting state of normal consciousness.

INTERVENTION: Cerebral blood flow distribution was examined in nine adults who were highly experienced yoga teachers during relaxation meditation (*yoga-nidrā*) and during normal resting state. In addition, cerebral blood flow was measured in two of the subjects. Spectral EEG analysis was performed during the examinations. Brain activity was measured using the H215O[792]-PET method, which was able to best visualise brain perfusion (cerebral blood flow distribution) in both the meditative state and the resting state of normal waking consciousness.

RESULTS: During *yoga-nidrā*, differentiated activity was observed in the posterior sensory and associative cortices involved in imagination tasks. In the resting state of normal consciousness (compared to *yoga-nidrā* as a baseline), activity was observed in specific brain structures thought to support an executive attention network. Mean

791 Kjaer, Troels, W., Lou, Hans, C., Friberg, L., Wildschiodtz, G., Holm, S., & Nowak, M. (1999). A 15O-H2O PET study of meditation and the resting state of normal consciousness. *Human Brain Mapping*, 7(2), 98–105. https://doi.org/10.1002/(SICI)1097-0193(1999)7:2<98::AID-HBM3>3.0.CO;2-M (accessed on 14.09.2023).

792 H215O is weakly radioactive labelled water.

cerebral blood flow remained unchanged in the two subjects examined throughout the examination.

CONCLUSION: Characteristic patterns of neuronal activity support both deep relaxation and conscious states. Neuronal activity and its changes can be measured. These results broaden our understanding of the neuronal basis of different aspects of consciousness.

Kjær, Lou et al. (2002)[793] were the first to provide evidence for the regulation of consciousness at the synaptic level and the connection between the release of endogenous neurotransmitters and conscious experience. The aim of this study at Hammersmith Hospital, London, was to investigate whether endogenous dopamine release increases during loss of control and self-regulation in the deep relaxation of *yoga-nidrā* practice.

INTERVENTION: Participants underwent two PET scans with the marker raclopride[794] as a selective antagonist of D2 dopamine receptors: Scan 1 was performed while they listened to a speech with their eyes closed and Scan 2 while they actively practised *yoga-nidrā*.

RESULTS: On the basis of the PET scans, metabolic processes could be mapped that corresponded to an increased dopamine release (by 65%) during the practice of *yoga-nidrā*. These processes correlated significantly with a simultaneous increase in theta activity on the EEG—a characteristic feature of *yoga-nidrā* practice. This theta increase is characterised by a dampened sense of urge to act, which is associated with reduced blood flow in specific brain structures that are thought to be organised in circuits and serve to control actions. All participants reported a reduced willingness to act during the practice, together with increased sensory imagery.

793 Kjaer, Troels, W., Lou, Bertelsen, C., Piccini, P., Brooks, D. & Alving, J. (2002). Increased dopamine tone during meditation-induced change of consciousness. Brain research. *Cognitive Brain Research*, 13(2), 255–259. https://doi.org/10.1016/s0926-6410(01)00106-9 (accessed on 14.09.2023)

794 Raclopride is an antipsychotic agent that can be used to obtain more accurate results in dopamine release PET scans.

CONCLUSION: During *yoga-nidrā* practice, there is an increased dopamine release coupled with the experience of reduced willingness to act.

Mandlik (2002)[795] used an electroencephalograph (EEG) to study the effect of *yoga-nidrā* on the brain activity of 20 subjects.

INTERVENTION: The subjects practised *yoga-nidrā* daily for one month. Each participant's EEG was recorded before the start of the study, during the *yoga-nidrā* practice and after one month.

RESULTS: The first EEG showed pronounced beta activity with intermittent alpha activity. As the *yoga-nidrā* practice progressed, the beta activity was replaced over time by even, well-formed alpha activity. After 30 *yoga-nidrā* sessions, the amplification of alpha activity was more pronounced, and with further *yoga-nidrā* practice, intermittent theta activity was observed mixing with the alpha activity.

CONCLUSION: Theta activity indicates a state of deep relaxation that can be achieved through continuous *yoga-nidrā* practice.

A study by **Roney-Dougal (2011)**[796] confirmed these results.

Lou, Kjær and Nowak (2005)[797] compared brain activity during *yoga-nidrā* with that during a state of conscious rest in a positron emission tomography study. Through *yoga-nidrā*, both the quality and the content of consciousness can be deliberately changed, which makes the method an obvious target in the search for the neural correlate of consciousness. Meditation is associated with relatively increased blood flow in the sensory-imaging system—hippocampus and higher-order sensory and associative regions—while blood flow

795 Mandlik Y. V., Jain P., & Jain K. (2002). Effect of Yoga Nidra on EEG. *Yoga Vidya Dham, Retrieved*, http://www.yogapoint.com/info/research5.htm (accessed on 14.09.2023).

796 Roney-Dougal, S. M. (n.d.). Altered States of Consciousness and Yogic Attainment in Relation to Awareness of Precognitive and Clairvoyant Targets, Psi Research Center, 2011. In Kamakhya Kumar (2013). *A Handbook of Yoga-Nidrā*, New Delhi: D. K. Printworld (P) Ltd., p. 81.

797 Lou, Hans C.; Kjaer, Troels W. & Nowak, Markus. (2005). The mental self. In *Progress in Brain Research*. 150, 197–204 & 594. https://doi.org/10.1016/S0079-6123(05)50014-1 (accessed on 14.09.2023.)

in the executive system—dorsolateral prefrontal cortex, anterior cingulate gyrus, striatum, thalamus, pons, and cerebellum—is reduced.

> **INTERVENTIONS AND RESULTS:** To identify regions that were active during both resting state and *yoga-nidrā*, an analysis of outcomes was performed. In this analysis, the blood flow data were divided into two groups of regions: one group corresponding to the executive system and the other to the systems that support sensory perception. A small group of regions contributed significantly to both networks: the medial parietal and medial prefrontal cortices, as well as the striatum, which is regulated by dopamine.

Subsequently, the neural networks supporting the retrieval of judgments about persons with varying degrees of self-relevance were examined, in descending order: self, best friend, and the Danish queen. It was found that a medial prefrontal precuneus[798] posterior cingulate cortex, thalamus, and cerebellum were activated under all conditions. This activation occurred together with the activation of the left lateral prefrontal/temporal cortex. The latter was dependent on the requirement to retrieve semantic information and was most pronounced in the 'queen' condition. Transcranial magnetic stimulation, which targeted the precuneus, was then applied to the medial parietal region to temporarily disrupt the normal functioning of the circuit. It was found that the efficiency of retrieving self-judgment decreased compared to the judgment about one's best friend.

Measurements showed that *yoga-nidrā* practice is accompanied by relatively increased blood flow in the sensory-imaging system (hippocampus and higher-order sensory and associative regions) and decreased blood flow in the executive system (dorsolateral prefrontal cortex, anterior cingulate gyrus, striatum, thalamus, pons, and cerebellum) and that the integrity of the function of the precuneus is essential for self-reference, but not for reference to others. This made it possible to visualise that specific brain regions show an alteration in their activity during the practice of *yoga-nidrā*.

---

798 The precuneus, a part of the medial cerebral lobe, plays an important role in visualisation. Furthermore, it is important for retrieving autobiographical memory content. This means that it is probably involved in the physiological trace that a stimulus leaves in the brain, the totality of which forms our memory.

CONCLUSION: The results are consistent with the assumption that self-awareness is an integral function of all conscious experiences and that it ties together conscious experiences into a single construct with a sense of unity of consciousness. Furthermore, it was shown which specific brain regions exhibited a change in activity during the practice of *yoga-nidrā*.

Roney-Dougal (2011)[799] observed in a study that the electroencephalography (EEG) of the subjects at the beginning of a *yoga-nidrā* session showed pronounced beta activity with intermittent alpha activity. As the practice progressed, the beta activity was slowly replaced by alpha activity and then by a steady, well-formed alpha activity. After thirty *yoga-nidrā* sessions, the increase in alpha activity was higher, and with further progression of the practice, intermittent theta activity was observed, which blended with the alpha activity, indicating a state of deep relaxation with awareness.

Immnik (2012)[800] presented an experiment that provided the first empirical test of *yoga-nidrā* for its potential to promote motor memory consolidation.

INTERVENTION: 12 adult residents of a yoga *āśrama* in Australia with an average of nine years of *yoga-nidrā* experience were trained to press a specific sequence of keys on a musical instrument. Three hours after this training, the *yoga-nidrā* group participated in a 30-minute *yoga-nidrā* session, while the control group performed light work for 30 minutes. The meditation was followed by a 4.5-hour waking phase, after which the participants took a test with trained and untrained sequences.

RESULTS: There was no significant difference in training performance between the two groups. However, a comparison of group

799 Roney-Dougal, S. M. (n.d.). Altered States of Consciousness and Yogic Attainment in Relation to Awareness of Precognitive and Clairvoyant Targets, Psi Research Center (2011). In Kamakhya Kumar (2013). *A Handbook of Yoga-Nidrā*. New Delhi: D. K. Printworld (P) Ltd., p. 81.

800 Immnik, M. A.(2012). Post-training Meditation Mediates Motor Memory Consolidation, Journal of Sport and Exercise Psychology, 7(11). Collection volume (2013). *Experience of Yoga, Golden Jubilee 1963–2013*. Bihar School of Yoga – Golden Jubilee. Bihar: Yoga Publication Trust, p. 171–172.

performance on the test showed that the *yoga-nidrā* group had an advantage in terms of the trained sequences, i.e., motor memory.

CONCLUSION: The fact that the *yoga-nidrā* group showed an advantage in performance specifically for the trained sequences after training is consistent with the assumption that *yoga-nidrā* promotes the stabilisation and consolidation of motor memory. However, there seems to be no general advantage in performance in motor tasks as a result of *yoga-nidrā*. These results represent the first evidence of consolidation of motor memory through *yoga-nidrā* and are consistent with a growing body of research demonstrating the benefits of *yoga-nidrā* for cognitive functions, including memory.

There are three main electrophysiological methods for measuring brain activity during sleep: electroencephalography (EEG), electromyography (EMG) and electrooculography (EOG). For a long time, there was no research on the electrophysiological characterisation of *yoga-nidrā*, so it was not possible to say whether it was a state of sleep or wakefulness.

Datta et al. (2022)[801] dedicated a study to the goal of electrophysiologically monitoring and characterising the *yoga-nidrā* method.

INTERVENTION: 30 subjects without experience of *yoga-nidrā* initially took part in five supervised *yoga-nidrā* sessions and then continued practising independently. They also kept sleep diaries for two weeks before and during the intervention. The electrophysiological examination was carried out after two weeks of *yoga-nidrā* practice using polysomnography for the period before, during and after *yoga-nidrā* practice. The polysomnographic data were evaluated according to standard criteria for the sleep-wake phases. The EEG data were grouped by brain area, namely central, frontal, prefrontal, parietal, temporal, and occipital areas in time segments. The parameters of the sleep diary before and after the *yoga-nidrā* training were also compared.

801 Datta, K., Mallick, H. N., Tripathi, M., Ahuja, N. & Deepak, K. K. (2022). Electrophysiological Evidence of Local Sleep During Yoga Nidra Practice. *Frontiers In Neurology*, 13, 910794. https://doi.org/10.3389/fneur.2022.910794 (accessed on 15.09.2023).

RESULTS: After two weeks of *yoga-nidrā* practice, wakefulness was observed throughout the entire session. Compared to before *yoga-nidrā* practice, there was an increase in delta wave power in the central brain area and a decrease in the prefrontal area during practice. The sleep diary showed improvements in sleep duration, efficiency, and quality, as well as in total waking time.

CONCLUSION: The results of the study suggest that the *yoga-nidrā* technique in beginners can be characterised electrophysiologically as a waking state with signs of slow waves, also known as 'local sleep'.

yoga-nidrā and distance learning during the COVID-19 lockdowns

During the COVID-19 lockdown, **Gulia and Sreedharan (2021)** conducted[802] an actigraphy[803]-based case study of a 56-year-old woman with menopausal symptoms to examine the therapeutic potential of *yoga-nidrā*, practiced using an online home-practice module.

INTERVENTION: Using M24-hour actigraphy and a sleep diary, the effect of the twenty-four-week intervention module on mood upon waking and during the day, BMI and body activity patterns was measured after a baseline of four weeks.

RESULTS: From the fifth week onwards, the results showed a significant improvement in mood, both on waking and during the day. However, total sleep time only improved after 16 weeks. The baseline BMI was lowered, the morning rising behaviour remained unchanged, but the subject no longer experienced menopausal symptoms or headaches.

---

802 Gulia, K. Kamalesh & Sreedharan, E. Sapna. (2021). Yogic sleep and walking protocol induced improvement in sleep and wellbeing in post-menopausal subject: a longitudinal case study during COVID lockdown. *Sleep and Vigilance*, 6(1), 229–233. https://doi.org/10.1007/s41782–021-00180–2 (accessed on 15.09.2023).

803 Actigraphy is a non-invasive procedure that uses a specialised device to measure a person's activity and rest cycles.

CONCLUSION: The researchers concluded that *yoga-nidrā* is a complementary method for improving the well-being of the older population that can also be easily practised at home.

Sharpe et al. (2021) conducted a study with 74 subjects who participated in 241 *yoga-nidrā* sessions via distance learning during the COVID-19 pandemic to investigate the effect of *yoga-nidrā* against insomnia and anxiety.

INTERVENTION: *yoga-nidrā* instruction via an online platform was delivered in real time at bedtime or asynchronously once a week for 16 weeks from April to July 2021 (during the first months of the COVID-19 pandemic).

RESULTS: 71% of the participants reported having subthreshold insomnia at baseline and 74% reported anxiety. 96% of the participants used the asynchronous online guidance. 52% of the respondents who completed the questionnaires both before and after the intervention reported an improvement in their sleep disorders. The overall anxiety level decreased by 41% in 32 participants.

CONCLUSION: *Yoga-nidrā* via distance learning is feasible and can help to improve anxiety and insomnia.

Gunjiganvi et al. (2021)[804] conducted a randomised control trial to examine the effectiveness of online or digitally delivered *yoga-nidrā* and supine relaxation exercises for healthcare workers during the COVID-19 pandemic.

INTERVENTION: The open-label study was conducted with healthcare professionals in a level III COVID care centre. Each online intervention lasted 30 minutes per day. All participants who completed more than nine days of practice were included in the study. The primary

804 Gunjiganvi, M., Mohan, G., Mishra, P., et al. (2021). Efficacy of Yoga Nidra vs Supine Relaxation Technique on Depression, Anxiety, Insomnia. In Frontline COVID-19 Health Care Workers: A Randomized Controlled Trial, PREPRINT (Version 1). *Research Square Journal*. https://doi.org/10.21203/rs.3.rs-486904/v1 (accessed on 15.09.2023).

outcome measures were the Physical Health Quality Index, the Generalised Anxiety Index and the Insomnia Severity Index (ISI).

RESULTS: The virtual *yoga-nidrā* sessions significantly improved subjects' depression, anxiety, and insomnia scores compared to the online-guided supine relaxation exercises.

CONCLUSION: *Yoga-nidrā* practices can also be taught via a digital platform and have been shown to be equally effective in treating insomnia and anxiety.

APPENDIX 3

Dictionary of Sanskrit Terms

Editor's Note:

Sanskrit terms come in three grammatical genders: masculine (m.), feminine (f.), and neuter (n.). Adjectives are marked by all three grammatical genders, since they may appear in any of the three forms, depending on the gender of the modified noun, like in German. Since the sequence of the Devanāgarī script and its predecessors used to write the Sanskrit language is different to that of the Latin alphabet and less familiar to anglophone readers, the sequence of terms follows the alphabetic order of the latter, rather than the traditional arrangement of the former. *Terms* included in this Glossary which appear in other entries are indicated accordingly. The transliteration used is the standard IAST (International Alphabet of Sanskrit Transliteration). Only proper names (such as Śaṅkara) are capitalised. All terms with the exception of proper names and terms which have become common in English (such as 'mantra' and 'yoga' more generally) have been rendered in italics. In certain cases (primarily with complex compound nouns, such as *yoga-nidrā*) a hyphen (-) has been added at internal word borders wherever possible or appropriate to aid readers. Terms which have other terms as their main constituent can be found under those terms, such as *antaraṅga-yoga* being filed under *yoga*.

Regarding meaning, it is poignant to point out that, like in many languages and cultures, different words were used in different contexts and across millennia by different cultures across the Indian Subcontinent in different ways. Thus, readers must by all means remain vigilant of the fact that the meanings of the terms reflected here are limited to the context of a few select traditions and texts in rather strictly defined periods of Indian history and should not be taken as exhaustive or conflatable into overarching terminological categories. Hence interested readers are advised to refer to well-established Sanskrit dictionaries such as the *Böhtlingk and Roth Grosses Petersburger Wörterbuch* or its anglophone version by Monier Williams, the *The Practical Sanskrit-English Dictionary* by Varman Shivaram Apte, as well as the newer online *Nachtragswörterbuch des Sanskrit* by the University of Halle and relevant scholarly literature pertaining to any particular question that may arise from the reading of this book.

A

Ādi Śaṅkarācārya—(c. 788—c. 820), proper n. Śaṅkara, was one of the most important philosophers and saints of India. He was the first to systematise the philosophy of Advaita-Vedānta or non-dual Vedānta

adhiṣṭhāna (n.)—consecration

advaita (mfn.)—non-duality, oneness

abhāva-pratyaya (m.)—'the cause of the absence of all impressions'—the stillness of the mind in the context of Patañjali's *Yoga-Sūtra* 1.10

abhyāsa (m.)—perseverance in practice, consistent practice, continuous practice

abhiniveśa (m.)—clinging [to life], fear of death

āgama (mfn.)—testimony, tradition, scriptural knowledge; knowledge acquired through the testimony of a trustworthy person or an authoritative text

agni (m.)—fire, fire as an element, the Vedic god of fire

ahaṃkāra (m.)—the principle of individuation, the I or ego, the I-consciousness or identity consciousness of a person

ahiṃsā (f.)—Non-violence, i.e. not harming others in thought, word or deed (esp. Buddhist)

ajapā-japa (m.)—a breath awareness technique within the Bihar Yoga system. *Ajapā-japa* means 'recitation of the non-recited', here understood to refer to continuous repetition, and includes the awareness of the flow of the natural breath between the navel and throat, as well as the awareness of the prāṇa and the vibrational power of the breath mantra *so 'ham*.

ājñā-cakra (n.)—the sixth *cakra* (prāṇic plexus) between the eyebrows, at the centre of the forehead or the third eye

ākāśa (mn.)—space; air space, sky; sometimes rendered as 'ether' (contentious)

ālambana (n.)—a support, hold; leaning on, holding on to something, aid to concentration; the original idea of the root cause; in immersive practice: the support of the practice: physical image, painting, visualised or experienced deity form

anāhata-cakra (n.) — psychic centre in the heart region, the heart *cakra*; '*cakra* of the unstruck [sound]'; location roughly corresponds to the cardiac plexus in the physical body

antaḥkaraṇa (n.) — the structure of the mind, inner functional structure of the psyche, inner organ, inner instrument

antaraṅga (mfn.) — relating to the interior, the inner part

antaraṅga-yoga (m.) — 'inner' branches of yoga

antar-mauna (n.) — 'inner silence', a *pratyāhāra* technique within the Bihar Yoga system

anuloma-viloma (m.) — lit. 'with the flow | against the flow': a mental alternate nostril breathing technique

amanaska (mfn.) — without mental capacity; without understanding; in the Haṭha-yoga-pradīpikā 4.4 synonym of *samādhi*; also refers to laya-yoga (practice of resorption)

Amanaska (m.) — abbreviation of 'Amanaska-yogavivaraṇa' (a medieval Sanskrit yoga text, unknown author)

amanaskatā (f.) — a term for the highest state; the prolonged, formless absorption in which cognitive thinking is transcended; a heightened, exalted state, the culmination of the *unmanī* state, synonym of *nirvikalpa-samādhi*, *yoga-nidrā* and *turīya* in particular contexts

ānandamaya-kośa (m.) — the sheath consisting of / relating to bliss (*ānanda*); see *pañcakośa*

annamaya-kośa (m.) — the sheath (*-kośa*) consisting (*-maya-*) of food (*anna-*); see *pañcakośa*

antaḥkaraṇa (n.) — inner organ, composed of *ahaṃkāra*, *buddhi*, *manas*, *citta*

antaraṅga (mfn.) — relating to the interior, the inner part

antar-mauna (n.) — the 'inner silence' technique

anumāna (n.) — logical reasoning; conclusion, inference

apāna-vāyu (m.) — one of the five main manifestations of the vital energy *prāṇa* usual to *haṭha-yoga* systems of subtle anatomy — its direction of movement is from top to bottom and it is responsible for excretion, sexuality, reproduction and creativity; see *prāṇa*

āpas (n.) — water; the water element

aparigraha (m.) — non-attachment, non-hoarding, lack of possessiveness

āsana (n.) — lit. 'seat'; in yoga: posture; in Patañjali: the third stage of his *aṣṭāṅga*-yoga

asmitā — (Vyāsa) the non-distinction between the power of the observer and that of the act of observation

asaṃprajñāta-samādhi (m.)—non-dualistic state of absorption; experience of unity

āśrama- (m. u. n.)—place of spiritual practice, phase of life

aṣṭāṅga-yoga (m.)—the eight-limbed path of yoga

asteya (n.)—integrity, truthfulness, non-stealing

asura (m.)—anti-gods, titans

ātman (n.)—the (highest) Self, being, nature

avidyā (f.)—incomprehension, ignorance

avyavahārya (m.)—the non-mundane; Transcendent (Consciousness)

B

bahiraṅga (mfn).—relating to the exterior, the outer part

bahiraṅga-yoga (m.)—'outer' branches of yoga

bandha (m.)—band, rope, shackle; the binding, connecting; (*haṭha-yoga*) contractions of specific muscle groups to direct the life energy in certain regions of the body, 'bindings', or 'holds'

bindu (mn.)—point, drop or dot

bhakti (f.)—devotion; (Bihar Yoga) non-dual, personal theistic stance emphasising devotion

bhakti-yoga (m.)—yoga of devotion; (Bihar Yoga) the path of emotional management

Bhāratī (f.)—name of a deity; one of the names of Sarasvatī; one of the ten orders of daśanāmī-saṃnyāsins

bhāvanā (f.)—active visualisation of a deity; see also *pratipakṣa-bhāvanā*

bhuvana (m.)—the different levels of existence of the Śaiva universe; see also *tattva*, *loka*

brahmacarya (n.)—restraint; celibacy; traditional twelve-year period of apprenticeship to a *guru*; (Bihar Yoga) being established in higher consciousness, right measure, self-control

brahman/ *Brahmā* (n.)—(Vedānta) the absolute, all-encompassing, universal; (Purāṇa) the creator god in several strands of Indic mythology

buddhi (f.)—(Sāṃkhya) reason, intellect; (Vedānta) one of the elements of the inner organ of mentation – the *antaḥkaraṇa*; (Patañjali) mind

C

cakra (n.)—wheel, disc, potter's wheel; throwing disc, discus; (*haṭha-yoga*/Tantra) the *cakras* in the human system are building networks, junctions or centres of consciousness and storage places for subtle energy forces. There are seven main cakras in the human subtle physiology, which are, in ascending order, as follows:

mūlādhāra-, svādhiṣṭhāna-, maṇipūra-, anāhata-, viśuddhi- and *sahasrāra-cakra.*

caturtha (adj.) — the fourth state, aside from waking, dreaming and sleeping; synonym of *turīya*

cetanā (f.) — (*Vedānta/Sāṃkhya*) the unmanifest aspect of cosmic intelligence with the ability to know, create and manifest

cidākāśa (mn.) — also *cittākāśa*: the space of consciousness; a space of consciousness perceived in front of or behind the forehead or also in the centre of the head

cin-mudrā (f.) — a hand gesture where the finger and thumb form a circle, with the palms facing upwards on the knees; said to stimulate the flow of energy to the lungs, promote vitality through prāṇa absorption there, conserving energy for the purpose of meditation

citta (n.) — paying attention; thinking, imagining; being thought, thought, remembrance; (*Patañjali*) mind; see *nirodha*

cittavṛtti (f.) — (*Patañjali*) movements/modifications of the mind

citta-viśrānti (m.) — a state of the absence of tension in the mind, regarded as a neutral prerequisite for certain yogic practices; centering the mind

D

darśana (n.) — philosophy, school of thought; point of view; ability to recognise, observation; vision of a deity

Daśanāmi Sampradaya (n.) — 'Tradition of Ten Names' — a Brahmanical monastic tradition of renunciation, which was established by *Ādi Śaṅkarācārya* in the 8th century CE. He organised ascetic Vedāntin monks into ten monastic orders assigned to the four cardinal monastic centers of the Advaita Vedānta tradition across the Indian Subcontinent.

devanāgarī (f.) — one of the official scripts of India and Nepal, which is used, among other things, for writing Sanskrit. The *Devanāgarī* script is composed of 48 primary characters, including 14 vowels and 34 consonants

devī (f.) — goddess, often *Durgā*; the universal energy (*śakti*), female principle

dhāraṇā (f.) — the practice of one-pointedness, focused awareness, binding the mind to a single object; the 6th limb of Patañjali's Yoga; see nirodha; see *yoga-nidrā*

dharma (m.) — depending on the context: law, justice, nature, quality; the ethics according to which people should behave, (innate) vocation, virtue

dhyāna (n.) — prolonged immersive focused awareness; the 7th limb of Patañjali's Yoga; generally deep states of immersion, colloquially often referred to as 'meditation'; (Tantra) visualisation; (Veda) 'invocation'

dīkṣā (f.) — initiation in a *Śaiva* or *Vaiṣṇava* context

dīrghakāla (adj.)—long-lasting

draṣṭā (m.)—Nom. Sg. of *draṣṭṛ*

draṣṭṛ (m.)—the seer, the observer

draṣṭā-bhāva (m.)—the observer stance, present, non-judgemental awareness

dṛṣṭi (f.)—observation, gaze

nāsikāgra-dṛṣṭi (f.)—focusing on the tip of the nose—one of the eye *mudrās*; see *dṛṣṭi*, *mudrā*

dvaita (n.)—twofoldness, duality

dveṣa (m.)—aversion; opposite of attraction (*rāga*)

Durgā (f.)—a popular Hindu goddess, subject of the *Durgā-saptaśatī*, considered goddess of perfection, the feminine force/energy of the universe, due to being born out of the power of all the gods for the sake of vanquishing evil forces

Durgā-saptaśatī—Later Sakta version of the Mārkaṇḍeya Purāṇa—one of the eighteen great *Purāṇas* (also Devīmāhātmya, c. 400–600 CE) from the Mārkaṇḍeya Purāṇa (c. 250–550 CE)

E

ekāgra (mfn.)—single-pointed (concentration)

ekāgratā (f.)—a state of 'one-pointedness', one of the stages or states of the mind; see *mūḍha*, *kṣipta*, *vikṣipta*, *niruddha*

G

guṇa (m.)—property, quality, also *tri-guṇa*, the three properties of primordial matter

H

hastamudrā (f.)—hand position/gesture; see *mudrā*

haṭha-yoga (m.)—tradition of yoga aimed at achieving liberation by means of the body, especially through physical yoga and manipulation of praṇa; one of the classical yoga branches according to Bihar Yoga—the yoga of balancing the subtle energies of the body

Haṭhayoga-pradīpikā—a 15th century classical text on *haṭha-yoga*, written by Svātmārāma

homa (m.)—fire offerings, often accompanying *pūjā* or a part of *sādhanas*; a central part of Vedic, but also Brahmanical and later tantric ritual

I

icchā (f.)—will; *-śakti*: the force and energy of will, willpower, volition *iḍā* (f.) — One of the three main pathways (*nāḍī*) for *praṇa* in the body; passive aspect of *praṇa* that manifests as a mental force; left energy channel; 'lunar' force that controls the subtle dimension

indriya (n.) — (*Sāṃkhya*) the ten organs/ faculties of perception and action, see also *indriya-pratyāhāra*

iṣṭadevatā (f.) — chosen personal tutelary deity

īśvara (m.) — Lord; designation of the highest personal God; cosmic will

īśvara-praṇidhāna (n.) — (*Patañjali*) complete surrender to the higher consciousness, surrender to God's will

J

jāgrat (mfn.) — wakeful; alertness, waking state; one of the four states of consciousness

japa (mfn.) — whispering, murmuring, half-loud recitation of a mantra or prayer; in later usage implies repetition

japamālā (f.) — a string of prayer beads with 27, 54 or 108 beads

jīvan-mukta (m.) — a self-realised person, a person who has achieved liberation while still in the living physical body

jīvātman (m.) — the individual Self residing in the body, the individual soul

jñānendriya (n.) — (*Sāṃkhya*) the five organs of perception, perceptive faculty — the ears/hearing (śrotra), the hands/touching (tvac), the eyes/seeing (cakṣus), the tongue/tasting (rasanā), the nose/smelling (ghrāṇa)

jñāna (n.) — cognition; knowledge, wisdom; refers to pure consciousness that is free of conceptual burdens

jñāna-mudrā (f.) — a hand gesture where the finger and thumb form a circle, with the palms facing downwards on the knees; said to stimulate the flow of energy to the large intestine, promote vitality through *prāṇa* absorption as well as detoxification on all levels, conserving energy for the purpose of meditation.

jñāna-yoga (m.) — the yoga of knowledge, study, self-knowledge

K

kalpataru (m.) — wish-fulfilling tree; also kalpavṛkṣa

kāraṇa (mfn.) — causal, the causal experience

karman (n.) — action, consequence; generally referred to as '*karma*' in the West

karma-yoga (m.) — the yoga path of action

karmendriya (n.) — (*Sāṃkhya*) organs of action — the vocal cords/speaking (vāc), the hands/grasping (pāṇi), the feet/motion (pāda), the sexual organs/procreation (upastha) and the excretory organs/evacuation (pāyu)

kāya-sthairyam (n.) — a *pratyāhāra* practice, or the first stage of every immersive practice, which induces steadiness of the body and prepares the body and the mind for further immersion. This is a technique whose modern version was established by Svāmī Satyānanda on the basis of tantric sources; see also *sthairya*

kaivalya — (*Patañjali*) isolation, liberation, autonomy

khecarī-mudrā (f.) — 'the seal of those who walk in the air realm'; the bending back of the tongue to press it against the palate

kīrtana (n.) — the practice of singing of mantras (as opposed to *japa*) and bhajans (hymns of adoration)

kleśa (m.) — (*Patañjali/Sāṃkhya*) affliction or tension causing suffering

kośa (m.) — (*Vedānta*) sheath or level of existence (also in other contexts 'treasury' or 'repository'); see *pañcakośa*

krama (m.) — step, sequence

kriyā (f.) — vigour, action

kriyā-yoga (m.) — (*Patañjali*) the process of purifying the mind through austerity (*tapas*), followed by scriptural self-study (*svādhyāya*), and ultimately surrender to the higher or cosmic will (*īśvara*); (Bihar Yoga) the yoga path of balancing the psycho-physiological movements of the mind

kṣipta (mfn.) — scattered, one of the states of the mind; see also *mūḍha*, *vikṣipta*, *ekāgra*, *niruddha*.

kumbhaka (mn.) — (*Patañjali*) the natural standstill somewhere in-between inhalation and exhalation; (Bihar Yoga) breath retention

kuṇḍalinī-śakti (f.) — (*Tantra/haṭha-yoga*) the dormant creative force in people, usually depicted as coiled snake at the lowest point of the subtle body.

L

loka (m.) — space, place, area, country, world, plane; also see *bhuvana*, *tattva*

M

Mahābhārata — the most famous and larges heroic epic and one of the most important philosophical works of India (ca. 400 BCE — 400 CE)

mahā-bhūta (n.) — (*Sāṃkhya*) the five (gross) elements — space (*ākāśa*), air/dynamism (*vāyu*), fire/form (*agni*), water/fluidity (*āpas*) and earth/solidity/stability (*pṛthvī*)

Mahāmāyā—(*Tantra*/*Purāṇa*) an epithet of the goddess *Yoganidrā*, as well as other supreme goddess figures in Indic religion; (Vedānta/Sureśvara) cosmic ignorance, delusion, illusory reality

mahāprāṇa (m.)—highest form of vital energy

mahat (mfn.)—great, wide, mighty; (*Patañjali*/*Sāṃkhya*) also the spirit (*buddhi*) as the first modification of *prakṛiti*

manaḥprasāda (m.)—happiness; (*Patañjali*) the first *yama*

maṇipūra-cakra (m.)—the third primary *cakra*, the Solar Plexus *cakra*, whose position is stated as being behind the navel; associated with the element fire and the power of transformation. It is said to govern digestion, metabolism, the *samāna-vāyu* vital energy, as well as the feeling of confidence, self-motivation and the a sense for purpose; see also *cakra*

manas (n.)—the inner sense, the interactive mind, see *mana-pratyāhāra*

maṇḍala (mn.)—(Vedic) cycle of hymns; (*Tantra*) disc, circle, circumference, ring; magic circle, diagram

Māṇḍūkya-upaniṣad (c. 100–200 CE)—one of the ten principle and most important Upaniṣads

manonāśa (f.)—dissolution of the mind; state of deep immersion

manomaya-kośa (m.)—the sheath consisting of / relating to mind (*manas*), the emotional sheath or mental sheath; see *pañcakośa*

mantra (m.)—(depending on context) a magical formula, sacred syllable, sacred word or sacred verse; (*Tantra*) in the sense of *vidyā*—a divine force that is supposed to manifest itself in this world through mostly repetitive recitation and affect the world in extraordinary ways

marma-sthāna (m.)—marma points are considered to be loci of concentrated *prāṇa*, stimulating those in the system of Āyurveda through touch or massage is thought to tap into the body's internal energy, promote healing, and balance the flow of *prāṇa*. The science of marma has been traditionally kept secret due to the dangers of abusing that knowledge to harm others

māyā (f.)—(Vedānta/Sureśvara,) illusion, world of appearance; (*Tantra*) multiplicity, evolved manifest level of reality, a goddess

mauna (n.)—silence, vow of silence

mokṣa (m.)—state of enlightenment, liberation from the cycle of rebirth (*saṃsara*)

mūḍha (mfn.)—deluded, one of the stages or states of the mind, see also *kṣipta*, *vikṣipta*, *ekāgra*, *niruddha*

mudrā (f.)—seal, mark; (*haṭha-yoga*) fixed bodily position; (iconography) symbolic and evocative gestures; see also hastamudrā *mūlādhāra-cakra* (m.) — the first primary cakra, the root cakra, whose position is stated as being situated at the base of the coccyx; associated with the element earth and the feeling of security and stability. It forms the border between animal and human consciousness and is linked to the unconscious mind, see *cakra*

muni (m.) — sage, ascetic, seer

N

nāḍī (f.) — channel (of a river), river; (*Tantra/haṭha-yoga*) tube, energy channel, energy pathway

nāḍi-śodhana (n.) — 'purification of the energy channels' technique, where the practitioner directs the flow of breath from one nostril to another in succession through closing and opening them with the help of a hand position (*mudrā*), see *śodhana*

nāmarūpa (n.) — 'name and form'

nairantarya (mfn) — uninterrupted

namaskāra (m.) — respectful greetings; (*Patañjali*) the first *niyama*

netī (f.) — yogic nose cleansing with a string or liquid; a kind of austerity

nidrā (f.) — deep sleep, non-consciousness; (metaphorical) immersive state

nirodha (m.) — dissolution, enclosure, siege, eradication

nirodha-dhāraṇā (f.) — the culmination of one-pointedness, the fixation of the mind on a point or a specific location, see *dhāraṇā*

nirodha-saṃādhi (m.) — the transcendental state of dissolution; see *saṃādhi*

pratyaya-nirodha (m.) — dissolution of the content of the mind, takes place after *saṃprajñāta-samādhi* — in the state in which one is still aware of the difference between knowledge, the object of knowledge and the knower

saṃskāra-nirodha (m.) — according to Patañjali, neutralisation or 'extinction' of *saṃskāra* only takes place in *asamprajñāta-samādhi* — the state of superconscious absorption

vṛitti-nirodha (m.) — dissolution of the impeding modifications of the mind, takes place in *dhyāna*; see *vṛtti*

niruddha (mfn.) — 'suppressed': one of the stages or states of the mind, see *mūḍha, kṣipta, vikṣipta, ekāgra*

nirvāṇa (n.) — (*Buddhism*) extinction, dissolution, release from *saṃsāra*; synonym of *mokṣa*

nirvikalpa-samādhi (m.) — highest level of samādhi — absorption beyond conceptual thinking.

niyama (m.) — (*Patañjali*) prescriptions for behavioural restrictions and observances; see also *yama*

nyāsa (m.) — sitting down, placing; inserting, inserting, placing, placing; the establishment and consecration of divine forms by means of *mantras* — see also *pratiṣṭhā*

P

pañcakośa (m.) — the five energy sheaths/bodies; The system was first mentioned in the Taittirīya Upaniṣad

annamaya-kośa (m.) — the sheath (*-kośa*) consisting of / relating to (*-maya-*) food/ physical substance (*anna-*)

manomaya-kośa (m.) — the sheath consisting of / relating to mind (*manas*), the emotional sheath or mental sheath

prāṇamaya-kośa (m.) — the sheath consisting of / relating to vital energy (*prāṇa-*)

vijnānamaya-kośa (m.) — the sheath consisting of / relating to wisdom/understanding (vijnāna-)

ānandamaya-kośa — (m.) — the sheath consisting of / relating to bliss (ānanda-)

pañcatanmātra (m.) — the five qualities of the *mahā-bhūtas*, which manifest themselves subtly in the mind as sound, touch, form, taste and smell

pañca-tattva (n.) — see *tattva*

pañca-prāṇa (m.) — (*haṭha-yoga*) the five vital energies: situated in the lower abdomen downward-flowing (*apāna*), situated in the lungs and heart inward- and upward-flowing (*prāṇa*), situated in the throat and head upward-flowing (*udāna*), situated in the navel sideways-flowing (*samāna*), all-pervasive outward-flowing (*vyāna*)

paramparā (f.) — continuous lineage of transmission of teachings from master to disciple over time

parā-vidyā (f.) — the highest science; knowledge, learning, scholarship; (*Tantra*) supreme goddess-mantra

parigraha (m.) — to take possession of, to encompass, to grasp

paramātman (m.) — the supreme Self

pavana-muktāsana (m.) — (*Bihar Yoga*) A group of *āsanas* which remove any blockages preventing the free flow of energy in the body and mind. Pavana-muktāsana is one of the most important groups of *āsana* practices in the yoga system of Svāmī Satyānanda for developing awareness of the body's movements and the subtle effects they have at the various levels of being. For details see *Asana, Pranayama, Mudra, Bandha* by Svāmī Satyānanda

piṅgalā (m.) — One of the three main pathways (*nāḍī*) for *praṇa* in the body; active aspect of *praṇa* manifesting as a vital force; the right energy channel; 'solar' force that controls the subtle dimension

prakṛti (f.)—(*Sāṃkhya*) the eternal, transcendent principle from which the manifest world evolves

prajñā (m.)—Wisdom, insight; in the Māṇḍukya Upaniṣad: the designation of the causal body, which is associated with the state of deep sleep

prāṇa (m.)—vital or life energy/force; see also *prāṇamaya-kośa, prāṇa-pratyāhāra*

prāṇa-vāyu (m.)—the vital energy situated in the lungs and heart inward- and upward-flowing, see *pañca-prāṇa*

prāṇa-vidyā (f.)—knowledge or mastery of *prāṇa*

prāṇa-yoga-nidrā (f.)—see *yoga-nidrā*

prāṇāyāma (m.)—(*Patañjali*) breath control via retention; (*haṭha-yoga*) various breathing techniques, control of vital energy;

pramāṇa (n.)—the right way of perception, one of the five *citta-vṛttis* of *Patañjali*

prāṇamaya-kośa (m.)—the sheath consisting of / relating to vital energy (*prāṇa-*); see *pañcakośa*

pratipakṣa-bhāvanā (f.)—(*Patañjali*) the discipline of 'cultivating the opposite view'; see also *bhāvanā*

pratiṣṭhā (f.)—the establishment and consecration of divine forms; see also *nyasā*

pratyāhāra (m.)—the withdrawal/uncoupling of the sense perception from the sense objects, fifth limb of Patañjali's Yoga

āsana-pratyāhāra (m.)—practicing *āsana* in full awareness, focusing on its different aspects in succession: for example, first focusing on the physical body, then proceeding with performing the *āsana* by adding focus on the breath/*prāṇa*, then on the energy centres (*kṣetras* and *cakras*), and finally on *mantra*.

indriya-pratyāhāra (m.)—control of the senses; see *indriya*

karma-pratyāhāra (m.)—control of action; see *karma*

prāṇa-pratyāhāra (m.)—control of the *prāṇa*; see *prāṇa*

mana-pratyāhāra (m.)—withdrawal of the mind from the senses; a process of purification of the mind in all its aspects such as *citta, buddhi, manas, ahaṃkāra* (cumulatively referred to as *antaḥkaraṇa*) in order to allow the more gross mind to merge into the subtle mind; see manas

śūnya-pratyāhāra (m.)—a state, in which all attachment to the material world is overcome and one is ready to connect with the transcendent; see also *śūnyatā*

prakāśatva-pratyāhāra (m.)—a state, where all ties to the material world dissolve and one can connect with the Higher Self, leading to infusion of light

pratyakṣa (n.)—apparent, visible; luminous; that which can be perceived directly, that which can be perceived with all five senses and the mind

pratyaya (m.) — conception, concept; experience, cognition; conviction, opinion, belief, certainty, mental experience of an object, content of the mind

pratyaya-nirodha — According to Vyāsa, neutralising or 'eradicating' pratyayas takes place after *saṃprajñāta-samādhi*

pravṛtti — tendencies and inclinations in attachment and behaviour

pṛthivī (f.) — earth; the earth element

pūjā (f.) — worship, veneration; a Hindu worship ritual consisting of a set of prescribed elements, such as five distinct offerings: light (fire), water, food, incense, and mantras/sound

pūraka (m.) — (*Patañjali*) breath retention after inhalation; (*haṭha-yoga*) inhalation

Purāṇa (m.) — or 'ancient histories' are among the most important sacred scriptures of India

puruṣa (m.) — man, human, humanity, person; (*Sāṃkhya*) one of the two primal separate principles of the cosmos, absolute, pure consciousness; (*Patañjali*) also the individual pure consciousness

R

rāga (m.) — desire, attraction; opposed to dveṣa

rajas (n.) — one of the three guṇas (aspects) of subtle matter (*prakṛti*), the dynamic and fighting element

rāja-yoga — (*haṭha-yoga*) the royal path, specifically equated with samādhi; (Bihar Yoga) one of the main paths of yoga; in later centuries used to refer to *Patañjali's* Yoga

recaka (m.) — (*Patañjali*) breath retention after exhalation; (*haṭha-yoga*) exhalation

ṛṣi (m.) — seer; mythical sage

S

sahasrāra-cakra (m.) — the seventh, crown *cakra*; see *cakra*

sādhaka (m.) — spiritual aspirant, practitioner

sādhana (n.) — regular practice with a particular (usually spiritual) goal. The practice can be ritual, mantric, or other, following a precise prescription

śakti (f.) — power, energy; (*Tantra*) the feminine force of the universe in contrast to consciousness (*Śiva*); also 'consort'

śaktipāta (m.) — transmission of energy by a master to the disciple during a rite of initiation

Śāṇḍilya-upaniṣad (f.) — a later text on yoga, attributed to the twenty Yoga-upaniṣads belonging to the Atharvaveda *samādhi* (m.) — (depending on context) superconscious absorption; collection, deep immersion; compound, connection, union; fourth state of consciousness; see *nirodha*

asaṃprajñāta-samādhi (m.) — (*Patañjali*) the highest *samādhi*

saṃprajñāta-samādhi (m.) — (*Patañjali*) the state of conscious absorption, still connected with an awareness of consciousness focussed on objects

samāna-vāyu (m.) — the vital force situated in the navel and flowing sideways; see *pañca prāṇa*

samarpaṇa (n.) — merging, devotion

śāmbhavī mudrā (f.) — one of the 'seals'; gaze pointed between the eyebrows; see *mudrā*

saṃkalpa (m.) — intention, resolve, violition, inner vow, imaginative willpower

saṃkalpa-vikalpa (m.) — thoughts and counter-thoughts; idea and counter-argument

saṃkalpa-śakti (f.) — willpower generated by strengthening one's own determination, see śakti

Sāṃkhya (n.) — one of India's oldest philosophical systems

saṃsāra (n.) — the cycle of reincarnation, the bonds of existence

saṃskāra (m.) — unconscious mental impression, impression in the subconscious; see *nirodha*

samyama (m.) — (*Patañjali*) *dhāraṇā, dhyāna, samādhi* are collectively referred to as *samyama*

sanātana-dharma (m.) — eternal order; name used by contemporary Hindus to describe the behavioural aspect of the religion as an expression of the eternal and divine order of the cosmos

saṅga (m.) — spending time with like-minded individuals

sat-saṅga (m.) — the gathering of people who listen to spiritual teachings and strive for the highest insight by listening, talking, reflecting and immersing themselves in the teachings together

santoṣa (m.) — contentment, modesty, simplicity, unpretentiousness

saṃnyāsin (m.) — an ascetic who has chosen the path of renunciation, or has been initiated into a monastic order; see *svāmin*

Sarasvatī (f.) — one of the principal goddesses in Hinduism, revered as the goddess of knowledge, education, learning, arts, speech, poetry, music, creativity, purification, language and culture

śarīra (n.) — body

kāraṇa-śarīra (n.) — the causal body

sūkṣma-śarīra (n.) — the subtle body

sthūla-śarīra (n.) — the gross body

śāstra (n.) — precept, rules, manual, compendium, book or treatise

satkārā (f.) — sincere reverence

sattva (n.) — one of the three aspects (*guṇas*) of prakṛti (*sattva*, *rajas* and *tamas*) or constituents of everything in creation and interpenetrating all beings; balance, knowledge, purity, control over the organs, practice of virtue; see *guṇa*

satya (m.) — truth; sincerity

śauca (n.) — purity of body, mind and thought, purity, cleanliness, cleanness

śava (mn.) — corpse

śavāsana (n.) — the corpse position, supine relaxation position

sevā (f.) — service; selfless engagement in all activities

siddhi (f.) — special supernatural powers and abilities which, according to tradition, are acquired through spiritual practice; these can be mundane (*laukika*) or supramundane (*lokottara*)

Śiva (m.) — the highest consciousness; the god Śiva; equanimity

smṛti (f.) — phenomenological recollection,'what is remembered', the name of a canon of Indian ritual and mythological literature

śodhana (n.) — the process or action of purification, cleansing; see *śuddhi*

śraddhā (f.) — trust, faith, belief, confidence

sthairya (m.) — firmness, stability, fixity, steadiness

sthūla (mfn.) — gross, the gross experience

śuddhi (f.) — purity, cleansing, purification; see *śodhana*

sukha (mfn.) — calmness, comfort; also pleasure, non-resistance, bliss

sūkṣma (mfn.) — subtle, subtle experience

sūkṣma vyāyāma — series of exercises which concentrate on the flow of *prāṇa* developed by Svāmī Dhīrendra Brahmacārī

śūnya (n.) — void; the sky

śūnyatā (f.) — state of being in the void; (*Buddhism*) emptiness (of own nature), principle of non-essentialism; see *śūnya-pratyāhāra*

sūtra (n.) — thread; treatise; aphorism

suṣumṇā (f.) — (*Tantra*/*haṭha-yoga*) one of the most important *nāḍis* (energy channels) of the subtle body, along which the seven main cakras are arranged

suṣupti (f.) — deep, dreamless sleep; deep sleep; synonym of *nidrā*

svādhyāya (m.) — the detailed study of your own self, which includes study of the entire structure of your personality, which includes the physical, mental, emotional and spiritual aspects; self-study; self-reflection; the recitation and study of the Vedas and other sacred texts

svāmin (m.)—an honorific title given to an ascetic who has chosen the path of renunciation (*saṃnyāsa*), or has been initiated into a monastic order; in this book rendered with the Nom. Sg. *svāmī*; usually spelled 'swami' in English

svapna (m.)—sleep; dream, dream state

svara (m.)—tone, scale, sound; (*Tantra*) breath

svara-yoga (m.)—(*Tantra*) achieving spiritual and worldly goals and powers via the science of manipulating the svara or 'breath'

T

tamas (n.)—torpor, torpidity, sloth; ignorance in the nature of mind; one of the three *guṇas* (aspects) of subtle matter (*prakṛti*)

tanmātra / *pañcatanmātra*—the five subtle elements—sound, touch, smell, taste, sight

tanoti—verb. 'to expand'

tantra (n.)—treatise; loom; fabric, continuum, interconnection, foundation; (*Tantra*) often deity-based ritual, initiatory and practice system aimed at achieving liberation; (Bihar Yoga) expansion of consciousness;

tāntrika (m.)—meaning someone who is relating to, e.g. is a practitioner of *Tantra*, see *tantra*

tattva (n.)—(true) essence, (true) nature; basic principle, the gross material elements—ether, air, fire, water, earth, also *mahābhūta* or *pañca-tattva* in the same sense; (Śivait) plane of existence; see *bhuvana*, *loka*

tapas (n.)—austerity, renunciation, asceticism; self-discipline as a purging fire

tāraka-yoga (m.)—a yoga path on which the deep dimensions of consciousness and the absolute can be experienced in various light phenomena

trāyate—verb. 'to release'

trāṭaka (n.)—one of the six cleansing techniques of *haṭha-yoga*, constant fixation on a point or object; (Bihar Yoga) the practice of gazing at a point, usually at the red tip of the ignited wick of a candle

turīya (f.)—the fourth state; a term for the highest state of consciousness

U

udāna-vāyu (m.)—the upward-flowing vital energy situated in the throat and head; see *pañca-prāṇa*

unmanī (f.)—'[the state] beyond the mind' (*manas*)

upaniṣad (f.) — short philosophical writings, part of the Vedas (usually from the late Vedic period)

V

vairāgya (n.) — non-adherence; the practice of non-attachment and letting go

vahana (n.) — vehicle

Vārāhī-tantra — ('Doctrine of the Boar-Goddess') A Śākta tantric text that focuses on Goddess Vārāhī belonging to the broader category of Śaiva Bhairava Tantras.

vāsanā (f.) — the thought of, the desire for; deep-rooted wish; unconscious mental impression; imagination, idea; behavioural tendencies; part of saṃskāra

vāyu (m.) — air; the air element

Vasiṣṭha (m.) — 'the most prosperous', one of the seven great sages in Brahmanism

Vedānta (m.) — alongside Sāṃkhya, one of the best-known schools of Indian philosophy today based upon upaniṣadic philosophy

vidhi (n.) — rituals and prescribed practices

vidyā (f.) — knowledge, wisdom, realisation; includes worldly and spiritual, theoretical and practical knowledge, sometimes used in the sense of 'science'; (*Tantra*) a power or Goddess, as embodyment/manifestation/emanation of mantric power; see *mantra*

vikalpa (m.) — thought, imagination, conceptual thinking; indecisiveness, doubt, indecision, hesitation; diversity, alternative, distinction; in contrast to saṃkalpa — 'counter-thought'

vikṣipta (mfn.) — partially distracted, one of the stages or states of the mind, see *mūḍha, kṣipta, ekāgra, niruddha*

vijnānamaya-kośa (m.) — the sheath consisting of / relating to wisdom/understanding (vijnāna-); see *pañcakośa*

viṣaya (m.) — sensory object

Viṣṇu (m.) — one of the most important forms of the divine in Hinduism, whose primary function is maintaining the Universe; (Vaiṣṇavism) the highest Godhead

viśuddhi-cakra (n.) — the fifth prāṇic plexus situated in the throat, the corresponding element is space (*ākāśa*), which suggests this space should be filled with energy. The *viśuddhi-cakra* is the starting point of *udāna-vāyu*. *Viśuddhi-cakra* is associated with the purification not only on the physical level, but also on the level of the psyche and mind; see *cakra*

viparyaya (m.) — false means of knowledge; falsely understanding something to be its opposite

viveka (m.) — correct discrimination

viveka-khyāti (f.) — discriminating knowledge

vyāna-vāyu (m.) — the all-pervasive outward-flowing vital energy; see *pañca-prāṇa*

Vyāsa (m.) — also known as Vedavyāsa was a mythical sage who is considered to be the collector or compiler of important ancient Indian scriptures

vrata (m.) — vow; observance

vṛtti (f.) — movement, behaviour; circular movement; see cittavṛtti

Y

yantra (n.) — derived from √yam — 'to support', 'to hold', and the suffix-tra — tool; diagrams used in the various Indic traditions. According to the Indian commentarial tradition, -tra refers to 'liberation'; see *trāyate*

yama (m.) — behavioural instructions for dealing with others; the first stage of *Patañjali's* Yoga

yoga (m.) — yoking, connection; ancient Indian philosophical teachings centred on the union of of the self with the divine or ultimate for the sake of liberation from the cycle of rebirth

yoga-nidrā (f.) — yogic sleep, conscious sleep, a state between sleep and waking, resp. hypnagogic/ hypnopompic state; a *pratyāhāra* technique

adhyātma-yoga-nidrā (f.) — sleep of union with the Supreme Self, from *Mahābhārata* 1.19.13

prāṇa-yoga-nidrā (f.) — advanced stage of *yoga-nidrā*, which involves becoming aware of the five vital energies, or *pañca-prāṇa*, where one has to withdraw the intensity of *prāṇa-śakti* from all parts of the body, from all marma points, and concentrate on the cakras. This technique leads to *prāṇa-pratyāhāra*

dhāraṇā-yoga-nidrā (f.) — when *pratyāhāra-yoga-nidrā* deepens with time and experience, it becomes possible to reach *dhāraṇā-yoga-nidrā*, which allows for focused, direct engagement with the subtle elements of the mind; see *dhāraṇā*

Yoganidrā (f.) — a Goddess from the *Mārkaṇḍeya-purāṇa* (*Durgā-saptaśatī*); see *Mahāmāyā*

Bibliography

A

Acharya, Narayan, Ram. (1987). *The Pañcadaśi of Vidyāraṇya Muni*. Delhi: Chaukhamba Sanskrit Pratishtan.

Agras W. S., Taylor C. B., Kraemer H. C., Allen R. A., & Schneider J. A. (1980). Relaxation Training: Twenty-four-Hour Blood Pressure Reductions. *Archives of General Psychiatry*, 37(8), 859–863. doi:10.1001/archpsyc.1980.01780210017001 (accessed on 13.09.2023).

Alter, J. S. (2004). *Yoga in modern India: The body between science and philosophy*. Princeton University Press.

Amita, S., Prabhakar, S., Manoj, I., Harminder, S., & Pavan, T. (2009). Effect of yoga-nidra on blood glucose level in diabetic patients. *Indian Journal of Physiology and Pharmacology*, 53(1), 97–101. https://pubmed.ncbi.nlm.nih.gov/19810584/ (accessed on 13.09.2023).

Anjana, K., Archana, R., & Mukkadan, J. K., (2022). Effect of om chanting and yoga nidra on blood pressure and lipid profile in hypertension—A randomized controlled trial. In *Journal of Ayurveda Integrative Medicine*, 13(4). https://doi.org/10.1016/j.jaim.2022.100657. (accessed on 13.09.2023).

Anderssen-Reuster, Ulrike. (2007). *Achtsamkeit in Psychotherapie und Psychosomatik*. Stuttgart: Schattauer Verlag.

Austin, Christopher, R. (2019). *Pradyumna: Lover, Magician, and Son of the Avatara*. Oxford: Oxford University Press.

Avalon, Arthur (Woodroffe, John G.). (1953). *Tantra of the Great Liberation* [*Mahanirvana Tantra*]—Translation and Commentary. Madras: Ganesh & Co. Ltd.

Ayyangar, TR Srinivasa. (1938). *The Yoga Upanishads*. Madras: Vasanta Press.

B

Bharati, Veda Swami. (2014). *My Experiments with Yoga Nidra*. [Kindle]. Himalayan Yoga Publications Trust.

Boyes, Denis. (1973). *Le yoga du sommeil éveillé. Méthode de relaxation—Yoga Nidra*. Paris: FeniXX réédition numérique (Épi).

Boyes, Dennis. (1986). *Autogenes Yoga—Tiefenentspannung im Liegen*. Düsseldorf: ECON Taschenbuch Verlag.

Bowers, Patricia. (1978). Hypnotizability, creativity and the role of effortless experiencing. *The International Journal of Clinical and Experimental Hypnosis*, 26(3), 184–202. https://doi.org/10.1080/00207147808409320.

Bowers, K. S. (1994). Dissociated control, imagination, and the phenomenology of dissociation. In D. Spiegel (Ed.), *Dissociation: Culture, Mind, and Body* (pp. 21–38). Washington DC. American Psychiatric Association.

Bräutigam, Uwe. (2006). Die Geschichte des Pratyahara. *VIVEKA. Hefte für Yoga*. Viveka Verlag, 37.

Brunner, Héléne; Oberhammer, Gerhard; Padoux, André (eds.). (2000). *Tantrikabhidhanakosa I: Dictionaire des termes techniques de la litterature hindoue tantrique—A Dictionary of Technical Terms from Hindu Tantric Literature—Wörterbuch zur Terminologie hinduistischer Tantren*. (BKGA 35.) Vienna: VÖAW.

Burkeman, Oliver. (2014). Therapy wars: the revenge of Freud. In *The Guardian News and Media*. https://www.theguardian.com/science/2016/jan/07/therapy-wars-revenge-of-freud-cognitive-behavioural-therapy (accessed on 10.01.2022).

C

Cade, C. Maxwell & Coxhead, Nona. (2011). *The Awakened Mind: Biofeedback and the Development of Higher States of Awareness*. USA: Element Books Ltd.

Chapple, Christopher, Key and Venkatesananda. (1984). *The Concise Yoga Vāsiṣṭha*. New York: SUNY Publishers.

Clark, John. H. (1983). A Map of Mental States. London: Routledge & Kegan Paul.

Collins, Charles Dillard. (1988). *The Iconography and Ritual of Siva at Elephanta: On Life, Illumination, and Being*. New York: SUNY Press.

Coburn, Thomas, B. (2002). *Devī Māhātmya, The Crystallization of the Goddess Tradition*. Delhi: Motilal Banarsidass Publications.

Cremerius, Johannes. (1990) Die hochfrequente Langzeitanalyse und die psychoanalytische Praxis. Utopie und Realität. *Psyche — Zeitschrift für Psychoanalyse*, 44A(1), 1–29. https://pep-web.org/browse/PSYCHE/volumes/44A?openNotificationModal=false (accessed on 13.10.2022).

D

De Michelis, Elisabeth. (2004). *A history of modern yoga: Patañjali and Western esotericism*. London & New York: Continuum.

Desai, Kamini. (2017). *Yoga Nidra — The Art of Transformational Sleep*. Twin Lakes: Lotus Press.

Desikachar, T. K. V. (1999). *The Heart of Yoga: Developing a Personal Practice*. (2nd edition). Rochester: Inner Traditions Bear and Company.

Dinsmore-Tuli, Uma & Tuli, Nirlipta. (2022) *Yoga Nidra Made Easy*. London: Hay House Publishing. (1st edition).

Dinsmore-Tuli, Uma. (2024). *Yogā Nidra — The Power of Rest*. Stroud: Sitaram and Sons Ltd. (1st edition).

Divanji, Prahlad, C. (1954). *Yoga-Yājñavalkya. A Treatise on Yoga as Taught by Yogī Yājñavalkya*. Vol. 3. B.B.R.A. Society Mongraph. Bombay: Bombay Branch of the Royal Asiatic Society.

E

Easwaran, Eknath (Hrsg.). (2008). *Die Upanischaden*. München: Wilhelm Goldmann Verlag.

Engler, Jack. (2003). Being Somebody and Being Nobody: A Reexamination of the Understanding of Self in Psychoanalysis and Buddhism. In Jeremy D. Safran (Ed.). *Psychoanalysis and Buddhism. An Unfolding Dialogue*. (pp. 35–79). Boston: Wisdom Publications.

Eliade, Mircea. (2009). *Yoga — Immortality and Freedom*. Princeton: Princeton University Press.

Eliade, Mircea. (2018). *The Myth of the Eternal Return: Cosmos and History*. Princeton: Princeton University Press.

F

Feuerstein, Georg. (2008). *The Yoga Tradition — Its History, Literature, Philosophy and Practice*. (3rd edition). Arizona: Hohm Press.

Feuerstein, Georg. (1990). *Encyclopedia Dictionary of Yoga*. Boston: Shambala Verlag.

Feuerstein, Georg. (1999). *Yoga Dictionary*. Boston: Shambala Verlag.

Flak, Micheline & de Coulon, Jacques. (1985). *Des enfants qui réussissent. Le yoga dans l'éducation*. Paris: Editions Desclée de Brouwer.

Flood, Gavin, D. (1996). *An Introduction to Hinduism*. Cambridge: Cambridge University Press.

Freud, Sigmund. (1925). Wege der psychoanalytischen Therapie. In Sigmund Freud, Anna Freud & A. J. Storfer (Hgs.). *Gesammelte Schriften von Sigmund Freud*, 6. Band. Leipzig, Wien, Zürich: Internationaler Psychoanalytischer Verlag.

Friedman, Joseph, H. Kelvin; Chou, L. (2007). Mood, Emotion, and Thought. In: Christopher G. Goetz. *Textbook of Clinical Neurology* (3rd edition), Amsterdam: Saunders Elsevier.

Fromm, Erich. (2020). *Zen-Buddhismus und Psychoanalyse*. Berlin. Suhrkamp Verlag.

G

Gerd, Rudolf. (2011). *Psychodynamische Psychotherapie. Die Arbeit an Konflikt, Struktur und Trauma*. Stuttgart. Schattauer Verlag.

Goldberg, Philip. (2013). *American Veda: From Emerson and the Beatles to Yoga and Meditation — How Indian Spirituality Changed the West*. New York: Random House Verlag.

Golden Jubilee Edition. (2013). *The Golden Collection 3* — A collection of original publications from the Bihar School of Yoga Tradition. Munger: Yoga Publication Trust.

Goodall, D. & Rastelli, M. (Eds.). (2013). *Tāntrikābhidhānakośa III, T–Ph: Dictionnaire des termes techniques de la littérature hindoue tantrique. A Dictionary of Technical Terms from Hindu Tantric Literature. Wörterbuch zur Terminologie hinduistischer Tantren*. (BKGA 76.) Vienna: VÖAW.

Gosh, A. K. (Mangalteertham, Sannyasi). (1988). Brain Electrical Activity Mapping During Yoda Nidra. In Yoga Research Foundation. (2015). *Volume One, YRF Journals 1989–1990*. Yoga Publication Trust & in Svami, Satyananda. (1976). *Yoga Nidra*. Chapter: Altered State of Consciousness. Bihar: Yoga Publication Trust.

Gruzelier, J. (1998). A working model of the neurophysiology of hypnosis: a review of evidence. *Contemporary Hypnosis*, 15(1), 3–21. https://doi.org/10.1002/CH.112 (accessed on 22.02.2022).

H

Haas, Dominik. (2018). Die Kaṭha-Upaniṣad (translation). In Master's Thesis: *Vom Feueraltar zum Yoga. Kohärenz und Konzept der Kaṭha-Upaniṣad*. https://doi.org/10.1007/S10781-019-09408-Y (accessed on 22.02.2022).

Hacker. Paul. (1950). Eigentümlichkeiten der Lehre und Terminologie Śaṅkaras: Avidyā, Nāmarūpa, Māyā, Īśvara. *Zeitschrift der Deutschen Morgenländischen Gesellschaft*. 100, N. F. 25, p. 246–286.

Halbfass, Wilhelm. (1988). *India and Europe: An Essay in Understanding*. New York: SUNY Press.

Hanegraaff, W. J. (1996). *New Age religion and Western culture: Esotericism in the mirror of secular thought*. Leiden: Brill.

Harrington, Anne, & John D. Dunne. (2015). When Mindfulness Is Therapy: Ethical Qualms, Historical Perspectives. *American Psychologist*. 70(7), pp. 621–631. http://nrs.harvard.edu/urn-3:HUL.InstRepos:25757884 (accessed on 07.11.2022).

———. (1994). Neodissociation theory. (pp. 32–51). In S. J. Lynn & J. W. Rhue (Eds.). *Dissociation: Clinical and Theoretical Perspectives*. New York: Guilford Press.

Hilgard, E.R. Eine Neo-Dissoziationstheorie des geteilten Bewusstseins. In *Zeitschrift Hypnose und Kognition* (HyKog). (1989)6(2).

Hilgard, E. R., Neodissociation Theory. In Lynn, S. J./Rhue, J. W. (Eds.). (1994). *Dissociation: Clinical and Theoretical Perspectives*. New York: Guilford Press.

Huchzermeyer, Wilfried. (2015). *Das Yoga-Lexikon*. Karlsruhe: Verlag W. Huchzermeyer.

I

Irschick, Eugene F. (1969). *Politics and social conflict in South India The non-Brahman Movement and Tamil Separatism 1916–1929*. Bombay: Oxford University Press.

J

Jacobson, Edmund. (1978). *You must relax: Practical Methods for Reducing the Tensions of Modern Living*. New York: McGraw-Hill Publications.

Janakānanda, Swami. (2022). *A deeper yoga and Yoga Nidra*. [eBook edition]. Hamneda: Bindu Publishers. https://yogameditationshop.com/products/a-deeper-yoga-and-yoga-nidra.

K

Kālī, Devadatta. (2003). *In Praise of the Goddess — The Devīmāhātmya and Its Meaning*. Maine: Nicolas-Hays Publication.

Kakar, Sudhir. (1991). *Shamans, Mystics and Doctors: A Psychological Inquiry into India and its Healing Traditions*. Chicago: University of Chicago Press.

Keller, Anandaratna, Urs. (2019). *Satyananda Yoga Nidra Ausbidungsmanual*. [Class handout]. Zürich: Samatvam Yoga-Schule.

Khanna, Madhu. (2003). *Yantra: The Tantric Symbol of Cosmic Unity*. Vermont: Thames & Hudson.

King, R. (1999). *Indian philosophy and Western intellectuals: The problem of Orientalism*. Oxfordshire: Routledge.

Kirsch, Irving & Lynn, Steven Jay. (1998). *Social-cognitive alternatives to dissociation theories of hypnotic involuntariness*. Psychological Bulletin. 2(1).

Kriz, Jürgen. (2014). *Grundkonzepte der Psychotherapie* (7th edition). Weinheim: Beltz.

Kumar, Kamakhya. (2013). *A Handbook of Yoga-Nidrā*. New Delhi: D. K. Printworld Ltd.

L

Laier, Michael. (2005). Hypnose. (pp. 1193–1195). In Werner E. Gerabek, Bernhard D. Haage, Gundolf Keil & Wolfgang Wegner (Hgs.). *Enzyklopädie Medizingeschichte*. Berlin, New York: De Gruyter Verlag.

Languani, Pittu. (2004). *Asian Perspectives in Counseling and Psychotherapy*. New York: Brunner-Rutlege Verlag.

Larson, G. J. (1969). *Classical Sāṃkhya: An interpretation of its history and meaning*. Delhi: Motilal Banarsidass.

——— & Bhattacharya, R. S. (1987). *Yoga: India's philosophy of meditation*. Delhi: Motilal Banarsidass.

Linehan, Marsha. (1996). *Dialektisch-Behaviorale Therapie der Borderline-Persönlichkeitsstörung*. München: CIP-Medien.

Lorenzer, Alfred. (2022). *Die Sprache, der Sinn, das Unbewusste*. Stuttgart: Klett-Cotta.

M

Maas, Philipp, A. (2013). A concise historiography of classical yoga philosophy. In K. Baier, P. Maas, & K. Preisendanz (Eds.). *Yoga in Transformation: Historical and Contemporary Perspectives* (pp. 57–87). Vienna: Austrian Academy of Sciences Press.

Mallinson, J. (2007). *The Shiva Samhita: A Critical Edition and an English Translation*. Woodstock: YogaVidya.com

——— & Birch, J. (2017). *The Yoga of the Haṭhapradīpikā: A critical edition and translation*. Oxfordshire: Routledge.

——— & Singelton, M. (2017). *Roots of Yoga*. London: Penguin Classics.

Miller, Richard. (2010). *Yoga Nidra — A Meditative Practice for Deep Relaxation and Healing*. Colorado: Sounds True Publications.

———. (2010). *Yoga Nidra — Eine meditative Praxis für Tiefenentspannung und Heilung*. Colorado: Sounds True Publications. 2nd edition.

———. (2015). *The iRest Program For Healing PTSD. A Proven-Effective Approach to Using Yoga Nidra Meditation and Deep Relaxation Techniques to Overcome Trauma*. Oakland: New Harbinger Publications.

Mitzinger, Dietmar. (2009). *Yoga in Prävention und Therapie. Ein Manual für Yogalehrer, Therapeuten und Trainer*. Köln: Deutscher Ärzte-Verlag.

Mohan, AG. (translation). (2000). *Yoga-Yājñavalkya*. Chennai: Ganesh & Co.

Muktibodhananda, Swami. (1999). *Swara Yoga*. Munger: Yoga Publication Trust.

Muñoz, Adrián. (2016). *Yogabīja: A critical transcription of a text on haṭha-yoga*. In: Nova Tellvs, 33/2.

N

Nakamura, Hajime. (2004). *A History of Early Vedānta Philosophy*. Part 2. Delhi: Motilal Banarsidass Publications.

Narasimhananda, Swami. (2019). *Yoga Taravali of Acharya Shankara*. Prabuddha Bharata, 124(1), 1–9. https://doi.org/10.17613/PHGE-X974.

Nataraja, Shanida. (2008). *The Blissful Brain — Neuroscience and proof of the power of meditation*. London: Octopus Publishing Group Ltd.

O

Olivelle, Patrick. (1998). *The Early Upaniṣads: Annotated Text and Translation*. New York/Oxford: Oxford University Press.

P

Panda, Nursing, Charan. (2011). *Yoga-Nidra*. (2nd edition). New Delhi: D.K. Printworld (P) Ltd.

Parker, S., Bharati, S. V. & Fernandez, M. (2013). Defining yoga-nidra: traditional accounts, physiological research, and future directions. *International Journal of Yoga Therapy*, 23(1), 11–16.

Pattanaik, Devdutt. (2014). *7 Secrets of the Goddess*. New Delhi: Westland Ltd.

Patañjali. (1998). *Patanjali's Yoga Sutras — with the Commentary of Vyāsa and the gloss of Vāchaspati Miśra, Prasāda, Rāma*. (translation). New Delhi: Munshirm Manoharlal Pub Pvt. Ltd.

R

Rama, Swami. (1982). *Enlightenment without God — Mandukya Upanishad*. Honesdale: Himalayan Institute Press.

———. (1988). *Path of Fire and Light*, Volume II. Honesdale: Himalayan Institute Press.

———. (2015). *Living With The Himalayan Masters*. Honesdale: Himalayan Institute Press.

Ramm-Bonwitt, Ingrid. (2010). *Yoga Nidra — Der Schlaf der Yogis*. Darmstadt: Schirner Verlag

Ranefeld, Johannes. (2012). Immer und überall. Die Suggestion. (pp. 199–210). In Peter, Geißler. *Stimme und Suggestion*. Die „musikalische Dimension' und ihre suggestive Kraft im psychotherapeutischen Geschehen. Psychosozial-Verlag.

Ranganathan, Shyam. (2009). *Patañjali's Yoga Sūtra*. Black Classics. Delhi: Penguin Black Classics.

Ratnākaraśānti. (1992). Mahāmāyātantram with Guṇavatī (Prof. Samdhong Rinpoche & Vrajavallabh Dwivedi, Eds.). *Rare Buddhist Text Series* (No. 10). Central Institute of Higher Tibetan Studies, Sarnath, Varanasi, India.

Reddemann, Luise. (2016). *Mitgefühl, Trauma und Achtsamkeit in psychodynamischen Therapien*. Göttingen: Vandenhoeck & Ruprecht.

Revenstorf, Dirk, Dr. & Burkhard, Peter, Dipl.-Psych. Dr. (Hsg.). (2009). *Hypnose in Psychotherapie, Psychosomatik und Medizin*. (2nd edition). Heidelberg: Springer Medizin Verlag.

Rilke, Rainer, Maria. (2011). *Letters to a Young Poet*. Penguin Edition Nr. 103. London: Penguin Classics.

S

Sabourin, M. E., Cutcomb, S. D., Crawford, H. J. & Pribram, K. (1990). EEG correlates of hypnotic susceptibility and hypnotic trance: spectral analysis and coherence. *International Journal of Psychophysiology: Official Journal of the International Organization of Psychophysiology*, 10(2), 125–142. https://doi.org/10.1016/0167–8760(90)90027-b (accessed on 20.04.2021).

Saraswati, Niranjanananda, Swami. (1997). *Yoga Sadhana Panorama*, Volume 2. Munger: Yoga Publication Trust.

———. (1997). *Yoga Sadhana Panorama, Volume 2*. Munger: Yoga Publication Trust.

———. (1999). *Yoga Sadhana Panorama, Volume 1*. Munger: Yoga Publication Trust.

———. (2002). *Yoga Darshan*. (1st edition, reprinted with corrections). Munger: Yoga Publication Trust.

———. (2008). *Samkhya Darshan*. Munger: Yoga Publication Trust.

———. (2013). *Tantra Darshan*. Munger: Yoga Publication Trust.

———. (2013). *Water the Roots 8* — The SWAN Principle. Bihar: Yoga Publication Trust.

———. (2014). *Prana und Pranayama*. Munger: Yoga Publication Trust.

———. (2015). *Yoga Chakra — The Wheel of Yoga*. Munger: Yoga Publication Trust.

———. (2017). *Raja Yoga Yatra 1 — Understanding Pratyahara*. Munger: Yoga Publication Trust.

———. (2018). *Progression of Pratyahara 1*. Munger: Yoga Publication Trust.

———. (2018). *Raja Yoga Yatra 2 — *Understanding Pratyahara. Munger: Yoga Publication Trust.

———. (2019). *Yoga Chakrodaya — Book 2/3*. Bihar: Yoga Publications Trust.

Saraswati, Satyananda, Swami. (n.d.). Yogic Concepts. *Yoga Magazine*. 2008(11/12). Munger: Yoga Publication Trust. http://www.yogamag.net/archives/2000s/2008/0811/0811ygcn.html (accessed on 12.01.2020).

———. (1979). The Path of Experience. Satsang (Lecture). *Yoga Magazine*. 1980(3). Munger: Yoga Publication Trust. http://www.yogamag.net/archives/1980s/1980/8003/8003paex.html (accessed on 30.07.2020).

———. (1982). Raja Yoga Sutras. In *Yoga Magazine*, 2016. From Swami Satyadharma & Swami G Saraswati (Eds.), *Teachings of Swami Satyananda Saraswati. Volume III*. Munger: Yoga Publication Trust. http://www.yogamag.net/archives/2010s/2016/1608/1608raja.html. (accessed on 28.07.2020).

———. (1989). *Teachings of Swami Satyananda Saraswati. Volume III*. In *Yoga Magazine*. Raja Yoga. 2016 (8). http://www.yogamag.net/archives/2010s/2016/1608/1608raja.html (accessed on 25.03.2020).

———. (2000). *Four Chapters on Freedom*. Munger: Yoga Publication Trust.

———. (2001). *Kundalini Tantra*. Munger: Yoga Publications Trust.

———. (2001). *Meditations from the Tantras*. (2nd edition). Munger: Yoga Publication Trust.

———. (2002). *Dynamics of Yoga — The Foundations of Bihar Yoga*. (reprint 2nd edition). Munger: Yoga Publication Trust.

———. (2006). *A Systematic Course in The Ancient Tantric Techniques of Yoga and Kriya*. (4th reprint). Munger: Yoga Publications Trust.

———. (2006). *Yoga Nidra*. (12th reprint). Munger: Yoga Publications Trust.

———. (2007). *Awakening the Vijnānamayakośa*. Munger: Yoga Publication Trust.

———. (2009). *Asana, Pranayama, Mudra, Bandha*. Munger: Yoga Publication Trust.

———. (2013). *Haṭha-Yoga-Pradīpikā*. Munger: Yoga Publications Trust.

———. (2013). *Yoga Nidra — Water the Roots* 4. Munger: Yoga Publications Trust.

Sarawati, Satyasangananda, Swami. (2004). *Sri Vijnana Bhairava Tantra — The Ascent*. Munger: Yoga Publication Trust.

———. (2005). *Tattwa Shuddhi*. Munger: Yoga Publication Trust.

———. (n. d.). Yogic Concepts. In *Yoga Magazine*. (2008). Munger: Bihar School of Yoga. (11/12). http://www.yogamag.net/archives/2000s/2008/0811/0811ygcn.html (accessed on 12.01.2020).

Satyadharma, Swami. (2013). *SWAN Meditation — Theory and Practice*. Munger: Yoga Publication Trust.

Saraswati, Shankardevananda, Swami. (n.d.). Sankalpa and Yoga Therapy. *Yoga Magazine*. 1999(9). Munger: Yoga Publication Trust. http://www.yogamag.net/archives/1990s/1999/9909/9909skyt.html (accessed on 22.05.2023).

Saraswati, Prakashananda, Swami. (2003). *Yoga Nidra — Neue Erkenntnisse*. Tettnang: Ananda Verlag.

Schopenhauer, Arthur. (2000). *Parerga and Paralipomena: Short Philosophical Essays (1976–1987)*. Volume II. (1st published 1974). Oxford: Oxford University Press.

Sharvananda, Swami. (1921). *Taittiriya-Upanishad*. Mylapore: The Ramakrishna Math.

Singleton, M. (2010). *Yoga body: The origins of modern posture practice*. Oxford University Press.

Singh, Jaideva. (1991). *The Yoga of Delight, Wonder, and Astonishment: A Translation of the Vijnana-bhairava with an Introduction and Notes*. New York: SUNY Publishers.

Solms, Mark & Kaplan-Solms, Karen. (2005). *Neuro-Psychoanalyse — Eine Einführung mit Fallstudien*. (2nd edition). Stuttgart: Klett-Cotta.

Strauss, S. (2005). *Positioning yoga: Balancing acts across cultures*. New York: Routledge.

Stowasser, J. M., Petschenig, M., Skutsch, F. (1979). *Lateinisch-deutsches Schulwörterbuch*. Wien: övb.

Svatmarama. (2002). *The Hatha Yoga Pradipika*. Akers, Brian Dana. (translation). New York: Yoga Vidya Publications.

SYAE. (2007). Yogic Studies 1. [*Class handout*]. Satyananda Yoga Academy Europe.

SYAE. (2009). Yogic Studies 2. [*Class handout*]. Satyananda Yoga Academy Europe.

T

Thieme, Paul. (1999). *Upanischaden*. Ditzingen: Reclam-Verlag.

Tokunaga, Muneo. (1999). *Mahabharata: Adiparvan*. Revised by John Smith, et al. [Electronic text]. Bhandarkar Oriental Research Institute, Pune, India, 1999 On the basis of the text entered by Muneo Tokunaga et al., revised by John Smith, Cambridge. http://gretil.sub.uni-goettingen.de/gretil/1_sanskr/2_epic/mbh/mbh_01_u.htm (accessed on 22.03.2022).

Torwesten, Hans. (1985). Vedanta: Herz des Hinduismus, Chapter: Maya, die indische Sphinx. Walter Verlag. Citated in *Vedanta-Heft*. 2, 2012. Wiesbaden: Vedanta-Zentrum.

U

Urban, H. B. (2003). *Tantra: Sex, secrecy, politics, and power in the study of religion*. Berkeley: University of California Press.

W

Walker, Matthew. (2017). *Why we sleep — unlocking the power of sleep and dream*. New York: Scribner.

Wallis, Christopher D. (2014). *To Enter, to be entered, to merge: The role of religious experience in the traditions of Tantric Shaivism*. Dissertation. Berkeley: University of California.

Walter, Michael. (1996). Jabir, the buddhist Yogi, Part Two: Winds and Immortality. In *Journal of Indian Philosophy* 24. Amsterdam: Kluwer Academic Publishers.

Wangyal, Tenzin, Rinpoche. (1998). *The Tibetan Yogas Of Dream And Sleep*. New York: Snow Lion Publications.

Warnke, Ulrich. (2017). *Quantenphilosophie und Spiritualität*. München: Goldmann Verlag.

Watzlawick, Paul., Beavin, Janet, H., & Jackson, Don. D. (1969). *Menschliche Kommunikation*, Stuttgart, Wien: Huber Bern Verlag.

Wolz-Gottwald, Eckard. (2016). *Yoga Philosophie-Atlas*. (5th edition). Petersberg: Verlag Via Nova.

Wujastyk, D. (2017). *The Yoga Texts Attributed to Yājñavalkya and their Remarks on Posture*. Asian Literature and Translation, 4(1)

Y

Yapko, Michael, PhD. (2018). *Trancework: An Introduction to the Practice of Clinical Hypnosis*. (5th edition). Oxfordshire: Routledge.

Yoga Research Foundation. (2015). *Volume One, YRF Journals 1989–1990*. Munger: Yoga Publication Trust.

Yoga Research Foundation. (2015). *Volume Two, Promotion Of Health 1998–2007*. Munger: Yoga Publication Trust.

Yoga Research Foundation. (2018). *Volume Three, Promotion of Health 1988–2007*. Munger: Yoga Publication Trust.

Internet Sources

B

Birch, Jason. & Hargreaves, Jaqueline. (2014). Yoganidrā. In *The Luminescent Blog*, https://www.theluminescent.org/2015/01/yoganidra.html (accessed on 16.01.2022).

F

Frawley, David. (n.d.). Pratyahara, Yoga's Forgotten Limb. *Yoga International*. https://yogainternational.com/article/view/pratyahara-yogas-forgotten-limb/ (accessed on 27.06.2020).

G

Gemeinsamen Bundesausschuss. (2020). *Richtlinie des Gemeinsamen Bundesausschusses über die Durchführung der Psychotherapie* (Psychotherapie-Richtlinie), p. 19. https://www.g-ba.de/downloads/62-492-2400/PT-RL_2020-11-20_iK-2021-02-18.pdf (accessed on 13.01.2022).

D

Desai, Kamini. (n.d.). https://www.kaminidesai.com/yoga-nidra (accessed on 24.01.2022)

Dharmachakra Translation Committee. (2013). *Śrī-mahāmāyā-tantrarājanāma*. Toh 425; Degé Kangyur volume 80, F.169.a; Translated by the Dharmachakra Translation Committee under the patronage and supervision of 84000: Translating the Words of the Buddhahttps://read.84000.co/translation/toh425.html?part=UT22084-080-009-chapter-2 (accessed on 22.03.2022).

H

Haas, Dominik (translation). (2019). *Die Māṇḍūkya-Upaniṣad* (revised version). https://www.academia.edu/40968181/Die_M%C4%81%E1%B9%87%E1%B8%8D%C5%ABkya_Upani%E1%B9%A3ad (accessed on 27.10.2022).

Haas, Dominik, A. (2025). *New Directions in Mantra Studies: Exploring the Emergence of Mantra Repetition*. ARGOS. https://doi.org/10.26034/fr.argos.2025.8033 (accessed on 28.10.2025)

Himalayan Tradition. (n.d.). https://www.himalayatradition.ch/home/die-himalaya-tradition/ (accessed on 10.12.2022).

I

iRest Yoga Nidra® Research Projects. (n.d.). https://www.irest.org/irest-research (accessed on 10.04.2020).

L

Lindemeier, Alexander. (2015). Neuropsychoanalyse. Modeerscheinung oder Rückkehr zu den Freud'schen Urkonzepten?. [online publication]. In *Springer*. Interview partners: Stephan, Doering & August, Ruhs. Neuropsychiatrie. (29). 39–42. https://doi.org/10.1007/s40211–015-0137-y (accessed on 11.01.2022).

M

Maas, Philipp, A. (2013). A Concise Historiography of Classical Yoga Philosophy. Pre-Print Version of the Article Published in: Eli Franco (Ed.), *Periodization and Historiography of Indian Philosophy*. Publications of the De Nobili Research Library, 37. Vienna: Sammlung De Nobili, 53–90. https://doi.org/10.5281/ZENODO.8055379 (accessed on 20.10.2022).

———. (2020). Sarvāstivāda Buddhist Theories of Temporality and the Pātañjala Yoga Theory of Transformation (pariṇāma). *Journal of Indian Philosophy*. 48.5: pp. 963–965. (accessed on 22.10.2023 https://doi.org/10.1007/s10781–020-09450–1).

———. (2021). YSP 21: What is Sāṅkhya Philosophy?. [*Yogic Studies*] https://www.youtube.com/watch?v=I1cnO7ADq3M&t=1829s (accessed on 10.10. 2022).

———. (n. d). *The Pātañjalayogaśāstra alias the Yogasūtra and the Yogabhāṣya. Sahapedia*. https://www.sahapedia.org/patanjalayogasastra-alias-yogasutra-and-yogabhasya (accessed on 22.10.2023).

———. (2022). The Yoga Sutras in Depth. [*Keen on Yoga Podcast*] https://www.youtube.com/watch?v=ZFkGCIhEmVw&t=265s (accessed on 30.10. 2022).

Mallinson, J. (2020). Haṭha Yoga's early history: From Vajrayāna to Śaivism. *Journal of the American Oriental Society*, 140(1), 1–28. https://doi.org/10.7817/jameroriesoci.140.1.0001 (accessed on 28.10.2025).

Mahabharata: Adiparvan. (1999). On the basis of the text entered by Muneo Tokunaga et al., revised by John Smith, Cambridge, et al. Electronic text. Pune: ©Bhandarkar Oriental Research Institute.http://gretil.sub.uni-goettingen.de/gretil/1_sanskr/2_epic/mbh/mbh_01_u.htm (accessed on 22.03.2022).

Miller, Richard. (2016). Developing Interoception — The Power of Body Sensing. [*YogaUOnline*] https://www.youtube.com/watch?v=EqdtKjukF7k&t=484s (Time: 11:16 min.) (accessed on 01.04.2019).

N

Nilsson, Robert. (n.d.) The relaxed State and Science. *Scandinavian Yoga and Meditation School.* https://www.yogameditation.com/reading-room/the-relaxed-state-and-science/ (accessed on 07.11.2022).

R

Reis, Jennifer. (n.d.). https://jenniferreisyoga.com (accessed on 01.04.2019).

S

Sovik, Rolf, PsyD. (2013). What is Yoga Nidra? [Video]. *Yoga International.* https://www.youtube.com/watch?v=4NBImrP0aPk (accessed on 20.01.2022).

———. (2013). Yoga Nidra: Introduction to the Complete Practice. [Video]. *Yoga International.* https://www.youtube.com/watch?v=6usuqKQOiqM (accessed on 01.04.2019).

Śrī-mahāmāyā-tantrarājanāma Toh 425; Degé Kangyur volume 80, F.169.a; Translated by the Dharmachakra Translation Committee under the patronage and supervision of 84000: Translating the Words of the Buddha / First published 2013).

Sternek, Katharina. (2014). Über den Einsatz und die Wirkungsweise von „Bildschirm-Techniken". Österreich: *Zeitschrift für Gestalttheoretische Psychotherapie.* 6(1). 20–29. /https://www.oeagp.at/cms/uploads/pdf/Fachartikel/Sternek2014Bildschirmtechniken.pdf (accessed on 02.03.2022).

T

The Sanskrit Project. (2020). *Göttingen Register of Electronic Texts in Indian Languages* (GRETIL). SUB Göttingen. https://gretil.sub.uni-goettingen.de/gretil.html (accessed 14.10.2024)

Total Yoga Nidra Network. https://www.yoganidranetwork.org (accessed on 20.12.2021).

Turnau, Narada, Marcel. (n.d.). Das Nirvana Shatakam von Shankara — Essenz des Advaita Vedanta. *Vedanta Yoga.* https://vedanta-yoga.de/advaita-vedanta/nirvana-shatakam-shankara-bedeutung/ (accessed on 30.04.2021).

U

Uma Dinsmore-Tuli.(n.d.). https://umadinsmoretuli.com (accessed on 21.12.2021).

Satyananda Yoga Nidra studies

A

Amita, S., Prabhakar, S., Manoj, I., Harminder, S. & Pavan, T. (2009). Effect of yoga-nidra on blood glucose level in diabetic patients. *Indian Journal of Physiology and Pharmacology*, 53(1), 97–101. https://pubmed.ncbi.nlm.nih.gov/19810584/ (accessed on 13.09.2023).

Anderson, Roberta et al. (2017). Using yoga nidra to improve stress in psychiatric nurses in a pilot study. *Journal for Alternative and Complementary Medicine*, 23(6). https://doi.org/10.1089/acm.2017.004 (accessed on 14.09.2023).

B

Bahrke, M., S. (1979). Exercise, meditation and anxiety reduction: A review, American Corrective Therapy Journal, 33(2). In Kamakhya Kumar. (2013). *A Handbook of Yoga-Nidrā*. New Delhi: D. K. Printworld (P) Ltd.

Bajpai, R., Rajak, C., & Rampalliwar, S. (2015). Effect of Bhramari Pranayama and Yoga Nidra on cardiovascular hyper-reactivity to cold pressor test. *International Journal of Medical Science Research and Practice*, 2(1), 24–26. https://www.ijmsrp.com/wp-content/uploads/2015/04/07_Ritu_Bajpai.pdf (accessed on 08.02.2023).

Bali, Lekh, Raj. (1979). Long-Term Effect of Relaxation on Blood Pressure and Anxiety Levels of Essential Hypertensive Males: A Controlled Study. Psychosomatic Medicine, 41(8), p. 637–646. In Kamakhya, Kumar. (2013). *A Handbook of Yoga-Nidrā*. New Delhi: D. K. Printworld (P) Ltd., p. 118.

Benson, H., Greenwood, M. M. & Klemchuk, H. (1975). The relaxation response: psychophysiologic aspects and clinical applications. *International Journal of Psychiatry in Medicine*, 6(1–2), 87–98. https://doi.org/10.2190/376W-E4MT-QM6Q-H0UM (accessed on 13.09.2023).

Bhalendu, Suriakant, Vaishnav, et al. (2019). Transformative effects of yoga nidra on hedonic and eudemonic dimensions of well-being: A qualitative study in trainee teachers. *International Journal of Yoga — Philosophy, Psychology and Parapsychology*, 7(1), p 17–23. http://dx.doi.org/10.4103/ijny.ijoyppp_14_18 (accessed on 12.09.2023).

Bhatia, T., Kumari, N., Yadav, A., Beniwal, R. P., Shah, G., Joel, W., Jones, J. R., Iyenger, S., Nimgaonkar, V. L., & Deshpande, S. N. (2022). Feasibility, acceptability and evaluation of meditation to augment yoga practice among persons diagnosed with schizophrenia. *Acta Neuropsychiatrica*, 34(6), 330–343. https://doi.org/10.1017/neu.2022.14 (accessed on 14.09.2023).

Bushan, Siddhartha. (2001). Yoga Nidra: Its Advantages and Applications. *Yoga Magazine*. http://www.yogamag.net/archives/2000s/2001/0103/0103ygnd.html (accessed on 14.09.2023).

———. (n.d.). Qualitative Transformation in Personality: A Function of Yoga Nidra, Journal of Indian Psychology, 24(1/2). In Kamakhya Kumar. (2013). *A Handbook of Yoga-Nidrā*. New Delhi: D. K. Printworld (P) Ltd., p. 64.

———. (n.d.). Yoga-Nidra as Intervenor to Promote Self-Confidence among Teenagers, Indian Journal of Psychometry and Education, 37(1). In Kamakhya,Kumar. (2013). *A Handbook of Yoga-Nidrā*. New Delhi: D. K. Printworld (P) Ltd.

Bhushan, S. & Sinha, P. (2001). Yoganidra and management of anxiety and hostility. Journal of Indian Psychology, 19(1–2), 44–49.

C

Carrington, Patricia, et al. (1980). The Use of Meditation–Relaxation Techniques for the Management of Stress in a Working Population. Journal of Occupational Medicine, 22(4). In Swami Satyananda Saraswati. (2006). *Yoga Nidra*. Bihar: Yoga Publications Trust. p.195.

Cascella, Marco; Bandyopadhyay, Susanta. (2023). Lambda Waves, 2022. In *Treasure Island* (FL): StatPearls Publishing LLC., 1. https://www.ncbi.nlm.nih.gov/books/NBK553088/ (accessed on 07.11.2022).

Chhetri, Praghosh et al. (2020). Immediate Effects of Yoga Based Relaxation Technique on Heart Rate Variability in Young and Healthy Volunteers. *Journal of Karnali Academy of Health Sciences*, 3(2), 65–72. https://doi.org/10.3126/jkahs.v3i2.30807 (accessed on 13.09.2023).

Chowdhary, Binod. (2019). Effect of yoga nidra and pranayama on selected physiological variables of tribal youths. *International Journal of Physiology, Nutrition and Physical Education*, 4(1), 2011–2015. https://www.journalofsports.com/pdf/2019/vol4issue1/PartAQ/4–2-105–195.pdf (accessed on 12.09.2023).

Christine, Michael (2017). Effect of Yoga Nidra on Stress among Nursing Students in Selected Colleges of Nursing. *Asian Journal of Nursing, Education and Research*, 7(3), 429–440. https://doi.org/10.5958/2349–2996.2017.00085.4 (accessed on 14.09.2023).

D

Das, Payel & Pandey, Vivek. (2020). Comparative Effect of Audio-Visual Biofeedback Therapy and Yoga Nidra on Lactate Clearance and Heart Rate during Recovery of Badminton Players. *International Journal of Science and Research* (IJSR), 9(5), pp. 158–164. https://www.ijsr.net/archive/v9i5/SR20501010219.pdf (accessed on 14.09.2023).

Datey, K. K. & Bhagat, S. J. (1977). Stress and Heart Desease and How to Control It with Biofeedback and Shavasana, Quart. Journal for Surgical Science, Banaras Hindu University, 13. In Kamakhya Kumar. (2013). *A Handbook of Yoga-Nidrā*, New Delhi: D. K. Printworld (P) Ltd., p. 55.

Datta, Karuna et al. (2021). Yoga nidra practice shows improvement in sleep in patients with chronic insomnia: A randomized controlled trial. In *National Medical Journal India*, 34(3), 143–50. https://

nmji.in/yoga-nidra-practice-shows-improvement-in-sleep-in-patients-with-chronic-insomnia-a-randomized-controlled-trial/ (accessed on 12.09.2023).

———., Bhutambare, A., V L, M., Narawa, Y., Srinath, R., & Kanitkar, M. (2023). Improved sleep, cognitive processing and enhanced learning and memory task accuracy with Yoga nidra practice in novices. *PloS one*, 18(12), e0294678. https://doi.org/10.1371/journal.pone.0294678 (accessed on 12.09.2023).

———., Mallick, H. N., Tripathi, M., Ahuja, N., & Deepak, K. K. (2022). Electrophysiological Evidence of Local Sleep During Yoga Nidra Practice. *Frontiers in Neurology*, 13, 910794. https://doi.org/10.3389/fneur.2022.910794 (accessed on 15.09.2023)

———., Tripathi, M. & Mallick, H.N. (2017). Yoga Nidra: An innovative approach for management of chronic insomnia—A case report. *Sleep Science Practice*, 1(7). https://doi.org/10.1186/s41606-017-0009-4 (accessed on 12.09.2023).

———., Tripathi, M., Verma, M., Masiwal, D., & Mallick, H. N. (2021). Yoga nidra practice shows improvement in sleep in patients with chronic insomnia: A randomized controlled trial. *The National Medical Journal of India*, 34(3), 143–150. https://doi.org/10.25259/NMJI_63_19 (accessed on 14.09.2023).

Datta K, Yadav N, Narawade Y, Mahajan U, Joseph T, Kumar A. (2022). Sleep Strategies for Sportsmen; What can they be? A Randomised Controlled Trial. *Sleep Vigilance*, 6(1), 165–171. https://doi.org/10.1007/s41782-021-00188-8 (accessed on 14.09.2023).

D'cunha, R.; Pappachan, B.; D'souza, O., Loyster; Tonse, R.; Saldanha, E. and Baliga, M. Shrinath (2021). Effectiveness of Yoga Nidra in Mitigating Stress. In Women Undergoing Curative Radiotherapy for Cervical Cancer. *Middle East Journal of Cancer*, 12(1), 117–127. https://doi.org/10.30476/mejc.2020.82648.1093 (accessed on 14.09.2023).

Deuskar, Megha. Poonawala, N. & Bhatewara, Sunit. (2006). Effect of Yoga Nidra and Applied Relaxation Technique on Steadiness and Performance of Archers. *Psychological Studies, University of Callicut*, 51(1), 64–68. https://www.researchgate.net/publication/285875486_Effect_of_Yoga_Nidra_and_Applied_ Relaxation_technique_on_steadiness_and_performance_of_archers (accessed on 14.09.2023).

Devi, Saraswati & Kala, Saraswati. (2015). Role of Yoga-nidra and Shirodhara on Hypertensive Patients. *International Journal of Yoga and Allied Sciences*, 4 (1), 22–27. http://indianyoga.org/wp-content/uploads/2015/05/v4-issue1-article4.pdf (accessed on 13.09.2023).

D'souza, O. L., Jose, A. E., Suresh, S., & Baliga, M. S. (2021). Effectiveness of Yoga Nidra in reducing stress in school going adolescents: An experimental study. *Complementary Therapies in Clinical Practice*, 45, 101462. https://doi.org/10.1016/j.ctcp.2021.101462 (accessed on 12.09.2023).

Dwivedi, Manish Kumar. (2022). Effectiveness of Yoga Nidra Intervention (Meditation) in Improving well-being of an Individual. *Indian Journal of Social Psychiatry*, 38(1):p 73–85, DOI: 10.4103/ijsp.ijsp_32_20 (accessed on 14.09.2023).

G

Ganpat, Tikhe, Sham. (2020). Yoga Nidra Practice Enhances Emotional Intelligence in University Students. In *Alternative and Complementary Therapies*, 26(5), 214–218. https://doi.org/10.1089/act.2020.29294.tsg (accessed on 12.09.2023).

Gawali, Minakshi, Haribhau. (2015). Effect of suryanamaskar and yoga nidra on menstruation problems of adolescent girls. *Semantic Scholar* https://www.semanticscholar.org/paper/Effect-of-suryanamaskar-and-yoga-nidra-on-problems-Gawali/739d6d988b7018a65484d-96915458c9ef81c0715 (accessed on 08.02.2023).

Gersten, D., J. (1978). Meditation as an Adjunct to Medical and Psychiatric Treatment. American Journal of Psychiatry, 135, 5. In Swami Satyananda Sataswati. (2026). *Yoga Nidra*. Bihar: Yoga Publication Trust. p. 196.

Gosh, A.K. (Mangalteertham, Sannyasi). (1988). Brain Electrical Activity Mapping During Yoda Nidra. In Yoga Research Foundation. (2015). *Volume One, YRF Journals 1989–1990*. Bihar: Yoga Publication Trust, p. 26–31 and Yoga Nidra: Altered State of Consciousness. In Swami Satyananda Saraswati. (2006). *Yoga Nidra*. Bihar: Yoga Publication Trust, p. 245–253.

Govardhan HB. et al. (2018). Developement of Comprehensive Yoga Program for Cervical Carcinoma. In *Journal for Inerative Oncology*, 7(1), 206. doi:10.4172/2329-6771.1000206 (accessed on 14.09.2023).

Graham, M. (2022). Effect of Yoga Nidra on Reducing Stress, Increasing Attention, Changing Behaviour and Increasing Happiness of School Students. *Journal of Inovation and Social Science Research*, 9(4), 239–245.

Gulia, Kamalesh, K. & Sreedharan, Sapna, Erat. (2021). Yogic sleep and walking protocol induced improvement in sleep and wellbeing in post-menopausal subject: a longitudinal case study during COVID lockdown. *Sleep and Vigilance*, 6(1), 229–233. https://doi.org/10.1007/s41782-021-00180-2 (accessed on 15.09.2023).

Gunjiganvi, Mallikarjun. Mohan, Gurjar. Mishra, Prabhakar et al. (2021). Efficacy of Yoga Nidra vs Supine Relaxation Technique on Depression, Anxiety, Insomnia in frontline COVID-19 Health Care Workers: A Randomized Controlled Trial, PREPRINT (Version 1). *Research Square Journal*. https://doi.org/10.21203/rs.3.rs-486904/v1 (accessed on 15.09.2023).

Gupta, K. S. S. (2004). Effect of Yoga Nidra on creativity in School Children. In Yoga Research Foundation: Volume three. (2018). *Promotion of Health 1988–2007*. Bihar: Yoga Publication Trust, pp. 242–249.

Madhu K. Gupta & Amool R. Singh. (2022). Exploring the Therapeutic Effect of Yoga to Enhance Psychological Well-Being Among Adolescent Girl Students. *Journal of Education, Society and Behavioural Science*, 35 (2), 13–19. https://doi.org/10.9734/jesbs/2022/v35i230402. (accessed on 12.09.2023).

H

Hari, R, Baillet, et al. (2018). IFCN-endorsed practical guidelines forclinical magnetoencephalography (MEG). In *Clinical Neurophysiology*, Volume 129(8), 1720–1747. https://doi.org/10.1016/j.clinph.2018.03.042 (accessed on 27.10.2022).

Hobson, J. A., & Pace-Schott, E. F. (2002). The cognitive neuroscience of sleep: neuronal systems, consciousness and learning. Nature reviews. *Neuroscience*, 3(9), 679–693. https://doi.org/10.1038/nrn915 (accessed on 28.10.2022).

I

Immnik, A. Maarten, Chan, W. & Hillier, S. (2012). Yoga and exercise for symptoms of depression and anxiety in people with poststroke disability: a randomized, controlled pilot trial. *Alternative Therapies in Health and Medicine*, 18(3), 34–43. https://pubmed.ncbi.nlm.nih.gov/22875560/ (accessed on 14.09.2023).

———., Hiller, Susan L. (2011). Yoga for Chronic Post-stroke Hemiparesis: a Pilot Randomized Controlled Trial. International Journal of Stroke. 6 (Suppl. 1), p. 17. In Collection volume. (2013). *Experience of Yoga*. Bihar School of Yoga — Golden Jubilee, Bihar: Yoga Publication Trust, p. 173.

———., Chan, Weili & Hiller, Susan L. (2011). Pilot Randomized Controlled Trial of Yoga Therapy Supplemented Excersise Interventions for Motor Function and Quality of Life Outcomes in Patients with Chronic Post-stroke Hemiparesis, Journal of Sport and Exercise Psychology. 34, p. 91. In Collection volume. (2013). *Experience of Yoga*. Bihar School of Yoga — Golden Jubilee. Bihar: Yoga Publication Trust, p. 172.

———., Garrett, R. & Hillier, S. (2011). Becoming connected: the lived experience of yoga participation after stroke. *Disability and Rehabilitation*, 33(25–26), 2404–2415. https://doi.org/10.3109/09638288.2011.573058 (accessed on 14.09.2023).

———., (2012). Post-training Meditation Mediates Motor Memory Consolidation, Journal of Sport and Exercise Psychology, 7(11). Collection volume (2013). *Experience of Yoga*. Golden Jubilee 1963–2013. Bihar School of Yoga — Golden Jubilee. Bihar: Yoga Publication Trust, p. 171–172.

———. (2013). Scientific Exploration into Satyananda Yoga Nidra™. In Collection volume (2013). *Experience of Yoga*. Golden Jubilee of Bihar School of Yoga. Bihar: Yoga Publication Trust. p. 150.

———., Hillier, S. & Petkov, J. (2014). Randomized controlled trial of yoga for chronic poststroke hemiparesis: motor function, mental health, and quality of life outcomes. Topics in *Stroke Rehabilitation*, 21(3), 256–271. https://doi.org/10.1310/tsr2103–256 (accessed on 28.10.2022).

———., Loudon, A., Barnett, T., Piller, N. & Williams, A. D. (2014). Yoga management of breast cancer-related lymphoedema: a randomised controlled pilot-trial. *BMC Complementary and Alternative Medicine*, 14, 214. https://doi.org/10.1186/1472–6882-14–214 (accessed on 14.09.2023).

J

Jaiganesh, D. K., Parthasarathy, D. S. & Mr. Duraisamy. (2022). Effect of Suryanamaskar Practices with and Without Yoga Nidra On Stress Among High School Students- A Randomized Controlled Trial: Life Sciences-Health. *International Journal of Life Science and Pharma Research*, 12(SP25), L28-L33. https://doi.org/10.22376/ijpbs/lpr.2022.12.6.SP25.L28–33 (accessed on 12.09.2023)

Jayshree, Kalita & Choudhury, Purujit. (2021) A pilot study on effect of yoga-nidra programme on depression, anxiety, and stress among patients with chronic kidney disease receiving haemodialysis. *International Journal of Applied Research*, 2022; 8(6), 346–349. https://doi.org/10.22271/allresearch.2022.v8.i6e.9893 (accessed on 12.09.2023).

Jensen, P. S. et al. (2012). Respiratory patterns in students enrolled in schools for disruptive behaviour before, during, and after yoga nidra relaxation. In *Journal of Child and Family Studies*, 21(4), 667–681. https://doi.org/10.1007/s10826–011-9519–3 (accessed on 12.09.2023).

K

Kanchibhotla, Divya et al. (2021). Enhancement of the Cognitive Abilities in Visually Impaired Children Following a Yoga Based Intervention. *Annals of Yoga and Physical Therapy*, 5(1), 1046. https://doi.org/10.26420/ANNYOGAPHYSTHER.2021.1046 (accessed on 08.02.2023).

Kim, Sang Dol.(2014). Effects of yogic exercises on life stress and blood glucose levels in nursing students. *Journal of Physical Therapy Science*, 26(12), 2003–2006. https://doi.org/10.1589/jpts.26.2003 (accessed on 14.09.2023).

Kisan, R., Sujan, M., Adoor, M., Rao, R., Nalini, A., Kutty, B. M., Chindanda Murthy, B., Raju, T., & Sathyaprabha, T. (2014). Effect of Yoga on migraine: A comprehensive study using clinical profile and cardiac autonomic functions. *International Journal of Yoga*, 7(2), 126–132. https://doi.org/10.4103/0973–6131.133891 (accessed on 12.09.2023).

Kjaer, Troels, W., Lou, Hans, C., Friberg, L., Wildschiodtz, G., Holm, S., & Nowak, M. (1999). A 15O-H2O PET study of meditation and the resting state of normal consciousness. *Human Brain Mapping*, 7(2), 98–105. https://doi.org/10.1002/(SICI)1097–0193(1999)7:2<98::AID-HBM3>3.0.CO; 2-M (accessed on 14.09.2023).

———, ———., Bertelsen, C., Piccini, P., Brooks, D. & Alving, J. (2002). Increased dopamine tone during meditation-induced change of consciousness. Brain research. *Cognitive Brain Research*, 13(2), 255–259. https://doi.org/10.1016/s0926–6410(01)00106–9 (accessed on 14.09.2023).

———, ——— & Nowak, Markus. (2005). The mental self. In *Progress in Brain Research*. 150, 197–204 & 594. https://doi.org/10.1016/S0079–6123(05)50014–1 (accessed on 14.09.2023).

Kohler, M., Rawlings, M., Kaeding, A.et al. (2017). Meditation is Effective in Reducing Sleepiness and Improving Sustained Attention Following Acute Sleep Restriction. *Journal of Cognitive Enhancement*, 1, 210–218, https://doi.org/10.1007/s41465-017-0032-5 (accessed on 12.09.2023).

Köksoy, S., Eti, C. M., Karataş, M., & Vayisoglu, Y. (2018). The Effects of Yoga in Patients Suffering from Subjective Tinnitus. *International Archives of Otorhinolaryngology*, 22(1), 9–13. https://doi.org/10.1055/s-0037–1601415 (accessed on 12.09.2023).

Kumar, Kamakhya. (2004). A Study on the Impact on Stress and Anxiety Through Yoga Nidra. In *Yoga Mimamsa, Indian Journal of Traditional Knowledge*, 36(3), 136–169. https://de.scribd.com/document/364474553/A-Study-on-Stress-Anxiety-Yoga-Nidra-Yoga-Mimansa (accessed on 12.09.2023).

———. (2004). Yoga Nidra and its Impact on Students' Well-Being. Yoga-Mimansa, In *Yoga Mimamsa, Indian Journal of Traditional Knowledge*, 36(1), 31–35. https://www.researchgate.net/publication/215451327_Yoga_nidra_and_its_impact_on_student%27s_well_being (accessed on 12.09.2023).

———. (2005). Effect of Yoga Nidra on Hypertension and other Psychological Co-relates. In *Yoga the Science Journal*, Yoga Publiations, Hubli, Karnataka, 3(7), 29–36. https://www.researchgate.net/publication/215451330_Effect_of_Yoga_nidra_on_hypertension_other_psychological_co-relates (accessed on 13.09.2023).

———. (2006). A Study on the Improvement of Physical and Mental Health Through Yoga Nidra. In *Dev Sanskriti Inter-disciplinary Research Journal*, 4(4), 39–46. https://www.researchgate.net/publication/215451321_A_study_of_the_improvement_of_Physical_and_Mental_Health_through_Yoga_nidra (accessed on 12.09.2023).

———. (2007). The Healing Sleep, Yoga Magazine Mind Body Spirit. 3(50), 42–44. In Kumakhya, Kumar. (2013). *A Handbook of Yoga Nidra*. New Delhi: D. K. Printworld (P) Ltd., p. 64.

——— & Pandya, Pranav. (2007). Yoga-Nidra and its Impact on Human Physiology. In *Yoga Vijñāna — The Science of Yoga Journal*, New Delhi, India, 1(1), pp. 1–18. https://www.researchgate.net/publication/260268130_Yoga_Nidra_Its_impact_on_Human_Physiology (accessed on 13.09.2023).

———. (2008). A study on the impact on stress and anxiety through Yoga Nidra. In *Indian Journal of Traditional Knowledge*, 7(3), 401–404. https://nopr.niscpr.res.in/bitstream/123456789/1700/1/IJTK%207%283%29%20401–404.pdf (accessed on 12.09.2023).

——— & Joshi, Bhanu. (2009). Reversing the Ischemic Heart Disease through Yoga Nidra. *Nature and Wealth*, 8(1), 453–454. https://www.researchgate.net/publication/215585754_Reversing_the_Ischemic_Heart_Disease_through_Yoga_Nidra (accessed on 13.09.2023).

——— & Joshi, Bhanu (2009). Study on the Effect of Pranakarshan Pranayama & Yoga Nidra on Alpha EEG & GSR. Indian Journal of Traditional Knowledge, 8(3), 453–454. In Kumakhya, Kumar. (2013). *A Handbook of Yoga Nidra*. New Delhi: D. K. Printworld (P) Ltd., p.65.

———. (2010). Psychological changes as related to Yoga Nidra. In *International Journal of Psychology: A Biopsychosocial Approach*. 6, 129–137. https://www.researchgate.net/publication/213341724_Psychological_changes_as_related_to_Yoga_Nidra (accessed on 12.09.2023).

——— & Pandya, Pranav. (2012). A study on the impact on ESR level through Yogic Relaxation Technique Yoga Nidra, Indian Journal of Traditional Knowledge. 11(2), 358–361. In Kumakhya, Kumar. (2013). *A Handbook of Yoga Nidra*. New Delhi: D. K. Printworld (P) Ltd., p.67.

——— & ———. (2012). Yoga Nidra and its Impact on Human Physiology. *Indian Journal of Traditional Knowledge*, Vol. 11(2), 358–361. https://nopr.niscpr.res.in/bitstream/123456789/13871/1/IJTK%2011%282%29%20358–361.pdf (accessed on 13.09.2023).

———. (2020). Role of Yoga-nidra in Immunity Development. *International Journal of Yoga and Allied Science*, 11(2), 358–61. https://www.researchgate.net/publication/350965226_Role_of_Yoga-nidra_in_Immunity_Development (accessed on 13.09.2023).

———, Pandi-Perumal, S. R., Spence, D. W., Srivastava, N., Kanchibhotla, D., Sharma, G. S., Gupta, R., & Batmanabane, G. (2022). The Origin and Clinical Relevance of Yoga Nidra. *Sleep and Vigilance*, 6(1), 61–84. https://doi.org/10.1007/s41782–022-00202–7 (accessed on 13.09.2023).

Kumari, Priyanka & Tripathi, J. S. (2020). A Pilot Study on Effect of Yoga Nidra in the Management of Stress. *International Journal of Science and Research* (IJSR), 9(1), 1101–1103.https://www.ijsr.net/archive/v9i1/ART20204197.pdf (accessed on 12.09.2023).

L

Lakshmipathy, Shalini & Easvaradoss, Veena. (2018). Impact of Yoga Nidra Meditation on Perceived Stress and Self Regulation in Teacher Trainees. *International Journal of Indian Psychology*, 6(3), 89–93. https://ijip.in/wp-content/uploads/2020/06/18.01.049.20180603.pdf (accessed on 12.09.2023).

Li, L., Shu, W., Li, Z., Liu, Q., Wang, H., Feng, B. & Ouyang, Y. Q. (2019). Using Yoga Nidra Recordings for Pain Management in Patients Undergoing Colonoscopy. *Pain Management Nursing: Official Journal of the American Society of Pain Management Nurses*, 20(1), 39–46. https://doi.org/10.1016/j.pmn.2018.04.005 (accessed on 13.09.2023).

Lustenberger, C.; Boyle, M. R., et al. (2015). Functional role of frontal alpha oscillations in creativity. In *Cortex Magazine*, 67, 74–82. https://doi.org/10.1016/j.cortex.2015.03.012 (accessed on 14.09.2023).

M

Macey, Jennifer. (2005). Stress in relation to immunity. *Journal of Experimental Medicine*, 02(11), pp. 1456–1482. https://www.researchgate.net/profile/Kamakhya-Kumar/publication/215451321_

A_study_of_the_improvement_of_Physical_and_Mental_Health_through_Yoga_nidra/links/0c9605390532ac1002000000/A-study-of-the-improvement-of-Physical-and-Mental-Health-through-Yoga-nidra.pdf (accessed on 13.09.2023).

Mandlik Y. V., Jain P., & Jain K. (2002). Effect of Yoga Nidra on EEG. *Yoga Vidya Dham, Retrieved*, http://www.yogapoint.com/info/research5.htm (accessed on 14.09.2023).

Manik, Ricardo & Gartia, Rajendra. (2016). A Comparative Study of Yoga Nidra and Nadisodhana Pranayam on Essential Hypertension. In *Advanced Science Letters*, 22(2), pp. 437–441(5), https://www.researchgate.net/publication/303808615_A_Comparative_Study_of_Yoga_

Nidra_and_Nadisodhana_Pranayam_on_Essential_Hypertension (accessed on 13.09.2023).

———, ———, Mahapatra, A. K., Bansal, S., & Patnaik, A. (2017). Effect of Selected Yogic Practices on Pain and Disability in Patients with Lumbar Spondylitis. *International Journal of Yoga*, 10(2), 81–87. https://doi.org/10.4103/0973–6131.205516 (accessed on 13.09.2023).

Markil, N., Whitehurst, M., Jacobs, P. L. & Zoeller, R. F. (2012). Yoga Nidra relaxation increases heart rate variability and is unaffected by a prior bout of Hatha yoga. *Journal of Alternative and Complementary Medicine* (New York, N.Y.), 18(10), 953–958. https://doi.org/10.1089/acm.2011.0331 (accessed on 13.09.2023).

Mathew, R. J., Ho, B. T., Kralik, P., Weinman, M. & Claghorn, J. L. (1981). Anxiety and platelet MAO levels after relaxation training. *The American Journal of psychiatry*, 138(3), 371–373. https://doi.org/10.1176/ajp.138.3.371 (accessed on 13.09.2023).

Mishra, Brajeshwar. (2013). Immunological Effect of Yoga Nidra on HIV/AIDS. In Collection volume. (2013). *Experience of Yoga*. Bihar School of Yoga — Golden Jubilee 2013. Bihar: Yoga Publication Trust, p. 183–186.

Monika, Singh, U., Ghildiyal, A., Kala, S. & Srivastava, N. (2012). Effect of Yoga Nidra on physiological variables in patients of menstrual disturbances of reproductive age group. *Indian Journal of Physiology and Pharmacology*, 56(2), 161–167. https://ijpp.com/IJPP%20archives/2012_56_2_%20Apr%20-%20Jun/161–167.pdf (accessed on 13.09.2023).

N

Nayak, K., & Verma, K. (2023). Yoga-Nidra as a mental health booster: A narrative review. *Journal of Ayurveda and Integrative Medicine*, 14(6), 100842. https://doi.org/10.1016/j.jaim.2023.100842 (accessed on 12.09.2023).

Nirmalananda, Swami. (n.d.). Research 1: Effect of Yoga on Blood Sugar in Diabetics. In Yoga Research Foundation. (2017). *Promotion of Health 1988–2007*, Volume Two. Bihar: Yoga Publication Trust.

———. (n.d.). Research II: Effect of Yoga on Blood Sugar and Cardiac Risk Factors in Diabetics. In Yoga Research Foundation: Volume two. (2017). *Promotion of Health 1988–2007*. Bihar: Yoga Publication Trust.

———. (n.d.). Research III: Effect of Satyananda Yoga on Hypertension. In Yoga Research Foundation: Volume two. (2017). *Promotion of Health 1988–2007*. Bihar: Yoga Publication Trust., p. 48–82.

———. (n.d.). Research IV: Effect of Yoga on Satyananda Yoga on Asthma and COPD. In Yoga Research Foundation: Volume two. (2017). *Promotion of Health 1988–2007*. Bihar: Yoga Publication Trust, p. 83.

O

Ozdemir, Ahmdet & Saritas, Serdar. (2019). Effect of yoga nidra on the self-esteem and body image of burn patients. In *Complementary Therapy in Clinical Practice*, 35(5), 86–91. https://doi.org/10.1016/j.ctcp.2019.02.002 (accessed on 12.09.2023).

P

Parasar Pandey A. O. & Dalal S. (2020). Effects of nadi-shodhan pranayama and yoga-nidra on emotional maturity and mental health of young adults. *International Journal of Indian Psychology*, 8(4), 1657–1668. doi:10.25215/0804.180 (accessed on 12.09.2023).

R

Reddy, Dhrithi B. et al (2018). Effect of Yoga Nidra on Mental Status Among Self-Employment Aspirants. *Journal of Emerging Technologies and Innovative Research*, 5(8), 412–419.https://www.jetir.org/papers/JETIR1808961.pdf (accessed on 14.09.2023).

Rajagopalan, A., Krishna, A. & Mukkadan, J. K. (2022). Effect of Om chanting and Yoga Nidra on depression anxiety stress, sleep quality and autonomic functions of hypertensive subjects - a randomized controlled trial. *Journal of Basic and Clinical Physiology and Pharmacology*, 34(1), 69–75. https://doi.org/10.1515/jbcpp-2022–0122 (accessed on 13.09.2023).

Rajpoot, Lata, Pushp & Sanwat, Singh. (2014). A study of the effect of Yoga Nidra on mental health of emotionally abused adolescents. In Academia: *An International Multidisciplinary Research Journal*, 4(12), 6–14. https://www.academia.edu/76315471/A_study_of_the_effect_of_Yoga_Nidra_on_mental_health_of_emotionally_abused_adolescents (accessed on 14.09.2023).

Rani, K., Tiwari, S., Singh, U., Agrawal, G., Ghildiyal, A. & Srivastava, N. (2011). Impact of Yoga Nidra on psychological general wellbeing in patients with menstrual irregularities: A randomized controlled trial. *International Journal of Yoga*, 4(1), 20–25. https://doi.org/10.4103/0973–6131.78176 (accessed on 13.09.2023).

———., Tiwari, S. C., Singh, U., Agrawal, G. G. & Srivastava, N. (2011). Six-month trial of Yoga Nidra in menstrual disorder patients: Effects on somatoform symptoms. *Industrial Psychiatry Journal*, 20(2), 97–102. https://doi.org/10.4103/0972–6748.102489 (accessed on 13.09.2023).

———., Tiwari, S., Singh, U., Singh, I., & Srivastava, N. (2012). Yoga Nidra as a complementary treatment of anxiety and depressive symptoms in patients with menstrual disorder. *International Journal of Yoga*, 5(1), 52–56. https://doi.org/10.4103/0973–6131.91715 (accessed on 13.09.2023).

———., Tiwari, S. C., Kumar, S., Singh, U., Prakash, J. & Srivastava, N. (2016). Psycho-Biological Changes with Add on Yoga Nidra in Patients with Menstrual Disorders: a Randomized Clinical Trial. *Journal of Caring Sciences*, 5(1), 1–9. https://doi.org/10.15171/jcs.2016.001 (accessed on 13.09.2023).

———., Kumar, A., Sharma, P. (2013). Effect of Yoga Nidra on Stress Level among B.Sc. Nursing first year students. *Nursing and Midwifery Research Journal*, (9), pp. 47–55. http://doi.org/10.33698/NRF0156 (accessed on 12.09.2023).

Rani, Monika., Singh, U., Agrawal, G. G., Natu, S. M., Kala, S., Ghildiyal, A. & Srivastava, N. (2013). Impact of Yoga Nidra on menstrual abnormalities in females of reproductive age. *Journal of Alternative and Complementary Medicine* (New York, N.Y.), 19(12), 925–929. https://doi.org/10.1089/acm.2010.0676 (accessed on 13.09.2023).

Reddy, Dhrithi B. et al. (2018). Effect of Yoga Nidra on Mental Status Among Self-Employment Aspirants. In *Journal of Emerging Technologies and Innovative Research*, 5(8), 413–19. https://www.jetir.org/papers/JETIR1808961.pdf (accessed on 14.09.2023).

Roney-Dougal, S. M. (n.d.). Altered States of Consciousness and Yogic Attainment in Relation to Awareness of Precognitive and Clairvoyant Targets, Psi Research Center (2011). In Kamakhya Kumar (2013). *A Handbook of Yoga-Nidrā*, New Delhi: D. K. Printworld (P) Ltd., p. 81.

S

Sachdeva, Sachi. (2018). To Study the Effects of Yoga Nidra on Reduction of Stress, Increase in Concentration, Changes in Behaviour and Increase in Happiness among School Going Students. In *International Journal of Science and Research* (IJSR), 7(12), 5–11.https://www.ijsr.net/archive/v7i12/ART20193216.pdf, (accessed on 12.09.2023).

Sandeep, C., Shivaprasad & Shetty, Prashant. (2016). Effects Of Yoga Nidra (Psychic Sleep) On Alcohol Dependent Individuals—A Randomized Control Trial. In *Journal of Dental and Medical Sciences* (IOSR-JDMS), 15(9), 8–13. https://www.iosrjournals.org/iosr-jdms/papers/Vol15-Issue%209/Version-11/C1509110813.pdf (accessed on 14.09.2023).

Selvam, A.S. & Elangovan, R. (2018). Effect of Brisk Walking with Yoga Nidra on Selected Psychological Variables among Obese College Boy. *Journal of Yoga, Physical Therapy and Rehabilitation*, 1(01), 1–4. http://doi.org/10.29011/YPTR-143.%20000043 (accessed on 13.09.2023).

Sethi, B. B., Trivedi, J. K. & Anand, R., (1981). A comparative study of relative effectiveness of biofeedback and Shavasana (Yoga) in tension headache. *Indian Journal of Psychiatry*, 23(2), 109–14. https://www.ncbi.nlm.nih.gov/pmc/articles/PMC3013159/pdf/IJPsy-23-109.pdf (accessed on 12.09.2023).

Sethi, Pramod, Kumar & Singh, Vikram. (2016). Effect of Yoga Nidra on reaction time and anticipation time of wrestlers. In *International Journal of Physical Education, Sports and Health*, 3(5), 504–7.https://www.kheljournal.com/archives/2016/vol3issue5/PartI/3-5-99-152.pdf (accessed on 14.09.2023).

Sharpe, E., Tibbitts, D., Wolfe, B., Senders, A. & Bradley, R. (2021). Qualitative Impressions of a Yoga Nidra Practice for Insomnia: An Exploratory Mixed-Methods Design. *Journal of Alternative and Complementary Medicine* (New York, N.Y.), 27(10), 884–892. https://doi.org/10.1089/acm.2021.0125 (accessed on 12.09.2023).

———., Butler, M. P., Clark-Stone, J., Soltanzadeh, R., Jindal, R., Hanes, D. & Bradley, R. (2023). A closer look at yoga nidra- early randomized sleep lab investigations. *Journal of Psychosomatic Research*, 166, 111169. https://doi.org/10.1016/j.jpsychores.2023.111169 (accessed on 12.09.2023).

Shashikiran, H. C., Shetty, P., Akshay, R., Venugopal, A. & Shetty, S. (2022). Effect of yoga nidra on the brain activity in individuals with migraine. *Yoga-Mimansa, Indian Journal of Traditional Knowledge*, 54(1), 18–23. DOI: 10.4103/ym.ym_35_22 (accessed on 12.09.2023).

Shealy R. C. (1979). The effectiveness of various treatment techniques on different degrees and durations of sleep-onset insomnia. *Behaviour Research and Therapy*, 17(6), 541–546. https://doi.org/10.1016/0005–7967(79)90097–4 (accessed on 12.09.2023)

Singh, I., Beena & Singh, H. (2016). To Study the Effect of Yoga Nidra on Anxiety and Stress in Medical Students. *European Journal of Biomedical and Pharmaceutical Sciences*, 3(2), 178–180. https://storage.googleapis.com/journal-uploads/ejbps/article_issue/volume_3_february_issue_2/1454068178.pdf/ (accessed on 12.09.2023).

T

Thangam, F. E. & Bharathi, A.D. (2019). Effect of Yoga-nidra on Blood Pressure among Elderly with Hypertension Residing at Selected Old Age Homes, Coimbatore. *International Journal of Nursing Education and Research*, 7(1), pp. 30–32. http://dx.doi.org/10.5958/2454–2660.2019.00006.1(accessed on 13.09.2023).

Tiwari, Vikash, K., Pandey, S. & Mishra, R. (2020). Yoga is an effective technique of stress reduction within the medical population: a biochemical study in MBBS students of BRD Medical College, Gorakhpur, Uttar Pradesh, India. *International Journal of Research in Medical Sciences*, 8(4), 1326–1330. https://doi.org/10.18203/2320–6012.ijrms20201318 (accessed on 12.09.2023).

Tripathi, R. C. (2018). Effects of yoga nidra on physical and psychological health. In M. Karasawa, M. Yuki, K. Ishii, Y. Uchida, K. Sato, & W. Friedlmeier (Eds.), *Venture into cross-cultural psychology: Proceedings from the 23rd Congress of the International Association for Cross-Cultural Psychology*. https://doi.org/10.4087/CVPP9404 (accessed on 12.09.2023).

Tseng, J. & Poppenk, J. (2020). Brain meta-state transitions demarcate thoughts across task contexts exposing the mental noise of trait neuroticism. *Nature Communications*, 11(1), 3480. https://doi.org/10.1038/s41467-020-17255-9 (accessed on 07.11.2022).

V

Vaishnav, S. B., Vaishnav, V. S. & Varma, J. R. (2018). Effect of Yoga-nidra on Adolescents Well-being: A Mixed Method Study. *International Journal of Yoga*, 11(3), 245–248. https://doi.org/10.4103/ijoy.IJOY_39_17 (accessed on 12.09.2023).

Vanitha, A., Pandiaraja, M., Maheshkumar, K. & Venkateswaran S. T. (2018) Effect of yoga nidra on resting cardiovascular parameters in polycystic ovarian syndrome women. *National Journal of Physiology, Pharmacy and Pharmacology*, 8 (11), 1505–1508. http://dx.doi.org/10.5455/njppp.2018.8.0411112082018 (accessed on 13.09.2023).

Verma, K., Srivastava, A. & Singh, D. (2022). Effects of Yoga on Psychological Health and Sleep Quality of Patients With Acute Insomnia: A Preliminary Study. *Advances in Mind-Body Medicine*, 36(4), 4–11. https://pubmed.ncbi.nlm.nih.gov/36351185/ (accessed on 15.09.2023).

Verma, Veena (Sannyasi Soumyashakti). (2004). Possibilities of Revolutionizing the Education System Through Yoga Nidra. *Yoga Magazine*. Bihar: Bihar School of Yoga, 5. http://www.yogamag.net/archives/2000s/2004/0405/0405pred.html (accessed on 15.09.2023).

Y

Yadav, Mahesh & Sardar, Sanjit. (2016). Comparative effect of yoga asana and yoga Nidra on the anxiety level of inter collegiate level football players. In *International Journal of Physical Education, Sports and Health*, (2), 148–150. https://www.kheljournal.com/archives/2016/vol3issue2/PartC/3-2-26.pdf. (accessed on 14.09.2023).

Lectures

Shavasana-3 (Swāmī, Niranjanānanda, Sarasvatī. Online-lecture. *Yoga-Chakra-Series*. May, 2021).

Figures

Tables

About the Author

Born in 1979 in Sofia, Bulgaria, and based in Vienna, Austria, for the last 28 years, Nadeshda Stürzebecher now divides her time between Sofia and Vienna. Holding two Master's degrees in Fine Arts and Pedagogy, she is an academic artist, high school art teacher, certified yoga teacher in the tradition of the Bihar School of Yoga, and practitioner specialising in sacred art, where creativity and spirituality intersect. She is currently deepening her expertise by pursuing a Master's degree in Clinical Art Therapy at the Sigmund Freud University in Vienna. In 2001, she met her *guru*, Svāmī Nirañjanānanda Sarasvatī, and was blessed to experience the presence of Svāmī Satyānanda Sarasvatī in person. She took her initiation into *saṃnyāsa* in 2005 from Svāmī Nirañjanānanda Sarasvatī. Since then, she has been practicing and studying and continuously deepening her knowledge and experience through further yogic trainings and courses in Europe, Australia, and India within the integral system of Bihar Yoga. She has been offering retreats and classes both across Europe and online. From 2011 to 2019, she co-founded and established in Vienna the only yoga centre teaching the Bihar Yoga system in Austria. Since 2017, she has been offering one-year-long in-person *yoga-nidrā* training courses in the method of Svāmī Satyānanda in German. For the past two years, Nadeshda has also been studying Indian iconography under the guidance of Drdha Vrata Gorrick further expanding her understanding of sacred art and its philosophical foundations.

Kontakt: yoganidraonlinecourse.com
Instagram: @yoga_nidra_vienna
YouTube: yoga_nidra_vienna

Yoga-nidrā Guided Audio Practices

According to the Method of Svāmī Satyānanda Sarasvatī

You will find the following three guided audio practices for download:

1. ***yoga-nidrā*** **for Beginners**
2. ***yoga-nidrā*** **with saṃkalpa**
3. ***yoga-nidrā*** **Full Practice**

yoganidraonlinecourse.com/audio

Printed in Dunstable, United Kingdom

78761200R00298